Slow Potentials and Microprocessor Applications

Documenta Ophthalmologica
Proceedings Series volume 37

Editor H. E. Henkes

1983 **Dr W. JUNK PUBLISHERS**
a member of the KLUWER ACADEMIC PUBLISHERS GROUP
THE HAGUE / BOSTON / LANCASTER

Slow Potentials and Microprocessor Applications

Proceedings of the 20th ISCEV Symposium
Iowa City, Iowa, U.S.A., October 25–28, 1982

dedicated to Hans Bornschein

Edited by Hansjoerg E.J.W. Kolder

1983 **Dr W. JUNK PUBLISHERS**
a member of the KLUWER ACADEMIC PUBLISHERS GROUP
THE HAGUE / BOSTON / LANCASTER

Distributors

for the United States and Canada: Kluwer Boston, Inc., 190 Old Derby Street
Hingham, MA 02043, USA
for all other countries: Kluwer Academic Publishers Group, Distribution Center
P.O.Box 322, 3300 AH Dordrecht, The Netherlands

Library of Congress Cataloging in Publication Data

I.S.C.E.V. Symposium (20th : 1982 : Iowa City, Iowa)
   Slow potentials and microprocessor applications.

   (Documenta ophthalmologica. Proceedings series ;
v. 37)
   Includes bibliographical references and index.
   1. Electroretinography--Congresses. 2. Electroculo-
graphy--Congresses. 3. Slow potentials (Electrophysiology)--Congresses. 4. Slow potentials (Electrophysiology)--Data processing--Congresses. 5. Optics,
Physiological--Congresses. 6. Optics, Physiological--
Data processing--Congresses. 7. Microprocessors--Con-
gresses. I. Bornschein, Hans. II. Kolder, Hansjoerg
E. J. W. III. Title. IV. Series.

RE79.E4 I17   1982   617.7'307547   83-9837
ISBN-13: 978-94-009-7277-3   e-ISBN-13: 978-94-009-7275-9
DOI: 10.1007/ 978-94-009-7275-9

ISBN 978-94-009-7277-3

Copyright

DEDICATION OF THE XXTH ISCEV SYMPOSIUM TO HANS BORNSCHEIN

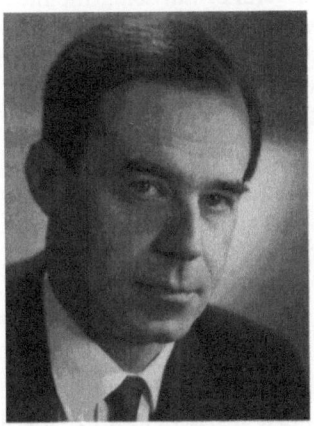

Hans Bornschein began his scientific career at the time when the foundation of this Society was laid. Riggs had pioneered the modern recording of the ERG and Karpe had published a monograph on that topic. Bornschein studied Medicine at the University of Vienna and later joined the Department of Physiology there.

A long tradition for research in sensory physiology had developed in Vienna starting with Brücke, and furthered by Exner, Kolmer, and Schubert (the latter himself a student of Tschermak-Seysenegg and Hering). Schubert recognized early Bornschein's talent for basic research. He encouraged him to visit with Ragnar Granit in Stockholm. Bornschein also spent time at the National Institute for Health in Bethesda, Maryland. On that occasion, he popularized the clinical recording of the ERG in the U.S.A. His technique is still used in several laboratories and clinics.

But Bornschein's interest was more fundamental. He analyzed ERG components in amphibian eyes and vertebrate eyes. He recorded ganglion cell potentials in the retina and action potentials from the optic nerve. He worked diligently to understand new concepts, like the Huxley-Hodgkins cable equation, and was able to apply new discoveries.

Bornschein was honored by a call to head the Institute for General and Comparative Physiology at the University of Vienna. He liked the city and its cultural environment. He preferred to stay there. Bornschein became the co-editor of Vision Research and published a profound text on the physiology of the retina. His scrupulously honest scientific mind would never settle for less than a perfect experiment. He published 161 original and review articles. In spite of hypertension which had led to complications, he continued with a rigorous teaching and research program for the benefit of several collaborators and many students. He was a critical reviewer and appointed discussant at several of our scientific meetings.

Hans Bornschein's work has benefited the goals of this Society in many ways. I am pleased to dedicate your work during this, the XXth Symposium of ISCEV, to the memory of Hans Bornschein and I am grateful to Mrs. Elsa Bornschein for sharing this time with us.

H. E. Kolder

REFERENCES

Obituary; Hans Bornschein by A. Kafka-Lützow
  Vision Res. 21:175–176 (1981)
Hans Bornschein, Nachruf mit Schriftenverzeichnis von W. Auerswald.
  Almanach der Österr. Akad. Wiss. 129:329–341 (1979).

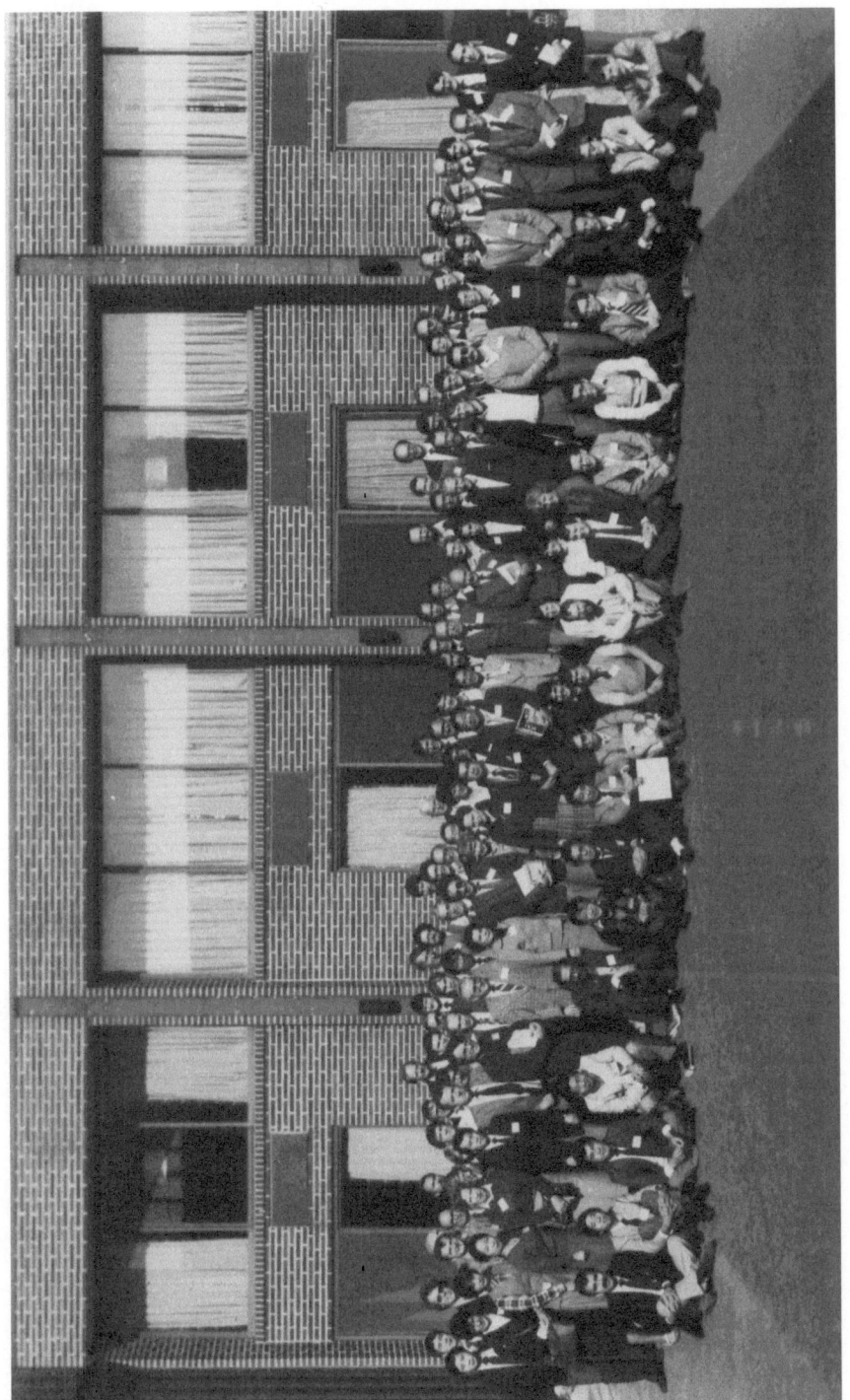

Participants of the XXth ISCEV Symposium, October 1982

PREFACE

Investigators and clinicians researching and applying electrophysiologic phenomena of the eye, met for the XXth Symposium of the International Society for Clinical Electrophysiology of Vision in Iowa City, Iowa, under the auspices of the University of Iowa and supported by the Department of Ophthalmology, headed by Professor Frederick C. Blodi.

Two main topics were discussed: 1) Electro-oculography and other slow potentials: the phenomenon, origin, analysis, and clinical diagnosis, and 2) Microprocessor applications for computer-assisted recording and analysis of electrovisual phenomena.

Unusual and challenging diagnostic problems were presented during one evening session. The interest and lively audience participation indicated a need for such an unrehearsed debate. Drs. H.W. Skalka, H. Nakano, H.S. Thompson, A.J. Packer, J.A. Parker, H.E. Kolder, V.M. Hermsen, M.L. Wolf, and Mr. A.I. Mallinson presented case reports and are herewith recognized for their contribution. No documentation is contained in the Proceedings. Several papers were read outside the main topics. Some material appears only as abstract. The highlight of the scientific program proved to be an improvised session on basic mechanisms of slow potentials from the eye. Dr. R.H. Steinberg and his collaborators, together with Dr. G. Niemeyer initiated this part of the program. It was enthusiastically received, provided an informal atmosphere, stimulated a lively discussion and exchanged profound information.

A novel feature of this volume is the addition of a cumulative index covering the Proceedings from the last ten ISCERG-ISCEV Symposia. Dr. J.R. Heckenlively furnished the computer program for the preparation of this — much needed — index.

No Symposium of the type customary for ISCEV participants can succeed without tangible and intangible support from many persons. The rural Midwestern environment lit up with Indian Summer weather. Excursions included a pig roast, a square dance, the John Deere tractor factory, a farm visit, and a dinner along the Mississippi River. The banquet was enhanced by the Stradivari Quartet playing A. Dvořák's American Quartet, opus 96; written when the composer, being homesick, escaped New York during the summer of 1893 to vacation in the Bohemian settlement of Spillville, Iowa.

X

The program could not have been successful without the competent, efficient, and cheerful help of my co-workers: Sara J. Putney, Jane R. Knoedel, and Joan E. Snyder. Special appreciation belongs to Sara, who typed and retyped the manuscript without despair.

May this volume keep alive the scientific exchange, the commitment for free communication of new and exciting discoveries, the spirit of cooperation between researchers from many countries, and the memory of Hans Bornschein to whom these Proceedings are dedicated in recognition of his invaluable contributions to the understanding of the electrophysiology of vision.

HEJWK
Iowa City, Iowa, March, 1983.

CONTENTS

PART THREE: MICROPROCESSOR APPLICATIONS

PART FOUR: PATTERN ERG

PART FIVE: ERG APPLICATIONS

PART SEVEN: MISCELLANEOUS TOPICS

THE CELLULAR ORIGIN OF THE LIGHT PEAK

R. H. STEINBERG, E. R. GRIFF and R. A. LINSENMEIER
(San Francisco, California, U.S.A.)

ABSTRACT

We studied the cellular origin of the light peak by DC electroretinography in two animal models — the intact cat and an *in vitro* lizard preparation (*Gekko gekko*). A change in the corneoretinal potential can originate from either or both the neural retina and retinal pigment epithelium (RPE). By recording the potential change across each of these tissues we learned that the light peak originates solely from the RPE, as an increase in the trans-epithelial potential (TEP). An increase in TEP can originate from either or both RPE cell membranes; i.e., from the apical membrane, facing the neural retina or from the basal membrane, apposed to the choriocapillaris. By recording the potential of each membrane we found that the light peak originates as a depolarization of the *basal* membrane. This contrasts with the c-wave whose RPE component originates as a hyperpolarization of the apical membrane. The c-wave is caused by a light-evoked decrease of potassium in the subretinal space, while the light peak does not appear to be directly related to any change in retinal potassium concentration. The light peak is, however, accompanied by a decrease in the electrical resistance of the RPE basal membrane. The events that lead to the basal membrane's depolarization and resistance change remain to be discovered.

INTRODUCTION

The purpose of this paper is to summarize our recent research using animal models to study the light peak (Griff and Steinberg, 1982; Linsenmeier and Steinberg, 1982). We chose the light peak for study because it is the first and most prominent of the slow oscillations of the human electrooculogram (EOG) (Marmor and Lurie, 1979), and because it is relatively easy to record in experimental animals (e.g., Kikawada, 1968). We have studied this response both in the intact cat eye and in *in vitro* preparations from the eye of a lizard, *Gekko gekko*. In cat the characteristics of the light peak of the DC ERG are very similar to those of the human EOG (and DC ERG) (Nikara et al., 1976; Täumer et al., 1976a; Niemeyer, 1980; Steinberg and Niemeyer, 1981). We developed *in vitro* preparations from the lizard eye in order to investigate the sequence of physiological events that cause the light peak.

Doc. Ophthal. Proc. Series, Vol. 37, ed. by H. E. J. W. Kolder
©1983 Dr W. Junk Publishers, The Hague/Boston: Lancaster

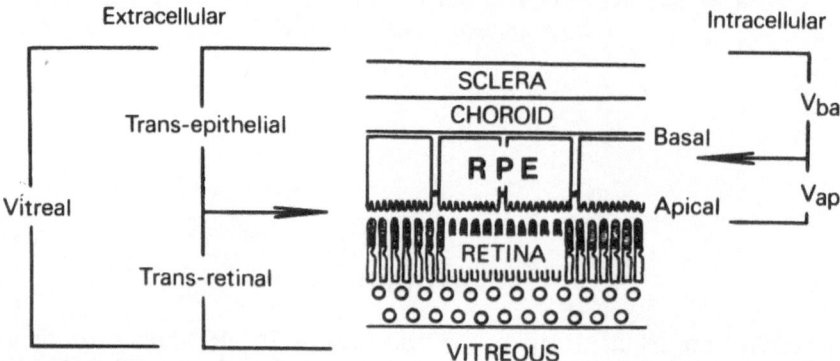

Fig. 1. Diagram of recording configurations. As shown, for cat, vitreal recordings were made between an electrode in the vitreous and a reference behind the eye. The arrow (left) represents a micro-electrode placed within the subretinal space that when referenced behind the eye recorded the trans-epithelial potential. The trans-retinal recording was obtained by subtraction (by computer) of the vitreal and trans-epithelial recordings. Intracellular recordings were obtained by placing the microelectrode in the cytoplasm of an RPE cell (arrow, right). The basal membrane potential, V_{ba}, was recorded between this micro-electrode and the reference behind the eye. The apical membrane potential, V_{ap}, was obtained from subtraction of a basal membrane respone from a trans-epithelial response obtained subsequently.

In gecko, the recording configurations were essentially the same. The trans-tissue potential was essentially equivalent to the vitreal recording in cat, while the trans-retinal and trans-epithelial potentials were simultaneously recorded. The apical and basal RPE membrane potentials also were simultaneously recorded.

One reason for our interest in the light peak was the possibility that it resulted from an interaction between the retinal pigment epithelium (RPE) and the neural retina (retina minus RPE). The results of previous investigations had implicated both the neural retina and RPE in its generation, but the role of each structure was not clear (Noell, 1953; Imaizumi et al., 1968; Täumer, 1976; Gouras and Carr, 1965; Lieberman, 1977; Madachi-Yamamoto, 1980). Our first goal was to determine the cellular origin of the light peak voltage. We found for both experimental preparations, cat and lizard, that the light peak voltage is generated only by the RPE, and this has also been shown by Valeton and van Norren (1982) for the monkey. We also more precisely located the generator to a depolarization of the RPE basal membrane. Further studies are in progress to work out the sequence of neural retinal and RPE events that lead to this potential change.

METHODS

We recorded from intact, anesthetised cats, paralysed and artificially ventilated. Recordings were made between a vitreal electrode and a reference electrode in the orbit behind the eye, and between a micro-electrode and this reference (see Fig. 1). Micro-electrodes used for intraretinal and intracellular recordings were advanced into the eye through a hypodermic needle. The DC ERG was recorded between the vitreal electrode and the reference behind the eye. The trans-epithelial recording was made between a micro-electrode in the sub-retinal space and the reference behind the eye. The trans-retinal recording was obtained from a subtraction (by computer) of the vitreal and trans-epithelial recordings. The basal membrane potential of RPE cells was recorded between an intracellular micro-electrode and the reference behind the eye. The apical membrane potential was obtained from subtraction of a basal membrane response from a trans-epithelial response obtained subsequently. The stimuli were provided by a dual-beam ophthalmoscope or a fiber-optic illuminator. Diffuse illumination of the retina always was used. (For more details see Linsenmeier and Steinberg, 1982).

In the gecko experiments a 3.0 mm square piece of tissue, consisting of the neural retina, RPE and choroid, was excised from the eye and mounted in a lucite chamber. The retinal and choroidal surfaces were each separately perfused by a modified Ringer's solution. The trans-tissue potential, equivalent to the vitreal recording in cat, was recorded between agar-Ringer bridges placed in the baths on each side of the tissue. The trans-epithelial and trans-retinal potentials were simultaneously recorded between a micro-electrode in the subretinal space and references in each of the baths. The apical and basal membrane potentials were obtained in a similar manner with an intracellular RPE micro-electrode. Voltage drops across the tissue or across the RPE cell membranes were obtained by passing constant current pulses between agar-Ringer bridges located on each side of the tissue. Diffuse illumination also was used in all experiments. (For more details see Griff and Steinberg, 1982).

RESULTS

Origin from Neural Retina or RPE

To determine the cellular origin of the light peak voltage, or of any other ERG component, it is first necessary to determine whether it can be recorded across the neural retina, the RPE, or across both structures. The experimental approach is to place extracellular electrodes that will record potentials originating either in the neural retina or in the RPE. The recording con-figuration for these experiments is diagrammed in Fig. 1. The arrow on the left side of the figure represents a microelectrode that has been placed in the subretinal space, i.e. between the neural retina and RPE (center of diagram). In an experiment the microelectrode penetrated the retina at its vitreal border – the internal limiting membrane, and passed through the entire thickness of the neural retina. It was then positioned accurately in the subretinal space by first penetrating an RPE cell and then withdrawing a few microns. By referring this electrode to the back of the eye, the potential across the RPE, the trans-epithelial potential (TEP), was recorded. By referring the electrode to the vitreous, the potential across the neural retina, the trans-retinal potential, was recorded. These recordings allow one to identify potentials generated by

3

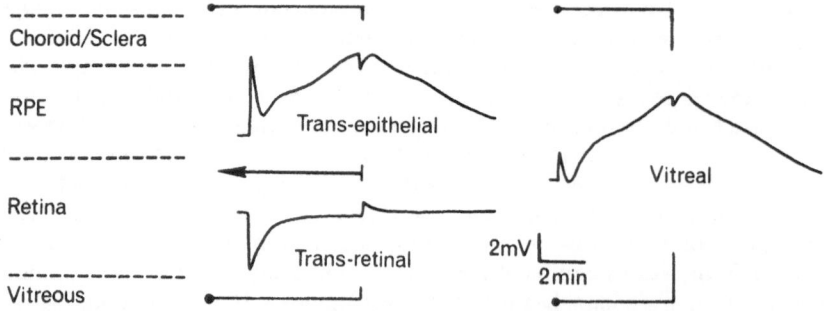

Fig. 2. The origin of the vitreal light peak (cat). Both the trans-epithelial and trans-retinal components are shown with a vitreal positive recording polarity. The light peak of the vitreal response was present in the trans-epithelial recording but not in the trans-retinal. Responses are to 5 min of illumination. All figures in this paper show tracings with the approximate time-courses and amplitudes of the actual responses.

either the neural retina or RPE provided that there are no passive voltage drops. This was not a problem in the study of the light peak, but is of importance in understanding the origin of other light-evoked responses. The vitreal response, which is larger in amplitude, but otherwise equivalent to responses from the cornea (Rodieck, 1973), was recorded between the vitreal electrode and the back of the eye.

Figure 2 shows an example of the DC ERG recorded from the vitreous in response to a 5 min stimulus. The light peak is the large and slow rise and fall of potential that follows the c-wave of the ERG. Although its time course is somewhat faster in cat than in human, it is similar in all other major respects. In cat, the light peak is graded in amplitude with illumination over a 5 log unit range and can be produced by rather brief flashes (10 sec), providing the intensity is sufficient (Linsenmeier and Steinberg, 1982).

Figure 2 also shows the trans-epithelial and trans-retinal recordings produced by an identical stimulus. In every case, there was a slow rise and fall of the TEP that followed the c-wave and had the time course of the vitreal light peak. By contrast, the trans-retinal recordings never showed a response of this type. We concluded that the light-peak voltage was generated by the RPE.

Origin from RPE Apical or Basal Membrane

The RPE has two cell membranes — the *apical* membrane, bordering the subretinal space and contiguous to the photoreceptors and the *basal* membrane, facing the choroid (Fig. 1). Since the TEP is determined by the potentials of both of these cell membranes, the light peak, which is a change in TEP, could originate from changes in either or both membrane potentials. Let us consider how the TEP is generated.

The TEP is the difference between the apical and basal membrane potentials. These membrane potentials are not the same because of differences in the passive and active ionic transport characteristics of the two cell membranes (Steinberg and Miller, 1979). In the circuit diagram of Fig. 3A, V_{ba}

4

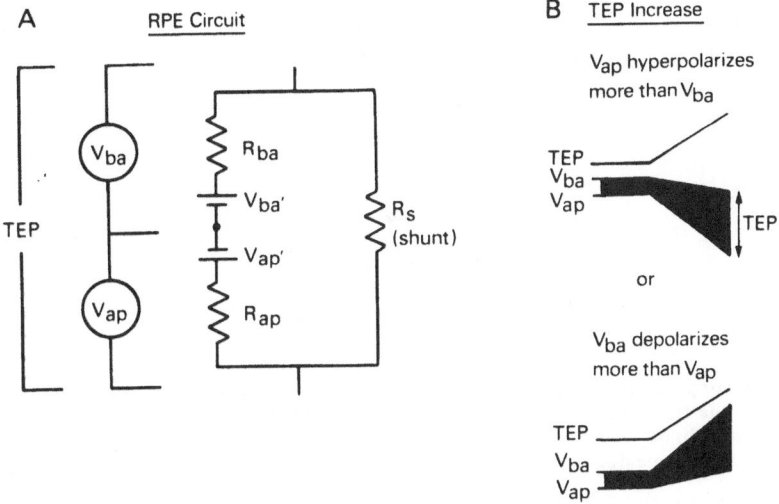

Fig. 3. Schematic circuit of the retinal pigment epithelium (A), and mechanisms for an increase in trans-epithelial potential (B). A. Circuit components: R_{ap} – apical membrane resistance; R_{ba} – basal membrane resistance; R_s – shunt resistance; V_{ap}' – apical membrane battery; V_{ba}' – basal membrane battery; V_{ap} – measured apical membrane potential; V_{ba} – measured basal membrane potential. TEP – trans-epithelial potential. B. TEP increase: A TEP increase may result either from a hyperpolarization of V_{ap} relative to V_{ba} (top) or from a depolarization of V_{ba} relative to V_{ap} (bottom).

represents the basal membrane potential and V_{ap} represents the apical membrane potential. In the dark, in cat, for example, the apical membrane potential is more hyperpolarized (more "inside negative") than the basal membrane potential. The difference is a TEP of about 12 mV whose polarity is apical side (or vitreal) positive.

The light peak starts with an increase in TEP and this can originate at the two cell membranes in one of only two ways (Fig. 3B). If it originates at the apical membrane, then the apical membrane must *hyperpolarize* with respect to the basal. If it originates at the basal membrane, then this membrane must *depolarize* with respect to the apical.[1] These two mechanisms clearly are quite different and finding out which one is responsible for the light peak is an important step towards understanding its mechanism.

If we are to interpret intracellular recordings from the RPE, then we must take into account the effects of passive voltage drops at the cell membranes, which result from current flow across the *shunt* resistances. Referring to the circuit diagram of Fig. 3A, it will be clear that the apical and basal membranes are connected through R_s, primarily the resistance of the tight junctions between cells. This means that current must flow around the circuit that will modify the apical and basal membrane potentials. More importantly this

---

[1] One additional possibility is that it originates as a diffusion potential across the paracellular shunt. In that case, the apical membrane would hyperpolarize and the basal membrane would depolarize.

5

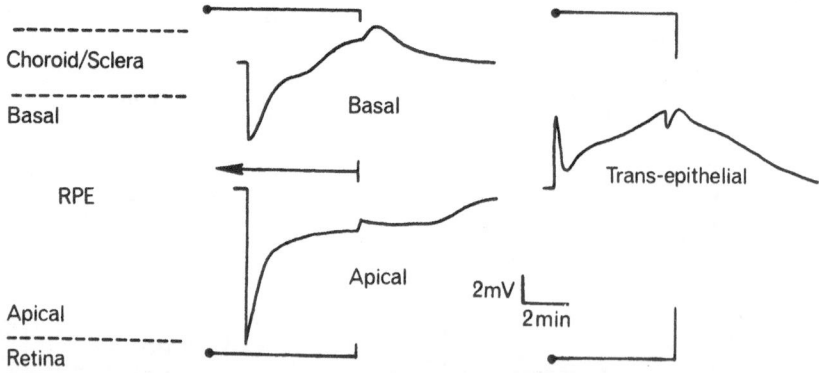

Fig. 4. The origin of the trans-epithelial light peak (cat). The intracellular RPE recordings show that the trans-epithelial light peak originates at the RPE cell as a depolarization of the basal membrane. Since there is little shunting from the basal to the apical membrane, the apical membrane does not depolarize. Responses are to 5 min of illumination.

current will change whenever a potential is initiated at either cell membrane. The size and relative importance of this effect will vary depending on the relative size of all three resistances in this circuit (R_{ap}, R_{ba}, R_s). The practical effect of shunting is to reduce the magnitude of the voltage at the membrane generating it and to produce a smaller voltage of the same polarity at the opposite membrane. Thus, as shown in Fig. 3B, top, a hyperpolarization initiated at the apical membrane is accompanied by a smaller hyperpolariz- ation of the basal membrane.

To find out which membrane generated the light peak, micro-electrodes were placed intracellularly in the RPE of both cat (Fig. 4) and gecko (Fig. 5) to record the apical and basal membrane potentials. In cat (Fig. 4) the response to light began with a large hyperpolarization of the apical membrane and because of "shunting" from the apical to the basal membrane, a smaller hyperpolarization, with the same time course, at the basal membrane (example in Fig. 3B, top). The hyperpolarization reached a peak at about 4.0 sec after the onset of light and then the apical membrane repolarized to a new plateau that was still more hyperpolarized than the dark-adapted level. This sequence of events is the response of the apical membrane to the light-evoked decrease of $[K^+]_0$ in the subretinal space and represents the RPE component of the c-wave (Steinberg et al., 1970; Oakley and Green, 1976; Oakley, 1977; Steinberg et al., 1980; Linsenmeier and Steinberg, this volume).

The c-wave response was followed by a depolarization of the basal mem- brane that had the time course of the light peak. In cat there is little shunting in the basal to the apical direction so the apical membrane does not appear to depolarize during the light peak in Fig. 4. The responses of gecko, however, show a large depolarization of the basal membrane and a smaller depolarization of the apical membrane during the light peak (Fig. 5). Here, there *is* shunting from the basal to the apical membrane, but as in cat, the depolarization is initiated at the basal membrane (example in Fig. 3B, bottom). The light peak, therefore, in both cat and gecko, originates as a depolarization of the basal membrane of the RPE.

6

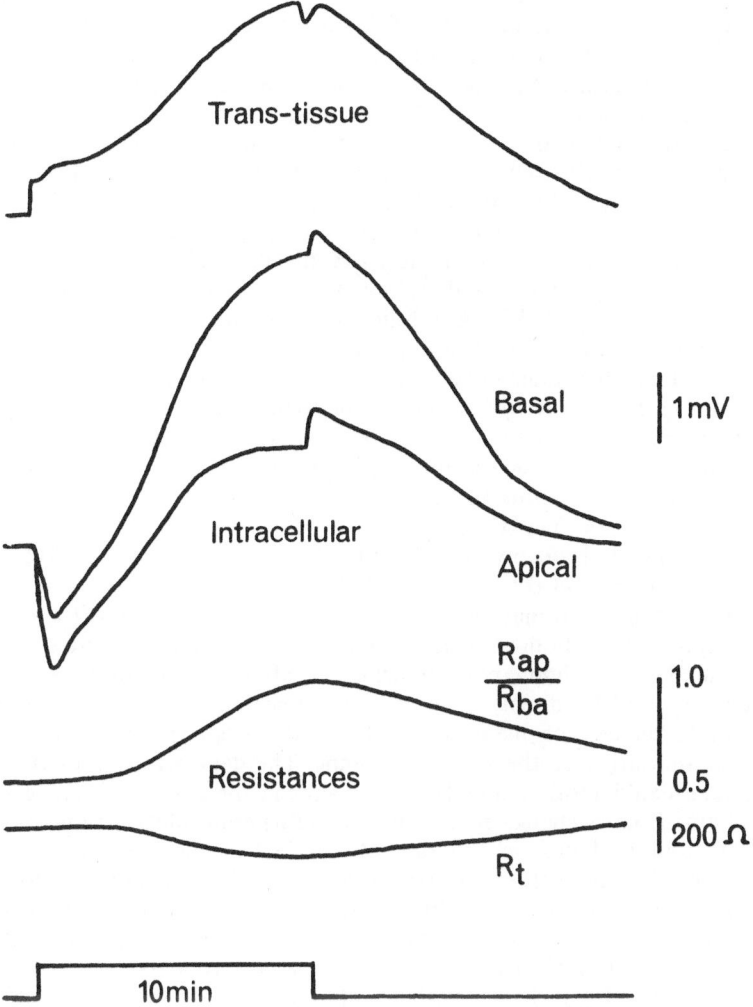

Fig. 5. Resistance changes during the light peak, and the RPE origin of the light peak in gecko. Intracellular RPE recordings (middle) show that the trans-tissue (top) light peak originates from the RPE cell as a basal membrane depolarization. Because of shunting the apical membrane also depolarizes with the same time course. Responses are to 10 min of illumination. To measure R_t, trans-epithelial resistance, and R_{ap}/R_{ba} (Fig. 3), 1.0 uA, 1.0 sec square current pulses were passed across the tissue and the iR drops were monitored across the tissue and separately across each RPE cell membrane. The iR drop across the tissue is proportional to R_t, while the ratio of the iR drops of the cell membranes gives R_{ap}/R_{ba}. These measurements show that R_{ap}/R_{ba} increases and R_t decreases with the time-course of the light peak. This is most consistant with a decrease in the resistance of the basal membrane, R_{ba}, during the light peak.

7

DISCUSSION

We have shown that the potential of the light peak originates at the RPE as a depolarization of the basal membrane. By contrast, it is preceded by the c-wave hyperpolarization, which originates at the apical membrane. Yet, the light peak, like the c-wave, depends upon light that is absorbed by the photoreceptors. It is intriguing, therefore, that the light peak originates from the other side of the RPE cell, at the membrane facing the choriocapillaris. What mechanisms produce this response?

Figure 6 shows a proposed sequence of events. From its spectral properties and sensitivity we know that the initial event must be absorption of light by the photoreceptors (Arden and Kelsey, 1962; Täumer et al. 1976b; Linsenmeier and Steinberg, 1982). But following this, until depolarization of the basal membrane, the sequence is hypothetical (brackets, Fig. 6). We speculate that a substance is produced (or consumed) by the neural retina and diffuses to (or away from) the *apical* membrane. This would resemble the $[K^+]_0$ change, which is intitiated by the photoreceptors (Oakley et al., 1979) and which then hyperpolarizes the apical membrane during the c-wave. Unfortunately, we do not yet know the nature of the "light-peak substance" or even where it originates. The time course of $[K^+]_0$ changes in the cat retina suggests that it is probably not K^+ (Steinberg and Niemeyer, 1981), while recent experiments on the *in vitro* gecko preparation suggest that our hypothetical substance still may originate in the photoreceptors (Griff and Steinberg, unpub. obs.). Following its change in concentration in the subretinal space the *basal membrane* must somehow be affected. The route to the basal membrane could be direct — the substance reaching there after being transported into the cell, or one or more intracellular messengers might be responsible for the effect at the basal membrane. The depolarization of the basal membrane could result either from a change in the concentration of a permeant ion, from a change in the membrane's permeability to one or more ions or from a change in the rate of an electrogenic ion pump. Current pulses can be passed across the RPE of gecko during the light peak to determine if there are changes in RPE resistances that might reveal a change in permeability at the basal membrane. Figure 5 shows that both the transepithelial resistance (R_t) and the ratio of apical to basal cell membrane resistances (R_{ap}/R_{ba}) change with the time course of the light peak. The direction of these changes is consistent with a decrease in basal membrane resistance (and increase in permeability) during the light peak (see legend Fig. 5 for more details), but this might be a voltage-dependent effect, and therefore a consequence of the basal membrane depolarization instead of its cause.

Does the light-peak mechanism, described here in animal models, also apply to the human response? As indicated above the cat and human light peaks are similar in form and in stimulus-response characteristics. The similarity extends, further, to the presence in cat of at least one additional slow oscillation following the light peak, which also has been shown to originate from a change in TEP (Linsenmeier and Steinberg, 1982). In addition, the resistance changes, just described for gecko, also have been found in cat where they are the basis for the changes in c-wave amplitude that occur

8

MECHANISM OF LIGHT PEAK

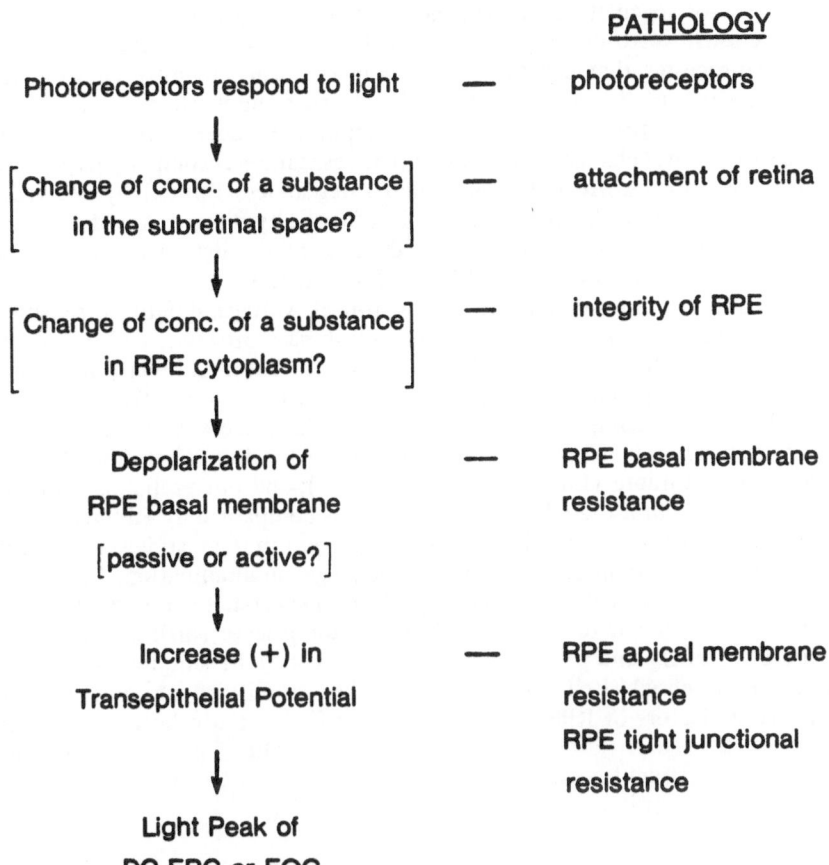

PATHOLOGY

Photoreceptors respond to light — photoreceptors

↓

[Change of conc. of a substance in the subretinal space?] — attachment of retina

↓

[Change of conc. of a substance in RPE cytoplasm?] — integrity of RPE

↓

Depolarization of RPE basal membrane [passive or active?] — RPE basal membrane resistance

↓

Increase (+) in Transepithelial Potential — RPE apical membrane resistance RPE tight junctional resistance

↓

Light Peak of DC ERG or EOG

Fig. 6. Mechanism of the light peak. A sequence of steps leading to the light peak of the DC ERG or EOG is outlined. Steps in brackets have yet to be demonstrated. Possible pathologies associated with each step are shown at the right.

during the light peak (Linsenmeier and Steinberg, 1983a and this volume pp. 21–28). Most strikingly, identical effects on the c-wave occur in the human retina, where they actually had been described much earlier (Skoog and Nilsson, 1974; Nilsson and Skoog, 1975). The c-wave effects indicate that similar changes in resistance occur also in the human RPE during the light peak. Thus, there is now very strong evidence that RPE participation in the light peak is very similar in lizard, cat and human.

Is knowledge of the cellular origin of the light peak voltage clinically useful? In Fig. 5 (right side) we suggest how pathological processes might disturb the light peak at each step in the generative sequence. The integrity of the neural retina, particularly the photoreceptors, the RPE, and their attachment all should be required for a normal response. What we need to

9

know, therefore, is the relative sensitivity of each of these steps to disease processes. More specifically, for effects of neural retinal pathology we can say little until the mechanisms there are better understood. For the RPE, however, we may speculate that the generation of the light-peak voltage should be quite sensitive to disease. The light-peak voltage will be changed by pathological processes that directly affect its mechanism and by processes that affect any one of the components of the electrical network of the tissue. It would seem that the latter should be a common consequence of RPE disease, as we suspect that changes in cell-membrane resistances accompany pathology of cell membranes. Also, the paracellular resistance, formed by the tight junctions between cells, might be readily affected by disease. Any disruption of these junctions, for example, would decrease the light-peak voltage by virtue of the decrease in shunt resistance (Fig. 3A, R_s).

We have just considered how the light-peak voltage should be sensitive both to direct attacks on its mechanism by disease processes and indirectly to events that alter any of the RPE resistances. These indirect effects also apply to other light-evoked RPE events such as the c-wave. We previously have shown, for example, that both the light peak and c-wave are exquisitely sensitive to hypoxia, changing at arterial oxygen tensions where the blood is still nearly saturated (Linsenmeier et al., 1983); and our preliminary observations indicate that these hypoxic effects are accompanied by RPE resistance changes. The sensitivity of the TEP also is present in the resting state, that is when the TEP is unmodified by previous changes in illumination. This "resting" TEP is the principal component of the corneal standing potential, which also has been shown to change its level in response to small alterations of blood PO_2, PCO_2 and pH (Linsenmeier et al., 1983). In sum, both the transepithelial potential itself, and its light-evoked modifications appear to be sensitive indicators of RPE function. We must find out now how *interactions* between the neural retina and the RPE alter the TEP. Only then may it be possible to distinguish whether the RPE *or* the neural retina is primarily affected by disease.

ACKNOWLEDGEMENT

We wish to thank A. Moorehouse for assistance with experiments. This work was supported by N.I.H. grants EY 01429 to R.H.S. and EY 05447 to E.R.G.

REFERENCES

Arden, G. B. and Kelsey, J. H. (1962). Some observations on the relationship between the standing potential of the eye and the bleaching and regeneration of visual purple. J. Physiol. 161, 205–226.

Gouras, P. and Carr, R. E (1965). Light-induced DC responses of monkey retina before and after central retinal artery interruption. Invest. Ophthalmol. 4, 310–317.

Griff, E. R. and Steinberg, R. H. (1982). Origin of the light peak: in vitro study of *Gekko gekko*. J. Physiol., 331, 637–652.

Imaizumi, K. Atsumi, K., Takahashi, F., and Toshida, G. (1968). In Clinical Value of Electroretinography. ISCERG Symp., 1966. pp. 74–82. S. Karger, Basel/N.Y.

Kikawada, N. (1968). Variations in the corneo-retinal standing potential of the vertebrate eye during light and dark adaptations. Jap. J. Physiol. 18, 687−702.

Lieberman, H. R. (1977). Origin of the ocular light-modulated standing potential in cat. Ph. D. Thesis, U. of Florida.

Linsenmeier, R. A., Mines, A. H., and Steinberg, R. H. (1983). Effects of hypoxia and hypercapnia on the light peak and electroretinogram of the cat. Invest. Ophthalmol. Visual Sci., 24, 37−46.

Linsenmeier, R. A. and Steinberg, R. H. (1982). Origin and sensitivity of the light peak in the intact cat eye. J. Physiol., 331, 653−673.

Linsenmeier, R. A. and Steinberg, R. H. (1983a). A light-evoked interaction of the apical and basal membranes of the retinal pigment epithelium: the c-wave and the light peak. J. Neurophysiol., in press.

Linsenmeier, R. A. and Steinberg, R. H. (1983b). Variations of c-wave amplitude in the cat eye. This volume. pp. 21−28.

Madachi-Yamamoto, S. (1980). Abolition of the light rise by aspartate. Societas Ophthalmol. Jap. 84, 607−616.

Marmor, M. F. and Lurie, M. (1979). Light-induced electrical responses of the retinal pigment epithelium. In The Retinal Pigment Epithelium, eds. Zinn, K. M. and Marmor, M. F. pp. 226−244. Harvard Univ. Press, Cambridge, Massachusetts.

Niemeyer, G. (1980). Electrooculography in isolated perfused mammalian eyes. Experientia 36, 699.

Nikara, T., Sato, S., Takamatsu, T., Sato, R., and Mita, T. (1976). A new wave (2nd c-wave) on corneoretinal potential. Experientia 32, 594−596.

Nilsson, S. E. G., and Skoog, K.-O. (1975). Covariation of the simultaneously recorded c-wave and standing potential of the human eye. Acta Ophthalmol. 53, 721−730.

Noell, W. K., (1953). Studies on the electrophysiology and metabolism of the retina. USAF School of Aviation Medicine Project 21-1201-0004.

Oakley, B., II. (1977). Potassium and the photoreceptor dependent pigment epithelial hyperpolarization. J. gen. Physiol. 70, 405−425.

Oakley, B., II and Green, D. G. (1976). Correlation of light-induced changes in retinal extracellular potassium concentration with the c-wave of the electroretinogram. J. Neurophysiol. 39, 1117−1133.

Oakley, B., II., Flaming, D. G. and Brown, K. T. (1979). Effects of the rod receptor potential upon extracellular potassium ion concentration. J. gen. Physiol. 74, 713−737.

Rodieck, R. W. (1973). The Vertebrate Retina. pp. 525−532, W. H. Freeman, San Francisco.

Skoog, K.-O. and Nilsson, S. E. G. (1974). The c-wave of the human D. C. registered ERG. II. Cyclic variations of the c-wave amplitude. Acta Ophthalmol. 52, 904−912.

Steinberg, R. H. and Miller, S. S. (1979). Transport and membrane properties of the retinal pigment epithelium. In The Retinal Pigment Epithelium, eds. Zinn, K. M. and Marmor, M. F. pp. 205−225. Harvard Univ. Press, Cambridge, Massachusetts.

Steinberg, R. H. and Niemeyer, G. (1981). Light peak of cat DC ERG: not generated by change in K^+. Invest. Ophthalmol. 20, 414−418.

Steinberg, R. H., Oakley, B., II. and Niemeyer, G. (1980). Light-evoked changes in $[K^+]_o$ in the retina of the intact cat eye. J. Neurophysiol. 44, 897−921.

Steinberg, R. H., Schmidt, R., and Brown, K. T., (1970). Intracellular responses to light from cat retinal pigment epithelium: origin of the electroretinogram c-wave Nature 227, 728−730.

Täumer, R. (1976). Electro-oculography: Its clinical importance, ed. R. Täumer. Bibl. Ophthalmol. 85.

Täumer, R., Hennig, J. and Wolff, L. (1976a). Further investigations conerning the fast oscillation of the retinal potential. Bibl. Ophthalmol. 85, 57−67.

Täumer, R., Rohde, N. and Pernice, D. (1976b). The slow oscillation of the retinal potential. Bibl. Ophthalmol. 85. 40−56.

Valeton, J. M. and van Norren, D. (1982). Intraretinal recording of slow electrical responses to steady illumination in monkey: retinal and pigment epithelial contributions. Vision Res. 22, 393−399.

Mailing address:
Department of Physiology, S-762
University of California, San Francisco
San Francisco, CA 94143,
U.S.A.

THE CELLULAR ORIGIN OF THE FAST OSCILLATION

E. R. GRIFF, R. A. LINSENMEIER and R. H. STEINBERG
(San Francisco, California, U.S.A.).

ABSTRACT

We studied the cellular origin of the fast oscillation of the DCERT in two animal models. In the intact anesthetized cat eye, a step of illumination evoked a DCERG similar in waveform and time course to that in the human. The fast oscillation was evident as a Rough between the c-wave and the light peak. By recording with microelectrodes directly across the retinal pigment epithelium (RPE), we demonstrated that a decrease in trans-epithelial potential (TEP) was the major source of the fast oscillation. Intracellular recordings from the RPE showed that this TEP decrease was accompanied by a hyperpolarization of the RPE basal membrane. In the lizard, *Gekko gekko*, a similar but slower sequence of potentials was recorded from an *in vitro* preparation of neural retina-RPE-choroid. As in cat, a decrease in TEP was generated primarily by a hyperpolarization of the RPE basal membrane. We have further studied this response in the isolated RPE of gecko where it can be produced solely by decreasing $[K^+]$ in the apical bathing solution. We conclude that the fast oscillation is initiated by a light-evoked decrease in subretinal $[K^+]$ that leads to an RPE basal membrane hyperpolarization.

INTRODUCTION

The purpose of this paper is to summarize our recent research on the fast oscillation of the cornea standing potential. The fast oscillation was first described by Kolder and Brecher (1966) in humans, and Kolder and North (1966) in rabbits and dogs in response to alternating periods of light and dark stimuli. One cycle of the fast oscillation can be evoked by maintained illumination, and it can be recorded indirectly in the electrooculogram (EOG) or directly in the DC electroretinogram (DCERG) (Täumer et al., 1976). In this paper, we describe the fast oscillation of the DCERG evoked by maintained illumination in the intact cat eye and *in vitro* preparations of the lizard, *Gekko gekko*. Responses to shorter or alternating stimuli are complicated by the summation of components at light on and light off.

There has been disagreement as to whether the fast oscillation is an individual event having a unique cellular origin or whether it is the sum of

13

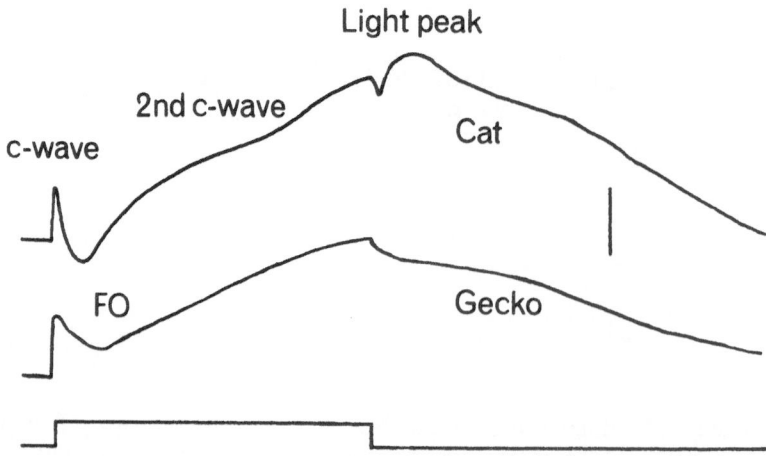

Fig. 1. DCERGs from the intact cat eye and the retina-RPE-choroid preparation of gecko. In both there is a dip in potential, the fast oscillation (FO), between the c-wave and the light peak; in cat, a 2nd c-wave is also present. The stimulus was 5 min in duration for cat and 10 min for gecko; the calibration is 1.0 and 0.7 mV, respectively. All figures in this paper show tracings with the approximate time courses and amplitudes of the actual responses.

previously described potentials that overlap in time. We will describe a new response of the retinal pigment epithelium (RPE), identified in both cat (Linsenmeier and Steinberg, 1983) and gecko (Griff and Steinberg, 1983). This response, termed the *delayed basal hyperpolarization*, is initiated by the light-evoked potassium decrease in the subretinal space and produces a decrease in the potential across the RPE. We will discuss the relative contributions of the neural retina and RPE to the fast oscillation and show that it is generated primarily at the RPE basal membrane.

RESULTS

Figure 1 presents examples of DCERGs recorded from the vitreous in cat and across the neural retina-RPE-choroid preparation in gecko (see Steinberg et al., these proceedings, for methods). The cat recording closely resembles the human DCERG, and the same responses can be observed in the EOG (Täumer et al., 1976). In cat there is a dip in potential to or below the baseline about 25 sec after light onset that is equivalent to the human fast oscillation (30 sec). This is followed by a small increase in potential to a shoulder, the 2nd c-wave (Nikara et al., 1976), and then a large increase to the light peak. These responses are also present in gecko, where they are considerably slower, as expected for a cold-blooded animal; for example, the dip following the c-wave occurs at 2 min. Thus, the fast oscillation, first described in the human eye, also can be recorded from cat and gecko, where it can be studied experimentally.

We first asked whether the fast oscillation was generated by the neural

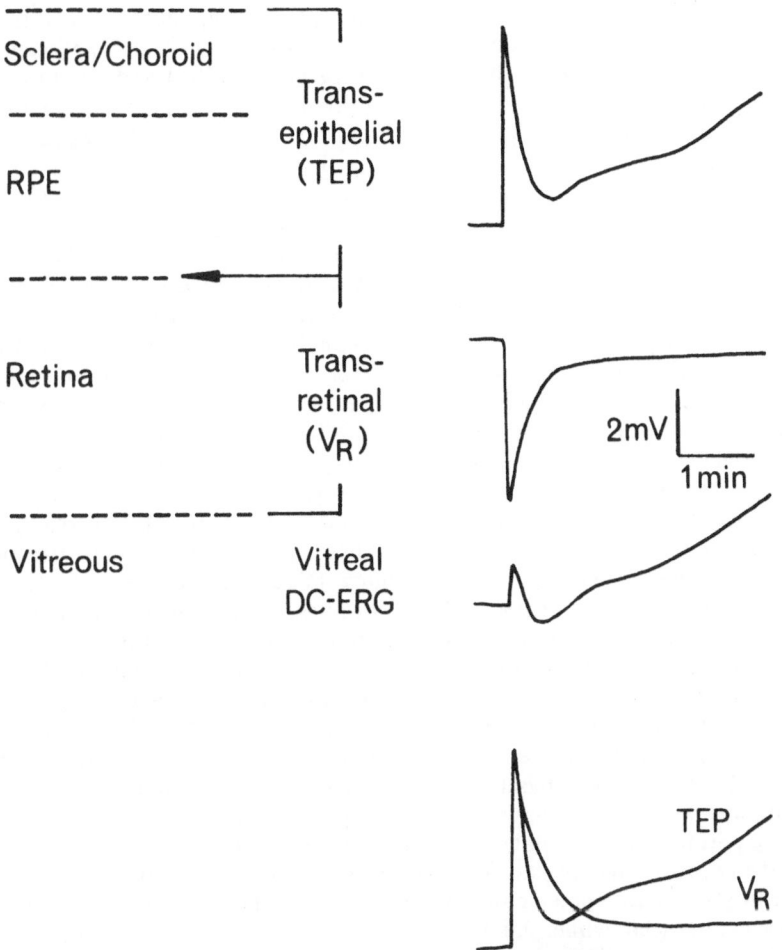

Fig. 2. Trans-epithelial and trans-retinal recordings (cat). A microelectrode was positioned in the subretinal space between the neural retina and RPE to record the trans-retinal potential, V_R, and the trans-epithelial potential, TEP. The vitreal response was recorded between the vitreous and a retrobulbar reference. All recordings are shown with a vitreal positive recording polarity. Below, V_R has been inverted and scaled to the TEP response.

retina, the RPE, or by both structures. Using the experimental approach described in the preceding paper (Steinberg et al., these proceedings), a micro-electrode positioned in the subretinal space recorded the potential across the neural retina, the trans-retinal potential (V_R), and the potential across the RPE, the trans-epithelial potential (TEP). Fig. 2 shows examples of these recordings in cat. The TEP response began with a vitreal positive component, the RPE c-wave, that added to a smaller vitreal negative component in the V_R response, called slow PIII (Faber, 1969), to produce the vitreal c-wave.

Previous work has shown that the TEP and V_R responses, until the c-wave peak, both result from the light-evoked decrease in subretinal potassium,

15

$[K^+]_0$ (Steinberg et al., 1980; Oakley, 1977; Griff, unpublished), and therefore follow the same time course. Following the c-wave peak, $[K^+]_0$ reaccumulated while the light was still on (Steinberg et al., 1980) and, as shown in Fig. 2, both V_R and REP returned toward their baselines. Their time courses, however, differed greatly, TEP returning *faster* and *further* than V_R; a dip in potential is evident in the TEP recording that corresponded in time to the vitreal fast oscillation. Superposition of an inverted V_R response, scaled to the TEP (Fig. 2, bottom), showed that this disparity began with the recovery from peak. We concluded from recordings of this type that the TEP contains a new component that is not present in V_R. In the *Discussion* we will show that this component is the principle source of the fast oscillation.

To determine whether the RPE apical or basal membrane generated the additional TEP component, we recorded each membrane potential as described in the previous paper (Steinberg et al., these proceedings). From previous work (Oakley, 1977; Steinberg et al., 1980), we expected that as $[K^+]_0$ decreased, the apical membrane would hyperpolarize to produce the TEP increase to the c-wave peak and then, as $[K^+]$ reaccumulated, the apical membrane would repolarize (depolarize) and produce the TEP decrease; the basal membrane would passively follow these apical changes due to electrical shunting (Steinberg et al., these proceedings; Miller and Steinberg, 1977). Fig. 3 shows examples of intracellular recordings during the c-wave and fast oscillation from gecko; similar results were obtained in cat (Linsenmeier and Steinberg, 1983). During the rise of the c-wave (period 1), the apical membrane hyperpolarized relative to the basal membrane, as expected. During period 2, however, the TEP decrease was not generated solely by an apical repolarization. Rather, the *basal membrane hyperpolarized relative to the apical*. In gecko, this basal hyperpolarization was shunted to the apical membrane where it was larger than the expected apical repolarization. Thus, during period 2, a hyperpolarization *generated* at the basal membrane dominated the recordings. In cat, where shunting from basal to apical is much less than in gecko (Linsenmeier and Steinberg, 1982), the apical membrane sometimes depolarized while the basal hyperpolarized. In both cat and gecko, therefore, the new TEP component began with a basal hyperpolarization.

We have further studied the mechanism of the basal hyperpolarization in an isolated RPE-choroid preparation (neural retina removed) of gecko (Griff and Steinberg, 1983). We produced RPE responses equivalent to the RPE c-wave and fast oscillation simply by decreasing the $[K^+]$ in the RPE apical bathing solution by an amount similar to the light-evoked $[K^+]$ decrease that occurred in the intact retina. In the isolated RPE, this $[K^+]_0$ decrease first hyperpolarized the apical membrane so that the TEP increased ("c-wave") and subsequently led to a basal hyperpolarization that produced a TEP decrease ("fast oscillation"). The apical hyperpolarization is the expected response due to a change in the potassium equilibrium potential (Miller and Steinberg, 1977). The basal hyperpolarization, recorded in isolation or evoked by light in the intact retina, is a *delayed* consequence of the decrease in apical (or subretinal) $[K^+]$, and we have termed this response the *delayed basal hyperpolarization*.

16

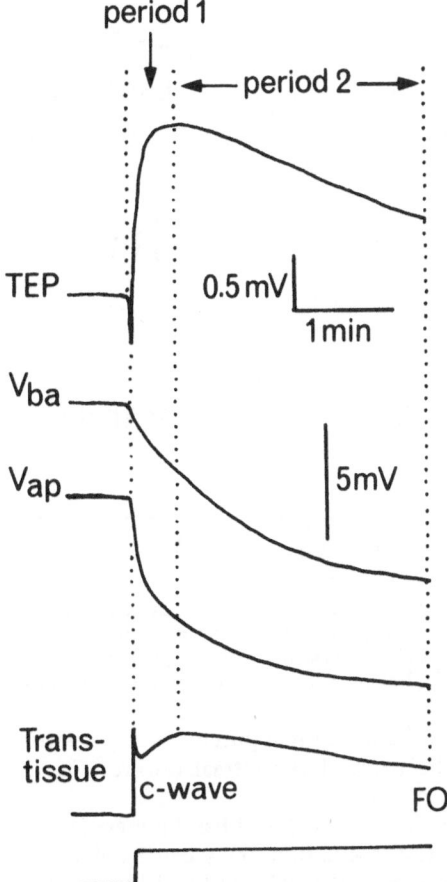

Fig. 3. RPE intracellular recordings (gecko). The trans-epithelial potential (TEP) was recorded as in Fig. 2. The basal membrane potential, V_{ba} was recorded between an intracellular microelectrode and an electrode in the choroidal bathing solution. The apical membrane potential, V_{ap} is the difference between TEP and V_{ba}. The trans-tissue recording across the retina-RPE-choroid is also shown. Responses to 3 min of illumination are shown: the c-wave (period 1) is followed by the fast oscillation, FO (period 2). During period 1, V_{ap} hyperpolarized more than V_{ba}; during period 2, V_{ba} hyperpolarized more than V_{ap}. See text for explanation.

DISCUSSION

We have described a new response of the RPE basal membrane that occurs during the fast oscillation of the DCERG in both cat and gecko. This delayed response is *generated* at the basal membrane and produces a *TEP decrease*. The TEP decrease from the peak of the c-wave also has another component, the repolarization of the apical membrane that follows the reaccumulation of $[K^+]_o$. Both events, therefore, tend to bring TEP back towards baseline following the c-wave. In addition to these potentials generated at the RPE

17

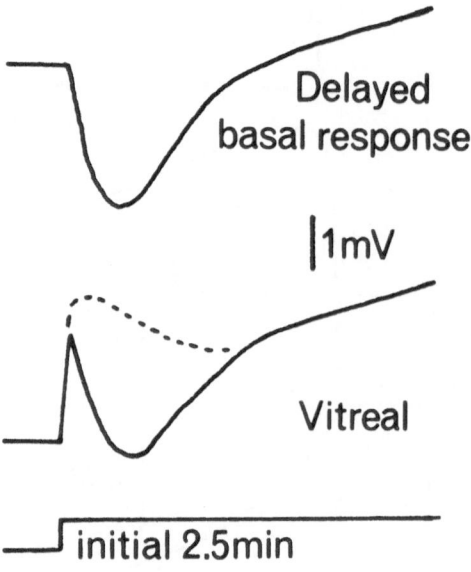

Fig. 4. The delayed basal response in the cat. The delayed basal response (top) was isolated by subtracting those potentials originating at the apical membrane which were shunted to the basal membrane (see text). When this response was, in turn, subtracted from the vitreal DCERG (bottom), the fast oscillation was absent (dotted line).

apical and basal membranes, retinal potentials also contribute to the decrease in potential from the peak of the vitreal c-wave (Fig. 2). What then is the source of the fast oscillation?

We will now show that the delayed basal hyperpolarization is the essential component of the fast oscillation. This can be illustrated by constructing DCERGs in the absence of the delayed basal hyperpolarization. To do this, we first had to determine its magnitude and time course, which is problematical since the potential change generated at the apical membrane during the delayed basal hyperpolarization is partially shunted to the basal membrane, and adds to the potentials that originate there. In cat, however, we were able to estimate how large these shunted potentials were, and to subtract them from the basal membrane potential.[1] Fig. 4 (top) shows the delayed basal component isolated by this subtraction. It began about 2 sec after light onset as a hyperpolarization that peaked in about 20 sec, and then recovered (depolarized) toward the baseline. This response gives not only an estimate of the delayed basal hyperpolarization, but also its contribution to the TEP, since, in cat, basal potentials are not significantly attenuated by shunting to the apical membrane (Linsenmeier and Steinberg, 1982). When this response

[1] Our analysis was possible in cat because the apical membrane potential is uncontaminated by basal potentials, whereas, in gecko, the delayed basal hyperpolarization is partly shunted to the apical membrane. In cat, we have simplified the analysis (but see Linsenmeier and Steinberg, 1983) by ignoring the passive iR drop of slow PIII across the RPE; pick-up of slow PIII, however, does not alter our conclusions.

MECHANISM OF FAST OSCILLATION

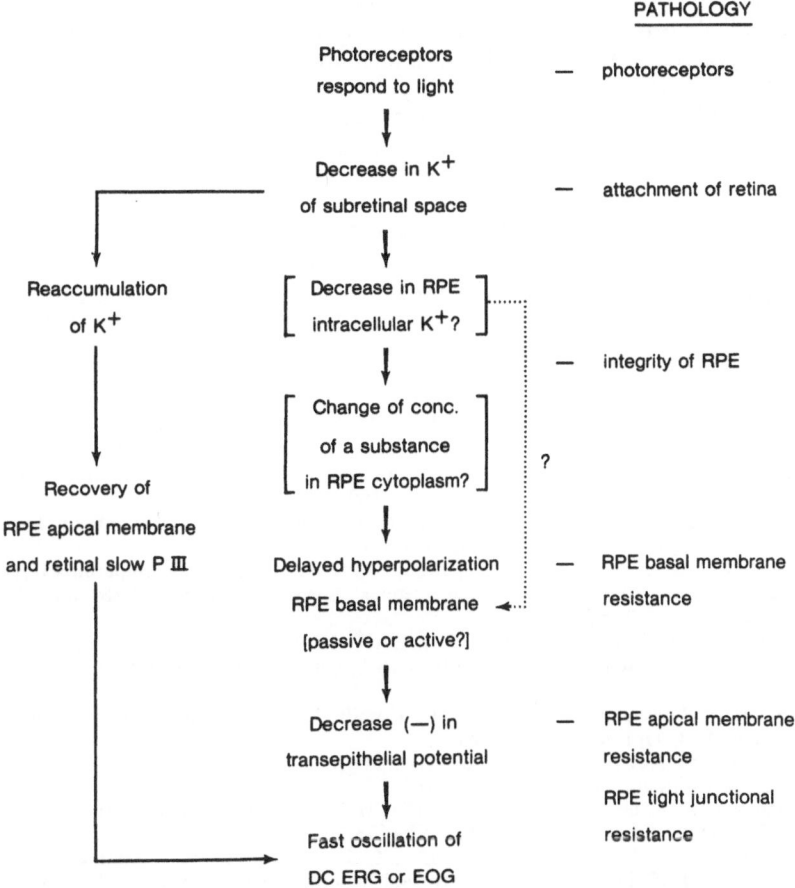

Fig. 5. Mechanism of the fast oscillation. A sequence of steps leading to the fast oscillation of the DCERG or EOG is outlined. Steps in brackets have yet to be demonstrated; the dashed line indicates an alternate path. Possible pathologies associated with each step are shown at the right.

was subtracted from the vitreal DCERG, little or no fast oscillation remained (Fig. 4, dotted vitreal response). We conclude, therefore, that the major source of the fast oscillation is a discrete event — the delayed basal hyperpolarization.

Figure 5 summarizes the mechanism of the fast oscillation and how it might be affected by disease at each step; the major pathway is shown in the center column. Light absorbed by the photoreceptors leads to a decrease in subretinal $[K^+]$ that initiates potentials in the neural retina and RPE, in particular a delayed basal membrane hyperpolarization that decreases TEP. The decrease in extracellular $[K^+]$ leads to a decrease in RPE intracellular $[K^+]$ that may be necessary to produce the basal response (Griff and Steinberg, 1982a). In the *isolated* RPE of gecko we have recently demonstrated

19

such a decrease using intracellular K+-selective microelectrodes (Griff and Steinberg, 1982b). The mechanism of the delayed basal hyperpolarization, however, and its relationship to intracellular [K+] are still unknown. The light-evoked decrease in subretinal [K+] also produces other retinal potentials. A hyperpolarization of the RPE apical membrane generates the TEP component of the c-wave and a proposed hyperpolarization of the Müller cells generates the slow PIII (Faber, 1969). These potentials occur during the fast oscillation and can, therefore, influence its amplitude and time course.

ACKNOWLEDGEMENT

We wish to thank A. Moorehouse for assistance with experiments. This work was supported by N.I.H. grants EY01429 to R.H.S. and EY05447 to E.R.G.

REFERENCES

Faber, D. S. (1969). Analysis of the slow transretinal potentials in response to light. Ph.D. thesis. State Univ. of New York at Buffalo.
Griff, E. R. and Steinberg, R. H. (1982a). Light evokes RPE basal membrane hyperpolarization. Invest. Ophthalmol. and Vis. Sci. 22 (suppl.), 280.
Griff, E. R. and Steinberg, R. H. (1982b). RPE basal membrane hyperpolarization follows light-evoked, K+-dependent, apical membrane hyperpolarization. Soc. Neurosci. Abstr. 7, 44.
Griff, E. R. and Steinberg, R. H. (1983). Delayed basal membrane polarizations: new potassium-dependent responses of the retinal pigment epithelium. J. Gen. Physiol. In press.
Kolder, H. and Brecher, G. A. (1966). Fast oscillations of the corneo-retinal potential in man. Arch. Ophthal. 75, 232–237.
Kolder, H. and North, A. W. (1966). Oscillations of the corneo-retinal potential in animals. Ophthalmologica, 152, 149–160.
Linsenmeier, R. A. and Steinberg, R. H. (1982). Origin and sensitivity of the light peak in the intact cat eye. J. Physiol. 331, 653–673.
Linsenmeier, R. A. and Steinberg, R. H. (1983). A delayed basal membrane hyperpolarization of the cat retinal pigment epithelium, and its relation to the fast oscillation of the DC electroretinogram. J. Gen. Physiol. In press.
Miller, S. S. and Steinberg, R. H. (1977). Passive ionic properties of frog retinal pigment epithelium. J. Membrane Biol. 36, 337–372.
Nikara, T., Sato, S., Takamatsu, R., Sato, R., and Mita, T. (1976). A new wave (2nd c-wave) on corneoretinal potential. Experientia 32, 594–596.
Oakley, B., II (1977). Potassium and the photoreceptor-dependent pigment epithelium hyperpolarization. J. Gen. Physiol. 70, 405–425.
Steinberg, R. H., Griff, E. R., and Linsenmeier, R. A. (1983). The cellular origin of the light peak. This volume. pp. 1–12.
Steinberg, R. H., Oakley, B. II, and Niemeyer, G. (1980). Light-evoked changes in [K+]_0 in retina of intact cat eye. J. Neurophysiol. 44, 897–921.
Täumer, R., Hennig, J., and Wolff, L. (1976). Further investigations concerning the fast oscillation of the retinal potential. Bibl. Ophthalmol. 85, 57–67.

Mailing address:
Department of Physiology, S-762
University of California, San Francisco
San Francisco, CA 94143,
U.S.A.

VARIATIONS OF c-WAVE AMPLITUDE IN THE CAT EYE

R. A. LINSENMEIER and R. H. STEINBERG

(San Francisco, California, U.S.A.)

ABSTRACT

C-wave amplitude changes as a result of a number of experimental manipulations, and presumably is affected in disease as well. The purpose of this paper is to describe the possible mechanisms that could account for these changes. The c-wave recorded at the cornea is the sum of two components, one generated in the neural retina and the other generated in the retinal pigment epithelium (RPE), and a change in either component will lead to a change in c-wave amplitude. Changes in the components could result from a change in the light-evoked decrease in $[K^+]$ in the subretinal space, from a change in the K^+ conductance of the membrane where the component originates, or, at least for the RPE component, from a change in the resistance of other parts of the epithelium. We show that changes in resistance alone account for at least one experimentally produced change in c-wave amplitude, the c-wave increase during the light peak.

INTRODUCTION

The c-wave is a relatively slow corneal-positive component of the ERG, peaking in 2 to 4 sec in mammals. Experimental work on both humans and experimental animals has shown that c-wave amplitude is quite sensitive to a large number of manipulations (Noell, 1953; Knave, Persson and Nilsson, 1975; Nilsson and Skoog, 1974; Skoog, 1974; Linsenmeier, Mines and Steinberg, 1983; Niemeyer, Nagahara and Demant, 1983) most of which are selective in that a- and b-wave amplitudes are not affected, or change in the opposite direction to the c-wave. This sensitivity of the c-wave to experimental manipulations suggests that it may also be selectively sensitive to certain diseases, and could be clinically useful, especially if the mechanisms for changes in c-wave amplitude were understood. As a step in improving the clinical value of the c-wave, this paper catalogs and explains the possible ways in which c-wave amplitude can change. This provides a foundation for investigating the mechanisms responsible for actual changes in c-wave amplitude in selected cases. In the cat we have studied one experimentally induced change in c-wave amplitude that also occurs in the human eye, and this will be presented as an example. The methods for recording from the cat eye

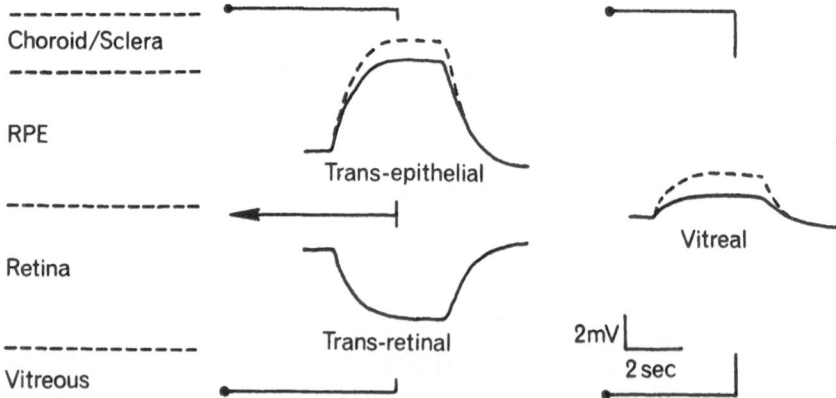

Fig. 1. The components of the cat vitreal c-wave. Both the trans-epithelial and trans-retinal (slow PIII) components are shown with a vitreal positive recording polarity. The TEP is recorded between a microelectrode in the subretinal space and an electrode behind the eye, and the trans-retinal recording is made between the microelectrode and a vitreal electrode. The solid lines show the normal maximum amplitudes of the potentials; the dashed lines show that a small increase in the TEP c-wave causes a large change in the vitreal c-wave. All figures show tracings with approximately the time courses and amplitudes observed. The c-wave is the only ERG component shown, and was evoked in all recordings in this paper by 4 sec flashes of diffuse white light.

have been described (Linsenmeier and Steinberg, 1982; Steinberg, Griff and Linsenmeier, these proceedings).

MECHANISMS FOR CHANGES IN C-WAVE AMPLITUDE

The c-wave as recorded at the cornea, or in the vitreous humor of animals, is the sum of two components (e.g. Rodieck, 1972). One component, generated by the retinal pigment epithelium (RPE) (Steinberg, Schmidt and Brown, 1970), is called here the 'TEP (trans-epithelial) c-wave.' The other component generated in the neural retina, is usually called 'slow PIII' (Faber, 1969). When measured with a vitreal positive recording polarity, the components are as shown in Fig. 1 (solid lines). The TEP c-wave in the cat has a maximum amplitude of about 6 mV, and slow PIII has a maximum of about 5 mV. The vitreal c-wave is the sum of these, so it is about 1 mV. Presumably, at least the relative sizes of these components are similar in the human eye.

Already we can see the complications that might arise in interpreting changes in c-wave amplitude. The vitreal c-wave will become larger if the TEP c-wave increases, slow PIII decreases or both, or if the TEP c-wave increases more than slow PIII. It is important to recognize that if only one component changes while the other is constant (Fig. 1 — dashed lines), the *percentage* changes in the vitreal response will be much larger than in the component that changes, although the absolute change is the same in both this component and in the vitreal c-wave. For instance, if the TEP c-wave increases from 6 to 7 mV, the vitreal c-wave will double. Thus the vitreal c-wave can magnify changes that occur in one component. On the other hand, if both components

22

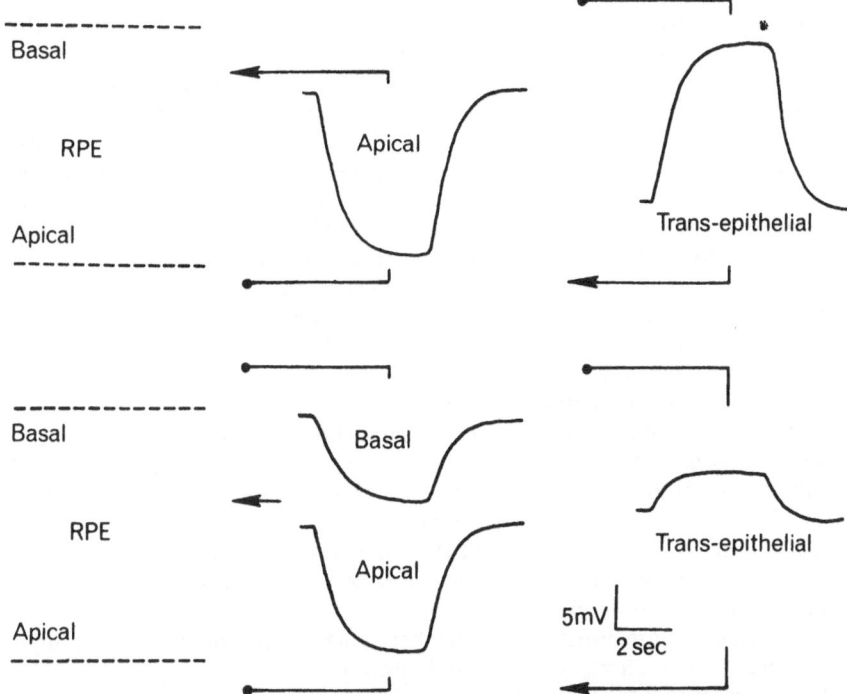

Fig. 2. The origin of the TEP c-wave. Upper: An apical membrane hyperpolarization leads to a TEP increase. Shunting has been ignored. Lower: A smaller TEP c-wave is actually observed, because part of the apical hyperpolarization is shunted to the basal membrane.

change, it is possible that the vitreal c-wave will be unaffected. For instance, if the TEP c-wave were reduced from 6 to 3 mV, and slow PIII were reduced from 5 to 2 mV, the vitreal c-wave would still be 1 mV.

Both c-wave components are thought to be responses to a light-evoked decrease in $[K^+]$ in the subretinal space (Oakley and Green, 1976; Steinberg, Oakley and Niemeyer, 1980), and both could change if the $[K^+]$ decrease were altered. The TEP c-wave is known to be generated by the hyperpolarization of the RPE apical membrane (Steinberg et al., 1970). This hyperpolarization is the expected response of the cell to the change in the K^+ equilibrium potential across the apical membrane, so the relative K^+ conductance of this membrane can also influence the c-wave. Details of the generation of slow PIII are less clear, but it is probably the extracellular sign of the hyperpolarization of Müller cells elicited by the same change in $[K^+]$ (Faber, 1969; Witkovsky, Dudek and Ripps, 1975; Karwoski and Proenza, 1977).

We can describe in detail how the RPE hyperpolarization gives rise to the TEP c-wave. As shown in Fig. 2 (upper), which temporarily neglects the basal membrane, the apical membrane potential is recorded with the intracellular microelectrode referenced to the subretinal space. The trans-epithelial potential, however, is recorded with essentially the opposite polarity, with the microelectrode in the subretinal space, and the reference behind the eye.

23

Therefore, the hyperpolarization of the apical membrane is inverted in the TEP recording, yielding an increase in TEP.

The lower part of Fig. 2 introduces shunting, a complication that is essential for understanding some changes in c-wave amplitude. As discussed in the preceding papers (Steinberg et al.; Griff, Linsenmeier and Steinberg, these proceedings), the apical membrane hyperpolarization leads to a change in current flow through the tight junctions between RPE cells and through the basal membrane, causing a basal hyperpolarization, also; in turn, the apical hyperpolarization is reduced by the current flowing out. Since the basal hyperpolarization effectively subtracts from the apical hyperpolarization, the TEP c-wave is reduced (compare upper and lower parts of Fig. 2). Clearly, factors that influence shunting can change the TEP c-wave. A circuit analysis of the RPE (Miller and Steinberg, 1977; also see Linsenmeier and Steinberg, 1983) shows that the electrical resistances of the apical and basal membranes, and of the paracellular pathway, are the important variables. (Each resistance is the reciprocal of the sum of ionic conductances.) If, for example, the basal membrane resistance decreased, then the shunted basal hyperpolarization would decrease, but the TEP c-wave would *increase*.

To summarize, these are the factors that could cause an increase in c-wave amplitude (a decrease would be produced in exactly the opposite ways):
(1) Decrease in slow PIII alone
    Detailed possibilities await further work on mechanism, but Müller cell conductances are probably important
(2) Increase in TEP c-wave alone
    (a) decrease in apical resistance (via an increase in an ionic conductance)
    (b) decrease in basal resistance
    (c) increase in paracellular resistance
(3) Increase in both components, but a larger change in TEP
    (a) increase in light-evoked change in $[K^+]_o$.

EXAMPLE

The example of c-wave changes considered here is the increase in c-wave amplitude that occurs during the light peak. Repeated flashes each elicit an ERG, and the summed energy of the flashes elicits a light peak. As Nilsson and Skoog (1975) first found in humans, the c-wave is larger at the peak of the light peak than before or after (Fig. 3). This effect also occurs in sheep (Calissendorff, Knave and Persson, 1974), and we have studied it in cats, where the vitreal c-wave amplitude can increase by up to a factor of three.

As illustrated in Fig. 4, recordings of the two c-wave components showed that only the TEP component changed during the light peak (Linsenmeier and Steinberg, 1983). Because of the magnification effect discussed above, a change of only about 20% in the TEP c-wave led to a doubling of the vitreal response. The finding that slow PIII was constant ruled out mechanisms (1) and (3) above, and led us to look for a change in resistance (mechanism 2) as the source of the change in the TEP c-wave. Based on the RPE circuit analysis,

24

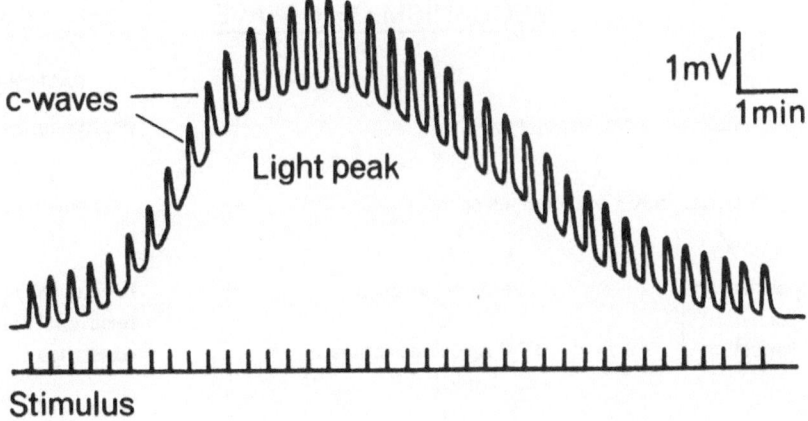

Fig. 3. DC ERG recording (vitreal) showing the variation of c-wave amplitude during the light peak. As shown in the stimulus trace, this response was evoked with a 4 sec flash of diffuse light presented every 30 sec.

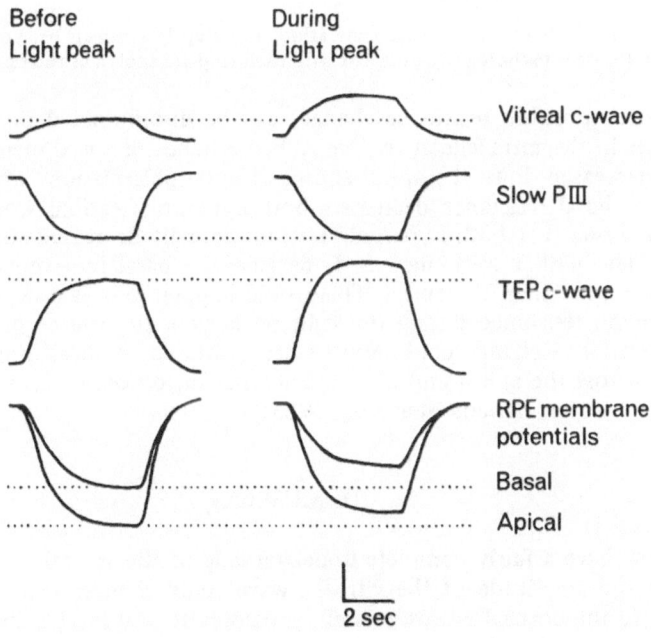

Fig. 4. The mechanism of the change in c-wave amplitude during the light peak, showing that slow PIII was constant while the TEP c-wave increased. The lower two traces show that the increase in the TEP c-wave was accompanied by a reduction in the hyperpolarization of both the apical and basal membranes. The voltage calibration bar is 2 mV for the extracellular recordings and 4 mV for the intracellular recordings.

MECHANISM OF C-WAVE

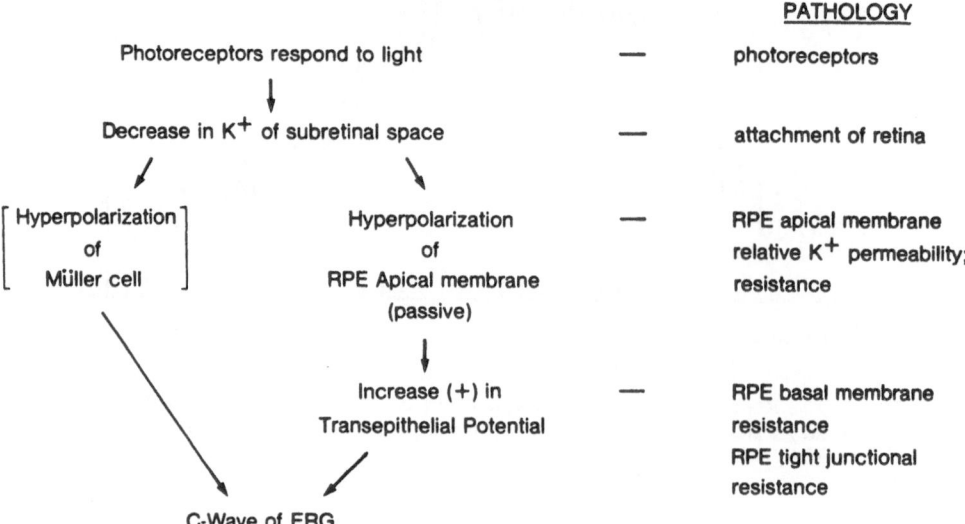

Fig. 5. The mechanism of c-wave generation. The step in brackets has yet to be demonstrated. Possible pathologies associated with each step are shown at the right.

the three possible resistance changes can be discriminated on the basis of changes in the intracellular responses. For instance, if apical membrane resistance decreased, both the apical and basal hyperpolarizations would increase, while if basal resistance decreased, both hyperpolarizations would decrease. Fig. 4 shows that both hyperpolarizations actually decreased during the light peak. The TEP c-wave increased, because the basal hyperpolarization was reduced more than the apical. This would happen only if a decrease in basal membrane resistance during the light peak were the source of the change. The resistance change could also be demonstrated by measuring the voltage drops across the apical and basal membranes in response to constant current pulses (Linsenmeier and Steinberg, 1983).

DISCUSSION

We now have a fairly complete understanding of the several possible ways in which the amplitude of the vitreal c-wave could change. These mechanisms apply to the corneal c-wave as well, and apply to any species, including man. It is not yet clear how many of these mechanisms are clinically important, but potentially all could be. Fig. 5 summarizes the stages in c-wave generation, and suggests how pathology could modify each stage.

In the example described, c-wave amplitude increased because the resistance of the basal membrane decreased during the light peak. We cannot rule out a small contribution from one of the other mechanisms, but this resistance change must be dominant. This is a rather subtle mechanism that would not have been considered without performing a careful circuit analysis of the RPE. An important piece of information gained by working out the mechanism of this c-wave change is that, since the human light peak is also accompanied by an increase in c-wave amplitude, there must be a basal membrane resistance change during the light peak in human, just as there is in cat and gecko (Steinberg, et al., these proceedings). This reinforces our confidence in the cat and gecko as good models for the study of the slow potentials generated by the human RPE, and it should be possible to determine, in gecko, the origin of the resistance change.

While it is too early to generalize, we have evidence that certain pharmacologically induced changes in c-wave amplitude are also a result of resistance changes. The basal membrane and the paracellular junctions form the blood-retinal barrier, and their electrical properties may be affected directly by changes in the composition of the blood.

It is important to realize that the change in c-wave amplitude in the example presented was not caused by a change in the K^+ response during illumination, nor by a change in the properties of the apical membrane, where the c-wave voltage originates. Other changes in c-wave amplitude, however, probably do result from changes in the light-evoked $[K^+]$ decrease. One example is the decrease in c-wave amplitude during light adaptation, where, because both c-wave components are affected (Linsenmeier and Steinberg, 1983), we assume that the K^+ response is changed (mechanism 3).

The mechanisms that explain experimentally induced changes in c-wave amplitude must also account for the variability of the c-wave in normal subjects. In fact, it seems likely that the relatively large interindividual variation in the normal human c-wave (Hock and Marmor, 1982) is a result of a very small variation in one of the c-wave components (Fig. 1), although this may be difficult to demonstrate directly.

ACKNOWLEDGEMENT

We thank Gerard Borgula and Anne Moorehouse for their assistance with data analysis and experiments, and Dr. E. R. Griff for comments on the manuscript. This work was supported by N.I.H. grant EY01429 to R.H.S.

REFERENCES

Calissendorff, B., Knave, B., and Persson, H. E. (1974). Cyclic variations in the c-wave amplitude of the sheep ERG. Vision Res. 14, 1141–1145.

Faber, D. S. (1969). Analysis of the slow transretinal potentials in response to light. Ph.D. thesis, State University of New York, Buffalo.

Griff, E. R., Linsenmeier, R. A. and Steinberg, R. H. (1983). The cellular origin of the fast oscillation. These Proceedings.

Hock, P. A. and Marmor, M. F. (1982). Variability of the normal human c-wave. Invest. Ophthalmol. Visual Sci. Suppl. 22, 138.

Karwoski, C. J. and Proenza, L. M. (1977). Relationship between Müller cell responses, a local transretinal potential, and potassium flux. J. Neurophysiol. 40, 244–259.

Knave, B., Persson, H. E. and Nilsson, S. E. G. (1974). A comparative study on the effects of barbiturate and ethyl alcohol on retinal functions with special reference to the c-wage of the electroretinogram and the standing potential of the sheep eye. Acta Ophthalmol. 52, 254–259.

Linsenmeier, R. A., Mines, A. H. and Steinberg, R. H. (1983). Effects of hypoxia and hypercapnia on the light peak and electroretinogram of the cat. Invest. Ophthalmol. Visual Sci., 24, 37–46.

Linsenmeier, R. A. and Steinberg, R. H. (1982). Origin and sensitivity of the light peak of the intact cat eye. J. Physiol., 331, 653–673.

Linsenmeier, R. A. and Steinberg, R. H. (1983). A light-evoked interaction of the apical and basal membranes of the retinal pigment epithelium: the c-wave and the light peak. J. Neurophysiol. In press.

Miller, S. S. and Steinberg, R. H. (1977). Passive ionic properties of frog retinal pigment epithelium. J. Memb. Biol. 36, 337–372.

Niemeyer, G., Nagahara, K. and Demant, E. (1983). Effects of changes in arterial PO_2 and PCO_2 on the ERG in the cat. Invest. Ophthalmol. Visual Sci., 23, 678–683.

Nilsson, S. E. G. and Skoog, K.-O. (1975). Covariation of the simultaneously recorded c-wave and standing potential of the human eye. Acta Ophthalmol. 53, 721–730.

Noell, W. K. (1953). Studies on the electrophysiology and metabolism of the retina. USAF School of Aviation Medicine, Project No. 21-1201-0004.

Oakley, B., II and Green, D. G. (1976). Correlation of light-induced changes in retinal extracellular potassium concentration with the c-wave of the electroretinogram. J. Neurophysiol. 39, 1117–1133.

Rodieck, R. W. (1972). Components of the electroretinogram – a reappraisal. Vision Res. 12, 773–780.

Skoog, K.-O. (1974). The c-wave of the human D.C. registered ERG. III. Effects of ethyl alcohol on the c-wave. Acta Ophthalmol. 52, 913–923.

Steinberg, R. H., Griff, E. R. and Linsenmeier, R. A. (1983). The cellular origin of the light peak. This volume. pp. 1–12.

Steinberg, R. H., Oakley, B., II and Niemeyer, G. (1980). Light-evoked changes in $[K^+]_0$ in the retina of the intact cat eye. J. Neurophysiol. 44, 897–921.

Steinberg, R. H., Schmidt, R. and Brown, K. T. (1970). Intracellular responses to light from the cat retinal pigment epithelium: origin of the electroretinogram c-wave. Nature 227, 728–730.

Witkovsky, P., Dudek, F. E. and Ripps, H. (1975) Slow PIII component of the carp electroretinogram. J. gen. Physiol. 65, 119–134.

Mailing address:
Department of Physiology S-762
University of California, San Francisco
San Francisco, CA 94143 U.S.A.

HYPEROSMOLARITY-INDUCED CHANGES IN THE TRANSEPITHELIAL POTENTIAL OF THE HUMAN AND FROG RETINAE

K. KAWASAKI, D. YONEMURA, S. MUKOH and J. TANABE

(Kanazawa, Japan)

ABSTRACT

The effect of hyperosmolarity on the transepithelial potential (TEP) was studied in the retinal pigment epithelium (RPE) − choroid preparations of the human and the frog. The osmolarity of the perfusing solution was increased 100 mOsmol above the control level by adding fructose. The TEP was increased by hyperosmolarity only in the apical chamber, and was decreased by hyperosmolarity in the basal chamber or by a simultaneous increase of the osmolarity in both chambers. Hyperosmolarity in the basal chamber changed the TEP more than hyperosmolarity in the apical chamber. The hyperosmolarity-induced changes in the TEP described above were reversible. The hyperosmolarity response in-vivo seems to depend mainly on the effect of hyperosmolarity on the basal side of the RPE.

INTRODUCTION

The c-wave in the electroretinogram (ERG) and the light rise in the electro-oculogram (EOG) are generally assumed to be indicative of the activity of the retinal pigment epithelium (RPE). The c-wave and the light rise, however, depend on the neural retina as well as on the RPE, since these waves are light-evoked responses. The standing potential of the eye was previously found to be changed by an intravenous injection of a hypertonic solution in the human, the monkey and the dog (1, 2). This phenomenon, which is called the hyperosmolarity response, was shown to originate mainly in the RPE (1−4). The hyperosmolarity response is useful as a specific electrophysiological test for the RPE function (1−4). The hyperosmolarity response is frequently abnormal in some chorioretinal diseases such as diabetic retinopathy, retinitis pigmentosa, fundus albipunctatus, Stargardt's disease, angioid streaks, coloboma of the choroid and retinal detachment (4).

The present study describes effects of hyperosmolarity on the potential across the in-vitro preparations of the RPE-choroid of the human and the frog.

Doc. Ophthal. Proc. Series, Vol. 37, ed. by H. E. J. W. Kolder
©1983 Dr. W. Junk Publishers, The Hague/Boston: Lancaster

METHODS

The isolated RPE-choroid preparations of the human and the bullfrog (Rana Catesbiana) were used. The human eye was obtained from a patient with an invasion of a malignant tumor into the orbit. The method of isolating the RPE-choroid preparations was similar to that described by Miller and Steinberg (5).

The isolated preparation was mounted between two lucite chambers, having 3 mm centered circular holes, so that the choroid and the apical surface of the RPE were immersed in separate solutions in the two chambers (40 ml each), named the basal chamber and the apical chamber. The bathing solution for the human eye was a modified Ringer's having the following composition (in mM): 119.50 NaCl; 3.60 KCl; 1.15 $CaCl_2$; 1.06 $MgSO_4$; 26.00 glucose; 25.10 $NaHCO_3$, 3.00 NaH_2PO_4. The composition of the solution for the frog (in mM) was 94.0 CaCl, 2.0 KCl, 1.0 $MgCl_2$, 1.8 $CaCl_2$, 15.0 $NaHCO_3$, 10.0 glucose. The solution was bubbled with 100% oxygen. The pH, the osmolarity and the temperature of the solution were respectively 8.02 ± 0.02, 3.0×10^2 mOsmol and $31 \pm 1°C$ for the human eye, and 8.05 ± 0.05, 2.2×10^2 mOsmol and $20 \pm 1°C$ respectively for the frog eye. The perfusion rate was maintained at 25 ml/min.

A pair of silver-silver chloride electrodes was placed in the bathing solutions to measure the transepithelial potential (TEP, the potential difference across the RPE-choroid). The potential was led to a DC-amplifier (Nihon Kohden, RDU-5, -3 dB at 200 Hz), and recorded on an ink-writing oscillograph (Riken, SP-J5V).

The osmolarity of the bathing solution was increased 100 mOsmol above the control level by adding fructose.

RESULTS

The RPE-choroid preparations of the frog and the human were used. The apical surface of the RPE was electrically positive with respect to the choroidal surface in all preparations tested. The TEP of three preparations of the frog was stabilized at 1.81, 5.24 and 5.59 mV after dark adaptation ranged from 30 to 90 minutes. When the osmolarity of the solution in the apical chamber was raised by adding fructose, the TEP increased by 0.07, 1.96 and 1.07 mV in the three frog preparations described above (Fig. 1). The hyperosmolarity by fructose in the basal chamber reduced the TEP of the three preparations by 0.24, 2.61 and 1.29 mV (Fig. 1). Thus, the hyperosmolarity in the basal chamber changed the TEP more than the hyperosmolarity in the apical chamber (Figs. 1, 2). The TEP was reduced by elevating the osmotic pressure by fructose in both chambers simultaneously (Fig. 3).

The TEP was stabilized at 2.0 mV after a dark adaptation of 60 minutes in a human RPE-choroid preparation obtained from the nasal peripheral part of the eye. The TEP increased by 0.75 mV, when the osmolarity in the apcial chamber was raised. The hyperosmolarity by fructose in the basal chamber

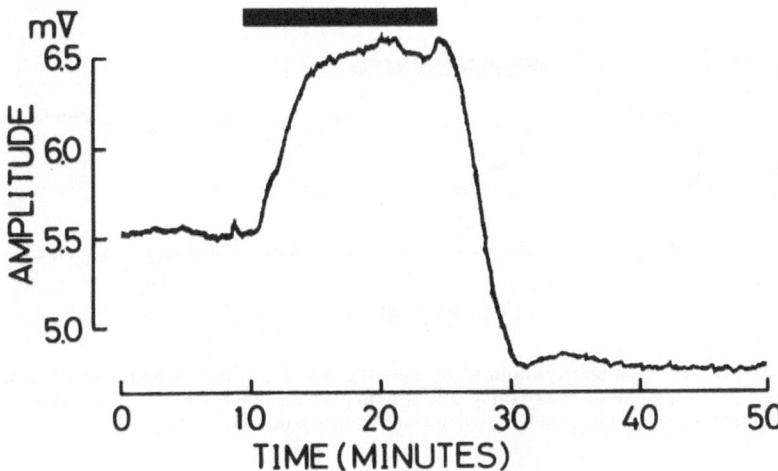

Fig. 1. The hyperosmolarity-induced change of the TEP in the frog RPE-choroid prepar-ation. The osmolarity of the bathing solution in the apical chamber was raised by fructose (black horizontal bar) 100 mOsmol above the control level. The apical surface of the RPE was electrically positive with respect to the choroidal surface. The TEP was increased (upward deflection) by the hyperosmolarity in the apical chamber.

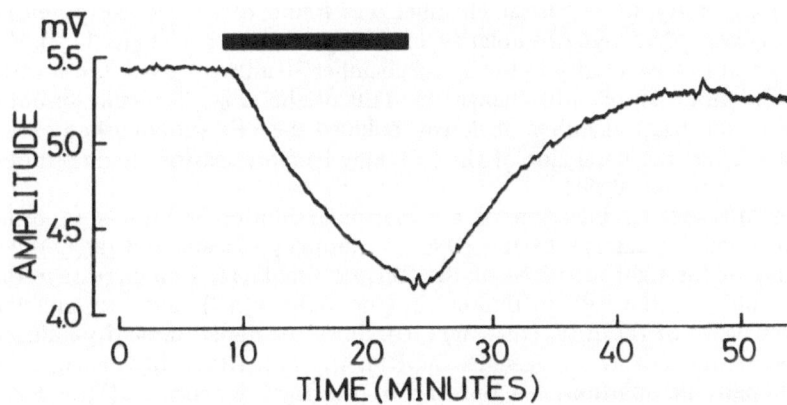

Fig. 2. The hyperosmolarity-induced change of the TEP in the frog RPE-choroid prepar-ation. The osmolarity of the bathing solution in the basal chamber was rasied by fructose (black horizontal bar) 100 mOsmol above the control level. The TEP was decreased (downward deflection) by the hyperosmolarity in the basal chamber.

reduced the TEP by 1.25 mV. In the human too the hyperosmolarity in the basal chamber changed the TEP more than the hyperosmolarity in the apical chamber. A simultaneous increase of the osmolarity in both chambers decreased the TEP in the human (not illustrated), as in the frog (Fig. 3).

The hyperosmolarity-induced changes in the TEP described above were reversible.

31

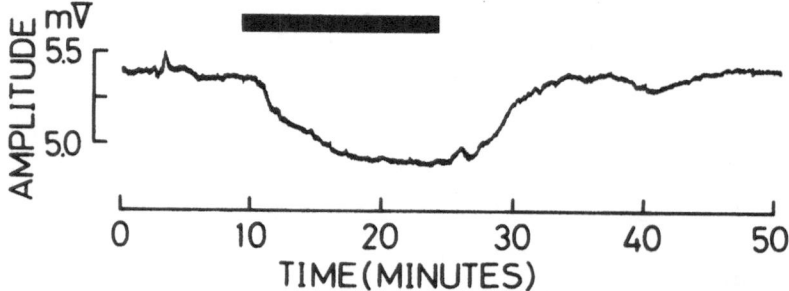

Fig. 3. The hyperosmolarity-induced change of the TEP in the frog RPE-choroid preparation. The osmolarity of the bathing solutions in both chambers was raised simultaneously by fructose (black horizontal bar) 100 mOsmol above the control level.

DISCUSSION

We previously reported that a hypertonic solution, perfusing both apical and basal chambers simultaneously, decreased the standing potential of the eye cups in-vitro in the human and the monkey (1, 2). The present study showed that the TEP was increased by hyperosmolarity only in the apical chamber (Fig. 1), and was decreased by hyperosmolarity in the basal chamber (Fig. 2) or a simultaneous increase of the osmolarity in both chambers (Fig. 3). Hyperosmolarity in the basal chamber was found to change the potential more greatly than hyperosmolarity in the apical chamber (Figs. 1, 2). An increase of the osmolarity in the apical chamber 30 mOsmol above the control level did not significantly change the TEP of the frog. The same osmotic stress in the basal chamber obviously reduced the TEP (unpublished observation). Thus, the basal side of the RPE may be more sensitive to an osmotic stress than the apical side.

An intra-arterial injection of a hypertonic solution is known to bring about a cellular damage of the RPE (the monkey (6) and the rat (7)), an opening of the tight junctions of the RPE (the rabbit) (8), an increase in the permeability of the RPE to fluorescein (the monkey) (9), and a suppression of the c-wave of the ERG (the cat) (10). Since the hyperosmolarity-induced change of the TEP was reversible, the RPE was not irreversibly damaged by our hypertonic solution. An opening of the right junctions of the RPE, which might occur during a perfusion with a hypertonic solution, may decrease the transepithelial electrical resistance. One might speculate that the changes of the TEP under study might be due to a possible reduction of the transepithelial electrical resistance. The change of the TEP, however, differed in polarity, depending on whether a hypertonic solution was given in the apical chamber or in the basal chamber (Figs. 1, 2). This polarity difference can not be explained by a hypothesized decrease of the transepithelial resistance. In fact, no significant change was detectable in the transepithelial electrical resistance of the frog RPE-choroid during an osmotic stress (+100 mOsmol by fructose, unpublished observation). It is unlikely that the hyperosmolarity-induced change in the TEP is due to an opening of the tight junction or a irreversible cellular damage of the RPE.

32

In general, the blood flow through the choroidal circulation is much greater than that through the retinal circulation. The mean blood flow through the retinal and choroidal circulations was reported 34 and 677 mg/min respectively in the monkey (11). Therefore, a hypertonic solution, injected intravenously, probably flows much more through the choroidal circulation than through the retinal circulation, and thus has more effect on the basal side of the RPE than on the apical side. Our previous study (1, 2) demonstrated that the standing potential of the eye in-vivo was reduced by an intravenous injection of a hypertonic solution (the hyperosmolarity response). The TEP in-vitro was found in the present study to decrease when a hypertonic solution was perfused to the basal side (Fig. 2). The potential changes in-vivo and in-vitro mentioned above coincide in polarity. The hyperosmolarity response in-vivo may reflect mainly the effect of a hypertonic solution of the basal side of the RPE.

REFERENCES

1. Yonemura, D. and Kawasaki, K.: New approaches to ophthalmic electrodiagnosis by retinal oscillatory potential, drug-induced responses from retinal pigment epithelium and cone potential. Doc. Ophthal., 48: 163–222, 1979.
2. Madachi, S.: Electrophysiological evaluation of retinal pigment epithelium for clinical use. (I) Hyperosmolarity response of the standing potential and its origin. Acta Soc. Ophthal. Jpn., 86: 374–384, 1982.
3. Madachi, S.: Electrophysiological evaluation of retinal pigment epithelium for clinical use. (II) Hyperosmolarity response in normal subjects. Acta Soc. Ophthal. Jpn., 86: 385–395, 1982.
4. Madachi, S.: Electrophysiological evaluation of retinal pigment epithelium for clinical use. (III) Clinical study in several chorioretinal diseases. Acta Soc. Ophthal. Jpn., 86: 396–413, 1982.
5. Miller, S. S. and Steinberg, R. H.: Passive ionic properties of frog pigment epithelium. J. Memb. Biol., 36: 337–372, 1977.
6. Okinami, S. and Ohkuma, M.: Ultrastructural alterations in the retinal pigment epithelial cells of the monkey after systemic urea injection. Acta Soc. Ophthal. Jpn., 81: 743–754, 1977.
7. Miki, H.: Ultrastructural studies on the blood-retina barriers under hyperosmotic agents. Acta Soc. Ophthal. Jpn., 81: 755–762, 1977.
8. Masuyama, Y.: Ultrastructural studies on the chorioretinal barrier of rabbit eye. Acta Soc. Ophthal. Jpn., 80: 585–597, 1976.
9. Laties, A. H. and Rapoport, S.: The blood-ocular barriers under osmotic stress. Studies on the freeze-dried eye. Arch. Ophthal., 94: 1086–1091, 1976.
10. Tornquist, P. and Ring, A.: The influence of hyperosmotic stress on the blood-retinal barrier. Effects on the electroretinogram. Acta Ophthal., 58: 707–711, 1980.
11. Alm, A., Bill, A. and Young, F. A.: The effects of pilocarpine and neostigmine on the blood flow through the anterior uvea in monkeys. A study with radioactively labelled microspheres. Exp. Eye Res., 15: 31–36, 1973.

Mailing address:
Department of Ophthalmology, School of Medicine
Kanazawa University
13–1 Takaramachi, Kanazawa 920,
Japan

EOG AND EXPERIMENTAL OPTIC NERVE TRANSECTION

J. JACKSON, H. E. KOLDER, L. D. HOMER and J. TIGGES

(Iowa City, Iowa, U.S.A.)

ABSTRACT

A series of experiments was performed on rabbits. One optic nerve was sectioned without compromising the blood supply to the globe. After 1–181 days the EOG was recorded, utilizing passive eye movements and electrodes sutured into the skin at the canthi. The animals were anesthetized initially and maintained on local anesthesia and Gallamine. A tracheotomy permitted passive ventilation. Endexpiratory CO_2 was maintained at normal levels. The unoperated eye served as control. The EOG light rise to a constant illumination was recorded following 90 minutes of dark adaptation. The data were plotted as light peak to dark trough ratio of the eye with optic nerve transection vs control eye. No deviation was found from a linear relationship. The coefficient of correlation was not significantly different from 1.0. It is concluded that the EOG response of the rabbit eye is independent of the intactness of the optic nerve. All globes were histologically evaluated and demonstrated a retrograde degeneration of the ganglion cell layer.

INTRODUCTION

Episodic evidence (K. W. McNeer, personal communication, H. E. Kolder, personal observation, Fig. 1) indicates that an accidental transection of the optic nerve in man does not alter the EOG response to light. The ERG after cutting the optic nerve has been investigated with some controversial findings (Jacobson and Suzuki, Gills, Horsten and Winkler). Part of the EOG response to light may be contributed by structures other than the pigment epithelium. A theoretical model of the oscillatory response of the EOG by Homer and Kolder postulates information transfer through three or four layers with feedback between adjacent layers. The experiments reported here were designed to 1) reproduce with rabbits the EOG recording conditions in man, and 2) to test for evidence of an effect of acute and chronic optic nerve transection on the light induced oscillation of the EOG.

Doc. Ophthal. Proc. Series, Vol. 37, ed. by H. E. J. W. Kolder
©1983 Dr W. Junk Publishers, The Hague/Boston: Lancaster

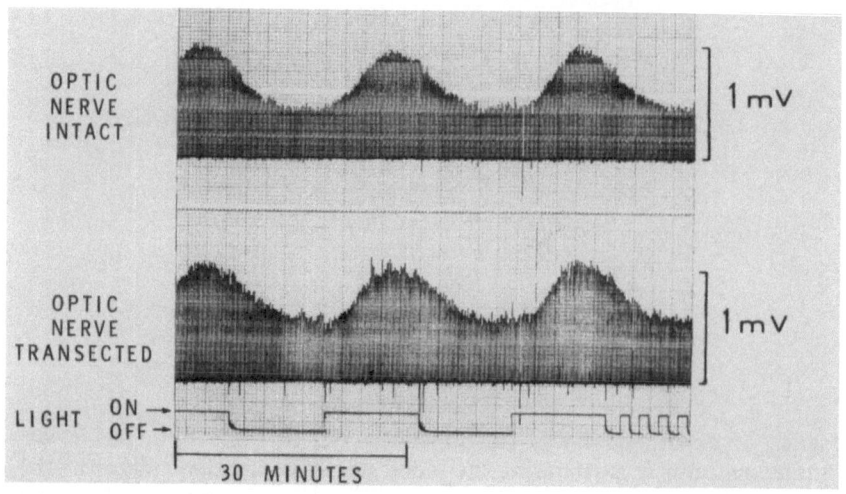

Fig. 1. Human EOG recorded five weeks after accidential optic nerve transection in one eye. 12.5 min on and off periods of light.

MATERIAL AND METHODS

Twenty-eight pigmented rabbits were used with a body weight between 1.7 and 3.3 Kg. Four animals served as controls, both optic nerves were intact. Five animals were used in acute experiments. Eleven rabbits had one optic nerve transected within the orbit, while thirteen had one optic nerve cut intracranially. The animals were initially sedated with 12.5 mg/Kg of Thorazine IM and anesthetized with Nembutal (10 mg/Kg IV) and maintained with local Xylocaine injections at the tracheotomy site and Tetracaine topically on the cornea. Gallamine was infused (2–3 mg per 30 minutes) and a respirator kept the minute volume at 1–1.5 l/min. The endexpiratory CO_2 concentration was adjusted to 3% (2.5–3.7%). The arterial blood pressure was recorded on a physiograph. The body temperature was kept constant. A pusher-rod device moved the globes every ten seconds over a constant angle of about 30 degrees (Kolder and North). The end of the rod was sutured to the limbus. The pupils were dilated using 2% Atropine. The indirectly recorded EOG potential was picked up by means of silver wire electrodes in the skin next to the canthi, DC amplified with an upper frequency roll-off at 10 Hz and recorded on paper moving at 2 mm/minutes. The amplitudes were manually read. The stimulus light was an incandescent bulb illuminating a diffusor in front of each eye. The illuminance at the eye level varied in different experiments between 270 and 807 Lux, but was kept constant for each eye of one animal. Ninety minutes of dark adaptation preceded the light stimulus which was either kept constant or turned on and off in twenty minutes intervals.

The left optic nerve was transected intraorbitally behind the entrance of the blood supply to the globe or intracranially in front of the chiasm. For the intraorbital approach two recti muscles had to be severed. The fundus

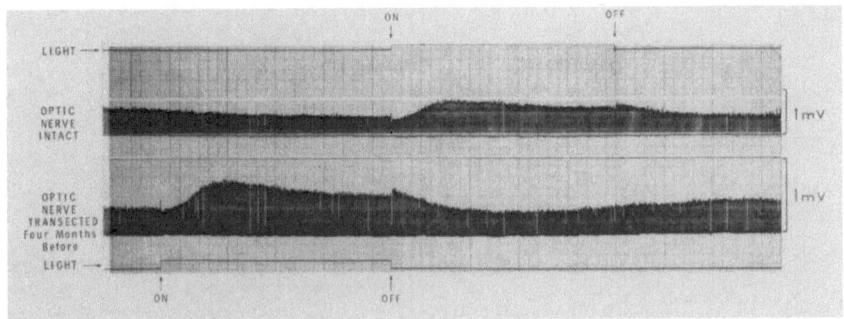

Fig. 2. EOG response to light in a rabbit. The left eye had the optic nerve cut four months previously. Ninety minutes of dark adaptation were followed by constant illumination with 270 Lux at the eye.

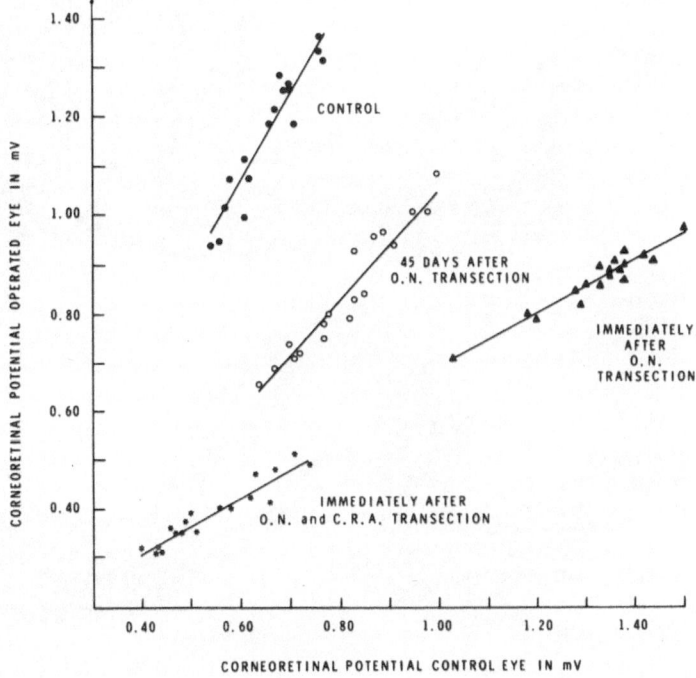

Fig. 3. Plot of the amplitude of the EOG light peak in a control eye against the amplitude from an eye whose optic nerve had been transected previously. Several lines indicate experiments done at different times after optic nerve transection.

was observed post-operatively to assure the intactness of the ocular blood supply. The direct pupillary response was absent in all optic nerve transected eyes, while the consensual response remained intact. The animals were sacrificed one to 181 days following the experiment by injecting Urethane

37

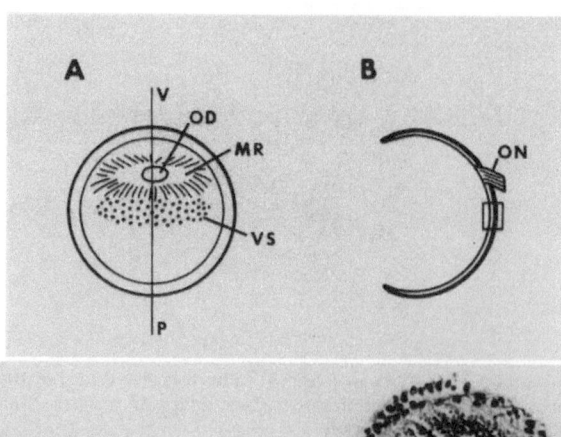

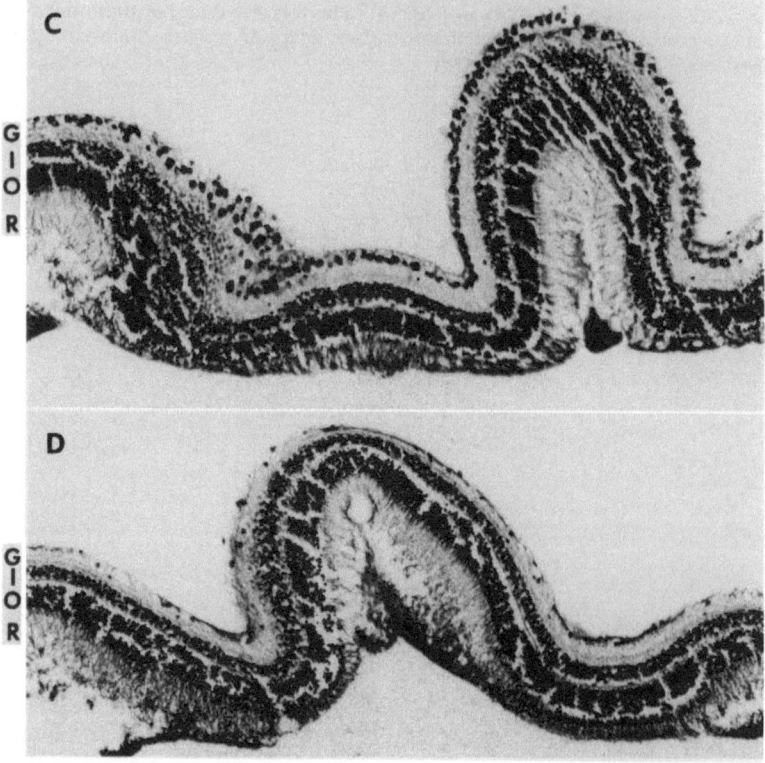

Fig. 4. (A) Schematic drawing of optic disk (OD), medullary rays (MR), and visual streak (VS). VP indicates the vertical plane through which the cuts were made. (B) Schematic drawing of a cut through the optic nerve (ON). (C) Photograph of the retina of a control eye taken from the area indicated by the rectangle in B. Note the large number of ganglion cells. (D) Same area as in C, but from an eye 125 days after the optic nerve had been cut. Only glial cells are left. G: ganglion cell layer; I: inner nuclear layer; O: outer nuclear layer; R: inner and outer segments of receptors. Magnification × 100.

intravenously. The optic nerves were checked for completeness of the transection. The eyes were enucleated, the cornea, lens and vitreous removed and the remaining part of the globe fixed in 10% Formaline. The specimen were embedded in paraffin and cut at 20u in the vertical plane. The sections were stained by the Nissl method. The retina of rabbits exhibits medullary rays which are bundles of myelinated axons of ganglion cells. Ventral to the medullary rays lies the visual streak containing the highest number of ganglion cells per area. Cuts through the visual streak were used for counting the ganglion cells (Prince and McConnell).

RESULTS

Fig. 2 shows the EOG response to light from an eye with an intact optic nerve and from the contralateral eye which had the optic nerve transected 120 days earlier. On and off responses are readily discernable. Fig. 3. summarizes for several experiments the relationship of the EOG light peak in the normal eye versus that of an eye with optic nerve transaction. A linear correlation is apparent. The correlation coefficient (r) varied between 0.97 and 0.99 for four control animals, between 0.94 and 0.99 for eleven animals with one optic nerve cut intraorbitally, and between 0.73 and 0.99 for thirteen animals with one optic nerve cut intracranially. An analysis of variance yielded no significant difference between groups (F 2.746).

The histologic examination revealed that the ganglion cells of eyes with a cut optic nerve had undergone practically complete degeneration. All ganglion cells measuring more than 10u in diameter had disappeared. The largest ganglion cell diameter in control eyes was 25u. The cells in the ganglion cell layer of the eye shown in Fig. 4D are glial cells. No alterations were found in the inner and outer nuclear layer.

DISCUSSION

The experimental procedure in rabbits simulates closely the technique used in man. No evidence was found that efferent information through the optic nerve contributes to the light induced slow oscillation of th EOG. Homer and Kolder's four layer model including the ganglion cells can therefore be rejected. The degeneration of the ganglion cells is in agreement with James's findings. He reported from 150 preparations that 120 days after transection of the optic nerve in rabbits all but two ganglion cells had disappeared. M. W. Dubin kindly supplied results from a preliminary study (personal communication). He cut the optic nerve of adult rabbits intraorbitally. Eight months later the ERG was normal. By light microscopy, not all of the ganglion cells had degenerated. Amacrine cells and horizontal cells were normal in all respects by light and electron micrscopy.

While newer experimental techniques permit the direct recording of potentials from the pigment epithelium, the results reported here eliminate heuristically a possible source for modification of the EOG on a macro scale.

ACKNOWLEDGEMENT

These experiments were performed at the Department of Physiology and the Yerkes Regional Primate Research Center of Emory University, Atlanta, Georgia, U.S.A.

REFERENCES

J. P. Gills: The electroretinogram after section of the optic nerve in man. Am. J. Ophthal. 62: 287–291 (1966).

L. D. Homer and H. Kolder: Mathematical model of oscillations in the human corneo-retinal potential. Pflügers Arch. 287: 197–202 (1966).

G. P. M. Horsten and J. E. Winkelman: Effect of section of the optic nerve on histological differentiation and electrical activity of the retina in dogs. Ophthalmologica 157: 293–300 (1969).

J. H. Jacobson and T. A. Suzuki: Effects of optic nerve section on the ERG. Arch. Ophthal. 67: 791–801 (1962).

J. R. James: Degeneration of ganglion cells following axonal injury. Arch. Ophthal. 9: 338–343 (1933).

H. Kolder and A. W. North: Oscillations of the corneo-retinal potential in animals. Ophthalmologica 152: 149–160 (1966).

J. H. Prince and D. G. McConnell: Retina and Optic Nerve. In: J. H. Prince, editor: The rabbit in eye research. Thomas, Springfield, 1964 p. 385–448.

B. S. Winkler: Analysis of the rabbit's electroretinogram following unilateral transection of the optic nerve. Exp. Eye Res. 13: 227–235 (1972).

Mailing Address:
Department of Ophthalmology
The University of Iowa
Iowa City, Iowa 52242,
U.S.A.

LIGHT MODULATION OF THE STANDING POTENTIAL IN THE PERFUSED MAMMALIAN EYE: CHARACTERISTICS AND RESPONSES TO ACIDOSIS

G. NIEMEYER

(Zürich, Switzerland)

ABSTRACT

Responses of the standing potential to light, analogous to the EOG, can be recorded from arterially perfused mammalian eyes (Niemeyer, Experientia 36: 699, 1980). In the dark adapted cat eye we recorded standing potentials of 5 to 6 mV; step increases in light elicit a-, b- c-waves of the DC ERG followed by a negative-positive fast oscillation with a peak time of about 1.2–2.2 min, and eventually a large light peak (LP), the first wave of a damped oscillation. The light peak is exquisitely sensitive to concurrent or to preceeding *hypoxia*.

Perfused dog eyes revealed absence of a positive c-wave and a longer (9–11 min) peaktime of the light peak as prominent features.

We tested effects of acidosis (pH 7.4 → 7.0) by either adding HCl to HEPES-buffered perfusate or by increasing pCO_2 in bicarbonate-buffered perfusate. In both cases the flow rate increased under low pH, and the b-wave was reduced by 30 to 40%. The light peak was greatly reduced only under elevated pCO_2. Corresponding measurements by ion-selective pH microelectrodes have demonstrated intraretinal changes in pH as predicted from the electrophysiological data (Weingart and Niemeyer, in prep.).

INTRODUCTION

The standing potential (SP) between cornea and sclera arises mainly from a difference in the potentials across the basal compared to the apical membrane of the retinal pigment epithelium (RPE; for review see Zinn and Marmor, 1979). The potential spreads through the retina, vitreous and anterior segment, acting as volume conductors, to the cornea. Clinically, this charge allows monitoring eye movements via skin-electrodes placed around the orbit. Potential changes, elicited by eye movements in a standardized angle, depend in size on the ambient illumination. This phenomenon is applied in ophthalmology as electrooculography (EOG) to test the functional state of the photoreceptor-RPE complex (Kolder, 1959; Arden et al., 1962; Täumer, 1976). The most prominent feature of the EOG is the change of the standing potential from a dark level to a "light peak" (Hauptschwingung) in response to a step increase in the ambient illumination. To study these mechanisms in vitro, we set out to record the SP in isolated, arterially perfused eyes of cats and of dogs and to study its modulation by light. In the anesthetized cat, Linsenmeier et al. (1982) observed depression of the light peak during hypercapnia. We tried to separate in vitro the effects of acidosis induced by HCl, from those induced by an increase in pCO_2. I will summarize results that are reported in full detail elsewhere (Niemeyer and Steinberg, Vision Res., in preparation).

METHODS

We enucleated eyes from adult cats and, in addition, 6 eyes from 6 dogs under general anesthesia and under anticoagulation. Their opthalmociliary arteries were connected to a gravity-driven perfusion system. The perfusate consisted of oxygenated, serum-enriched and HEPES- or bicarbonate-buffered tissue culture medium. This method was introduced by Gouras and Hoff (1970) and modified by the author (Niemeyer, 1975, 1981). The DC-recording was done via AgAgCl salt bridge-electrodes which touched the center of the cornea and the surface of the sclera near the optic nerve. The eye-chamber was connected to ground by a third, identical electrode. The saline-metal interface of each electrode was shielded from light in small glass chambers placed above the preparation. The electrodes were connected to a differential input DC preamplifier, and the data were recorded and stored using conventional electronic equipment. Electroretinograms (ERG) were monitored to assess the adequacy of the perfusion, maintaining the functional state of the neuro-retina throughout the experiment. Stimulation by light (150 W Xenon source and a modified fundus camera, Funkhouser and Niemeyer, 1982) consisted of brief pulses of 620 nm, 2–3 log units above dark adapted threshold for the b-wave. To trigger oscillations of the standing potential, mainly a light peak, steps of "white" light, 0.6–4.0 log units above dark adapted b-wave-threshold were applied for durations from 0.05 to 10 minutes.

For experiments involving changes in pH we used two different procedures. In the case of 'HCl acidosis' 0.1 N HCl was injected at 0.04 to 0.08 ml/min into the stream of the HEPES-buffered perfusate. This resulted in a decrease in pH by 0.3 to 0.4 units as monitored on line by a small pH electrode (Dr. Bühler, Ingold, Zürich). A similar step decrease in pH in 'hypercapnia' experiments was generated by using two bicarbonate-buffered perfusates: the control perfusate pH7.4) was equilibrated with 5% CO_2 and 95% O_2, and the test-perfusate (pH 7.0) was equilibrated with 10% CO_2 and 90% O_2 (pH 7.0). Further details will be published (Niemeyer and Steinberg, Vision Res., in preparation).

For preretinal measurements of pH, glass micropipettes, the tip of which was filled with a proton-sensitive resin, were introduced through the pars plana and guided under visual control towards the central retina. The electrode was positioned within 30 to 300 μ in front of the retina and, together with a vitreal AgAgCl electrode as reference, connected to a WPI-F 233 A electrometer. The electrometer provided digital display of a voltage corresponding to the pH value, which was recorded on a 4-channel oscillographic recorder, synchronously with the pH of the perfusate and electrophysiologic signals. Prior to and after each intraocular recording series all electrodes were calibrated in test solutions of various pH values.

RESULTS

Standing potential

Following an inevitable period of anoxia (4 to 12 minutes) between enucleation and connection of the eye to the perfusion system a cornea-positive potential grew during about 30 minutes to 5.4 mV (cat) and 3.7 mV (dog). The standing potential remained near this level as long as steady state perfusion and dark adaptation were maintained.

Arrest of the perfusion induced a transient increase of about 1 mV and a subsequent linear decay to zero mV within approximately 7 min.

MODULATION BY LIGHT

Arterially perfused cat eyes in this study exhibited typical ERGs with prominent c-waves and characteristic slow potential changes with a large light peak that was followed by oscillations of diminishing amplitude (Fig. 1 and lower traces in Fig. 2 a.3). Preparations that were exposed to extended or repeated periods of *hypoxia* prior to onset of *adequate* perfusion often failed to generate large LPs upon standard stimulation. Fig. 1 represents a typical signal from an invitro perfused cat eye comparable to the invivo situation (Steinberg and Niemeyer, 1981). The maximum amplitudes of the LPs recorded in vitro measured 3–4 mV. The time from the onset of the stimulus to the light peak was 5–6 minutes at 37°C. This signal could be elicited consistently with stimuli of an intensity of 1 log unit below rod saturation or higher, and of at least 1 min in duration. The responses to step increased in light in *perfused dog eyes* (German shepherd) were essentially similar to those described for cat eyes, except for absence of a positive c-wave and a time to the peak of 9 to 11 minutes (Fig. 4).

Responses to stimuli of a constant duration of one minute and of increasing intensity are shown in Fig. 2. At low intensity (top trace) the *fast oscillation*, also referred to as 'second c-wave' (Nikara et al., 1976) followed the early components of the ERG. At low intensity, the LP can just be recognized at time 4–5 min, but grows with increasing intensity. High stimulus intensity typically triggers DC responses in which the fast oscillation occurs just as a shoulder (hump) in the rising phase of the LP (see also Fig. 1 and bottom trace in Fig. 3). Another procedure to separate the fast oscillation is varying the stimulus duration. In Fig. 3, the early components of the DC ERG are followed by the fast oscillation, that is most clearly separated from the LP in the top trace. The constant stimulus intensity was above that required for rod saturation, and therefore the OFF effects at the terminations of the stimuli were positive.

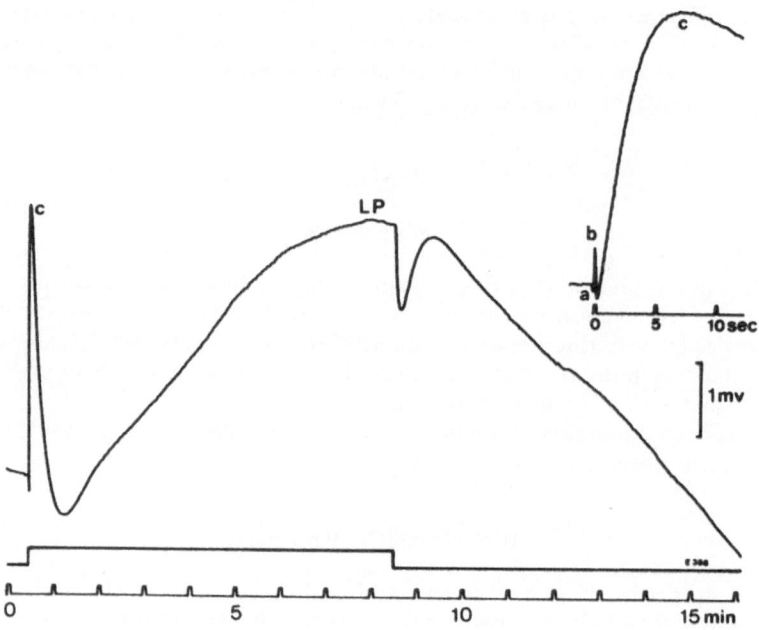

Fig. 1. Typical DC-ERG and light peak of a perfused cat eye. The stimulus consisted of a step increase from almost full dark adaptation by 4 log units of white light, 3 min duration. The a-, b- and c-waves are followed by a negative wave, by a hump in the rising phase (fast oscillation) at 2 min, and by the light peak (LP). Note the negative off-effect coinciding with the termination of the stimulus, indicating an intensity below rod saturation. The inset illustrates the a-, b- and c-waves of this ERG at a faster time base.

Perfused dog eyes in dark adaptation typically exhibit DC ERGs with a slow negative component following the b-wave instead of a positive c-wave (Rodieck, 1972; Niemeyer, 1981). This is illustrated in Fig. 4A. In Fig. 4B a response to maintained illumination reveals a larger negativity, referred to as the trough of the fast oscillation (Griff, et al., 1983). The following positive component reaches maximum amplitude at about 2.5 min and often merges with the rising phase of the light peak. In the dog eye the light peak reaches its maximum at 9–11 min after onset of illumination. In the example of Fig. 4B termination of the sitmulus results in a brief positive OFF-effect, indicating a stimulus intensity well above rod saturation.

The *time course* of the fast oscillation was practically unchanged under stimulation with different intensities (Fig. 2). Changes in the duration of the stimulus, however, shifted the peak time of the fast oscillation in the perfused dog eye in the range of 1.1 to maximally 2.5 min, as plotted in Fig. 5.

HCl-acidosis

A transient decrease of the pH from about 7.4 to 7.0 consistently induced the following combination of changes: the *flow rate* of the perfusate increased,

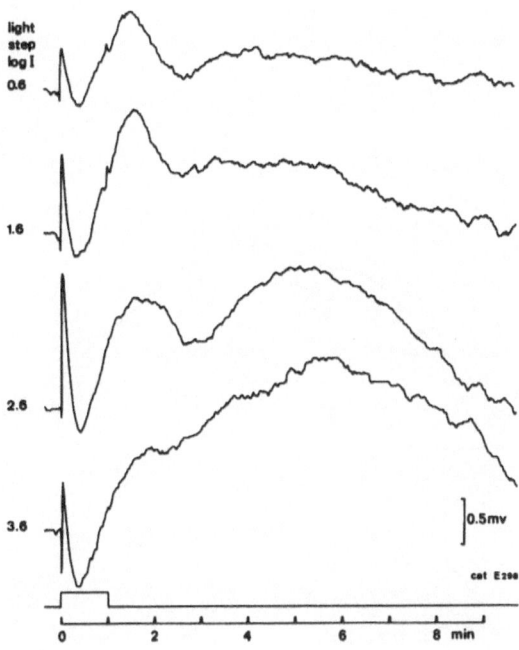

light
step
log I
0.6

1.6

2.6

3.6

0.5mv

cat E298

0   2   4   6   8 min

Fig. 2. Intensity series for a one-minute flash of white light, revealing distinct fast oscillation and LP. Note an effect of partial light adaptation at relative intensity of 3.6 log units (bottom signal), where the fast oscillation merged with the rising phase of the LP.

indicating decrease of vascular resistance in the isolated eye. The b-wave decreased by 30–40% and the c-wave generally increased in amplitude. The amplitudes of the fast oscillation and of the LP were essentially unaffected; sometimes the light peak was slightly smaller and a little delayed under low pH (Niemeyer and Steinberg, 1981).

Hypercapnia

In order to induce tissue acidosis by an increase in pCO_2 we recorded the DC ERG, fast oscillation and light peak with control bicarbonate-buffered perfusate (pCO_2 38 mm Hg; pH 7.4) and subsequently with a test perfusate at a pCO_2 of 78 mm Hg and pH 7.0. Under elevated pCO_2 we obtained the following changes: the flow rate of the perfusate increased more than observed during HCl-acidosis. The b-wave decreased, whereas the c-wave showed no consistent change. The fast oscillation was little, if at all affected. The light peak, in contrast, was *greatly reduced* under hypercapnia. These effects were reversible upon return to the control perfusate (Niemeyer and Steinberg, 1981).

In order to test if the experimentally induced decreases in pH pass the blood-retina barrier we performed measurements of preretinal pH by means of H^+ ion-selective microelectrodes. Preliminary results reveal that the HCl

45

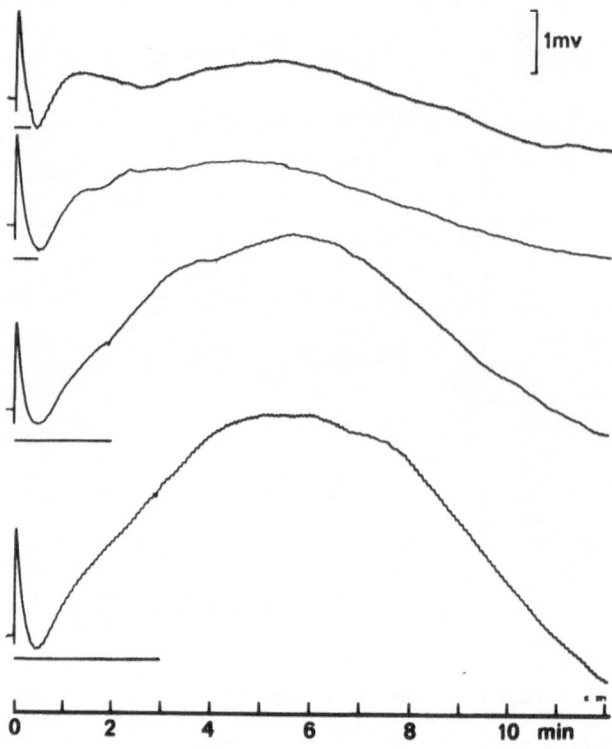

Fig. 3. DC-ERG and light peak at various stimulus durations, as indicated by the horizontal bars. The LP increases in amplitude, but changes only little in its time course. The fast oscillation is most clearly separated in the upper traces. The stimulus intensity was at rod saturation.

acidosis as well as the hypercapnia induce decreases in pH within $300\,\mu$ vitread of the retina. These are similar in time course and polarity, but smaller in extent than the synchronously recorded changes in pH in the perfusate.

DISCUSSION

Differences in standing potential, c-wave and time course of the light peak among various vertebrates have been noted before (Kikwada, 1968; Miller and Steinberg, 1977; Griff and Steinberg, 1982) and became apparent in this study. Variations among the species in passive and active conductances of the basal and apical membranes of the RPE may contribute to those differences. However, step increases in light induced the sequence of a-, b- and c-wave, fast oscillation and light peak in vitro, that is typical for the anesthetized cat (Niemeyer, 1980; Steinberg and Niemeyer, 1981; Linsenmeier et al., 1982). The fast *oscillation* could be separated from the light peak in this study by applying stimuli of short duration and/or low intensity. These data extend evidence for the functional integrity of the retina-pigment epithelium complex in the perfused eye (Niemeyer, 1976; 1981).

46

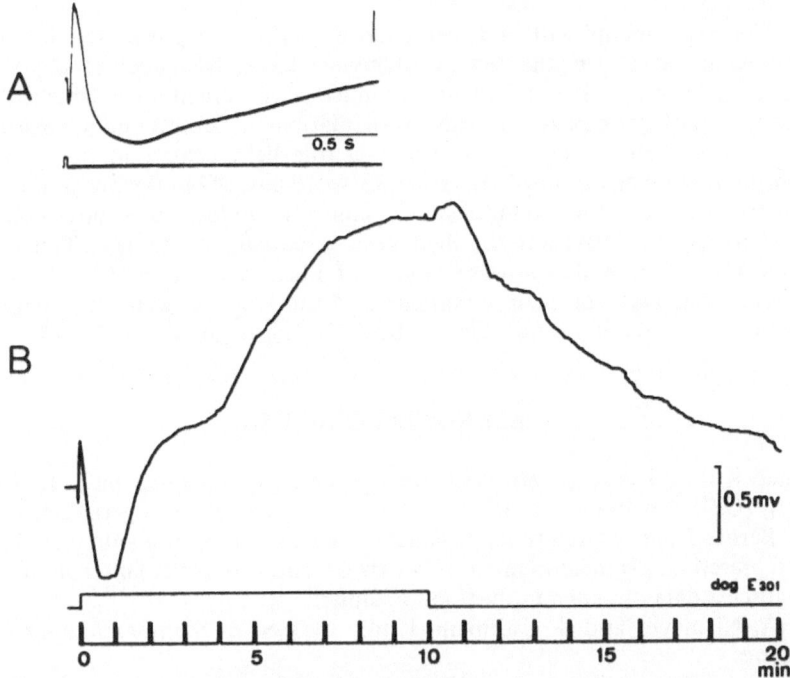

Fig. 4. Light-evoked signals from a dark adapted, perfused dog eye (German shepherd). —A: The DC-ERG consists of an a- and b-wave, followed by a slow negative component instead of a positive c-wave. The stimulus was a pulse of white light, 20 msec in duration and of intensity that saturates the b-wave. Calibration: $200\,\mu V$. —B: DC-ERG and light peak elicited by diffuse white light, presented for 10 min. The b-wave is followed by a large negative component and a positive wave, corresponding to the "fast oscillation". The positive wave is superimposed on the rising phase of the light peak. The light peak in perfused dog eyes reached maximum amplitude typically 9 to 11 min after stimulus onset.

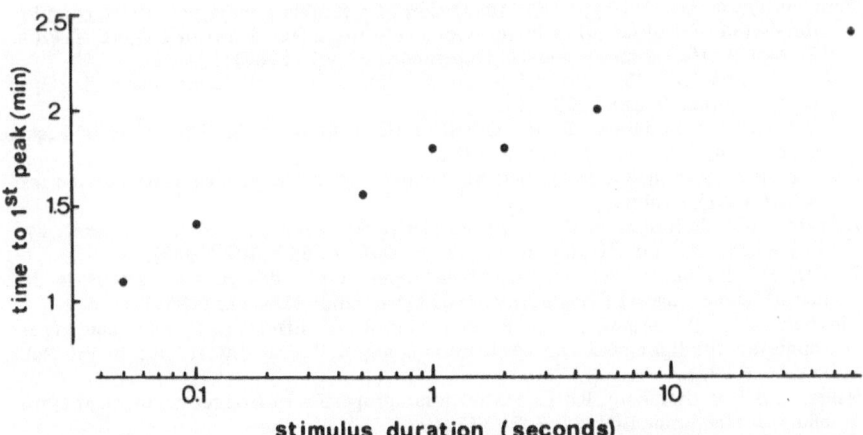

Fig. 5. Peak time of the fast oscillation (perfused dog eye) plotted against duration of the stimulus (from 50 msec to 1 min). The stimulus intensity was 0.6 log units below rod saturation.

47

The experiments with induced acidosis confirm its previously described depressing effect on the b-wave (Winkler, 1972; Niemeyer et al., 1982; Linsenmeier et al., 1982). The data on the c-wave were more variable and are therefore not yet conclusive. The fast oscillation has been found less sensitive to acidosis than the light peak. However, the light peak exhibited distinct sensitivity to increase in pCO_2 (from 38 to 78 mm HG in the perfusate) that almost abolished this component. In contrast, increase in proton concentration (HCl acidosis) left the light peak essentially unchanged. This result confirms and extends the observations of Linsenmeier et al. (1982) on the anesthetized cat: the main component of the EOG is exquisitely sensitive to elevated pCO_2 and is not affected by acidosis brought about by HCl.

ACKNOWLEDGEMENTS

Dr E. Korach-Demant assisted in some of these experiments. Drs R. H. Steinberg (U.C. San Francisco, Dept. of Physiology) and R. Weingart (University of Berne, Dept. of Physiology) collaborated in the experiments on acidosis and preretinal pH measurement, respectively, and I appreciate their permission to discuss data obtained in these joint studies.

A. Niemeyer and S. Hoffmann kindly assisted in the preparation of the figures.

This study was supported by grant 3.239.77 (to G.N.) from the Swiss National Science Foundation and by the EMDO foundation, Zürich.

REFERENCES

Arden, G. B., Barrada, A. and Kelsey, J. H.: A new clinical test of retinal function based upon the standing potential of the eye. Brit. J. Ophthalmol. 46: 449–467 (1962).

Funkhouser, A. and Niemeyer, G: Adaptation of a fundus camera permitting complex stimulation and observation in the visible and the infrared. Docum. Ophthal. Proc. Ser. Vol. 31 (G. Niemeyer and Ch. Huber, eds.) 39–42 (1982).

Gouras, P. and Hoff, M.: Retinal function in an isolated, perfused mammalian eye. Invest. Ophthal. 9: 388–399 (1970).

Griff, E. R. and Steinberg, R. H.: Origin of the light peak: in vitro study of gecko gecko. J. Physiol. (Lond.), in press, 1982.

Griff, E. R., Linsenmeier, R. A. and Steinberg, R. H.: The cellular origin of the fast oscillation. This volume, (1983).

Kikiwada, N.: Variations in the corneo-retinal standing potential of the vertebrate eye during light and dark adaptations. Jap. J. Physiol. 18: 687–702 (1968).

Kolder, H.: Spontane und experimentelle Aenderungen des Bestandspotentials des menschlichen Auges. Pflüger's Arch. ges. Physiol. 268: 258–272 (1959).

Linsenmeier, R. A., Mines, A. H. and Steinberg, R. H.: Effects of hypoxia and hypercapnia on the light peak and electroretinogram of the cat. Invest. Ophth. Vis. Sci., in press (1982).

Miller, S. S. and Steinberg, R. H.: Passive ionic properties of frog retinal pigment epithelium. J. Membrane Biol. 36: 337–372 (1977).

Niemeyer, G.: The function of the retina in the perfused eye. Docum. Ophthalmol. 39: 53–116 (1975).

Niemeyer, G.: C-waves and intracellular responses from the pigment epithelium in the cat. Bibl. Ophthal. Vol. 85 (R. Täumer, ed.) Karger, Basel, 68–74 (1976).

Niemeyer, G.: Electrooculography in isolated, perfused mammalian eyes. Experientia, 36: 699 (1980).

Niemeyer, G.: Neurobiology of perfused mammalian eyes. Neurosci. Meth. 3: 317–337 (1981).

Niemeyer, G. and Steinberg, R. H.: Effects of low pH and high CO_2 on the b-wave and light peak of the DC ERG in the perfused cat eye. Invest. Ophthal. Vis. Sci. (ARVO Suppl) 20: 43 (1981).

Niemeyer, G., Nagahara, D. and Demant, E.: Effects of changes in arterial PO_2 and PCO_2 on the electroretinogram in the cat. Invest. Ophthal. Vis. Sci. in press (1982).

Nikara, T., Sato, S. and Takamatsu, T., Sato, R. and Mita, T.: A new wave (second c-wave) on corneoretinal potential. Experientia 32: 594–596 (1976).

Rodieck, R. W.: Components of the electroretinogram – A reappraisal. Vision Res. 12: 773–780 (1972).

Steinberg, R. H. and Niemeyer, G.: Light peak of the cat DC ERG: not generated by change in K^+. Invest. Ophthal. Vis. Sci. 20: 414–418 (1981).

Täumer, R.: Electro-oculography – its clinical importance. Bibliotheca Ophthalmol. Vol. 85, Karger, Basel, (1976).

Winkler, B. S.: The electroretinogram of the isolated rat retina. Vision Res. 12: 1183–1198 (1972).

Zinn, K. M. and Marmor, M. F.: The retinal pigment epithelium. Harvard University Press, Cambridge and London (1979).

Mailing Address:
Department of Ophthalmology
Universitätsspital
CH-8091 Zürich,
Switzerland

CHANGES IN THE ELECTRORETINOGRAM OF ALBINO RABBITS AFTER INTRAVITREAL INJECTION OF DL-α-AMINODIPIC ACID

S. E. G. NILSSON, O. TEXTORIUS and E. WELINDER

(Linköping, Sweden)

ABSTRACT

Four albino rabbits were studied with registration of the D.C. electroretinogram 13.5–15 h after injection of 0.1 ml of 0.15 M DL-α-aminoadipic acid (α-AAA) into the vitreous body of one eye and the same volume of saline into the contralateral, control eye. In the α-AAA-treated eye the amplitudes of the *a*- and *c*-waves were increased and that of the *b*-wave markedly reduced compared with those of the control eye. Since α-AAA is known to damage the Müller cells, the present findings support the notion that these cells are related to the generation of the *b*-wave and to the negative slow PIII-potential, which modifies the *c*-wave.

INTRODUCTION

Some of the potentials underlying the electroretinogram (ERG) are of non-neuronal origin. The main positive component of the *c*-wave is generated by the pigment epithelium (Noell 1953; Brown and Wiesel 1961; Steinberg et al., 1970; Schmidt and Steinberg 1971). It is modified by negative potentials, e.g., slow PIII, which presumably originates in the Müller cells (Witkovsky et al., 1975; Oakley 1977). Also the *b*-wave is thought to arise passively in these cells (Faber, 1969; Miller and Dowling, 1970; Kline et al., 1978; Dick and Miller 1978; Newman 1979, 1980). Thus, an injury to the Müller cells should be expected to change the ERG. It has been observed that DL-α-aminoadipic acid (α-AAA) selectively affects the Müller cells after subcutaneous administration to infant mice (Olney et al., 1979) or intravitreal injection in rats (Lund Karlson, 1978; Pedersen and Lund Karlsen, 1979). The drug caused changes ranging from vacuolization of the cytoplasm and decrease in electron density to necrosis of the Müller cells 4 h after intravitreal administration of 100 µg. However, the cell injury was reversible (Lund Karlsen 1978; Pedersen and Lund Karlsen 1979).

The aim of the present experimental study on rabbits was to evaluate the ERG-changes following intravitreal injection of α-AAA and thus to test the Müller cell hypothesis on the origin of the above-mentioned potentials.

MATERIAL AND METHODS

Four albino rabbits were examined. During short-term general anaesthesia 0.1 ml of a freshly prepared 0.15 M solution of DL-α-aminoadipic acid in isotonic saline (2.4 mg of the active substance) was injected intravitreally into one eye and 0.1 ml of isotonic saline into the fellow, control eye. Maximal dilatation of the pupils preceded the injections, which were made transsclerally, just behind the ciliary body, and under direct visual control (surgical microscope and contact lens).

The DC ERG was registered under general anaesthesia (pentobarbital i.v.) 13.5–15 h after the injections. The recording procedure and the preparation of the animals were described in detail previously (Skoog and Nilsson 1974a, b; Skoog 1975; Nilsson and Skoog 1975; Textorius et al., 1978; Textorius and Welinder 1981), and included scleral suction contact lenses connected with saline-agar bridges to calomel half cells, D.C. amplification and low-pass filtering (220 Hz cut-off, 18 dB/octave). Stimulus light was produced by a 150 W Xenon lamp and transmitted equally to both eyes through quartz fibre optics. The light intensity was measured at the corneal surface of the contact lens.

After about 45 min of dark-adaption the eyes were exposed to a series of repeated 10 s light stimuli of increasing intensity: 12 cd/m^2 – 8 stimuli, 1 per 2 min; 120 cd/m^2 – 8 stimuli, 1 per 3 min; 1200 cd/m^2 – 6 stimuli, 1 per 4 min; 12000 cd/m^2 – 4 stimuli, 1 per 5 min. After the ERG registration the animal obtained a lethal dose of pentobarbital. However, one rabbit was reexamined two weeks after the injections.

ERG responses from each eye at each intensity level were averaged. The a-wave was measured from the iso-electric line, the b-wave from the trough of the a-wave when present or otherwise from the iso-electric line, and the c-wave from the iso-electric line. Statistical significances were assessed with Student's t-test.

RESULTS

In Fig. 1 a typical ERG registrations 13.5 h after intravitreal injection of α-AAA into one eye (lower traces) and saline into the contralateral eye (upper traces) are shown. In the right pair of registrations the time scale is expanded to show the a- and b-waves more clearly. The increased c-wave, the extinguished b-wave and the increased a-wave of the eye injected with α-AAA are evident.

These changes are quantified in Figs. 1b and 1c. In Fig. 1b the c-wave amplitudes from four eyes injected with α-AAA and the corresponding control eyes are plotted against stimulus intensity. The c-wave of the eyes treated with α-AAA was about twice as large as that of the control eyes, and this difference was statistically significant (p < 0.001). The relation between the a- and b-wave amplitudes from the same four animals and stimulus intensity is shown in Fig. 1c. The b-wave amplitude of the eyes treated with α-AAA was much less (p < 0.001), and the a-wave amplitude much larger (p < 0.001) than those of the control eyes.

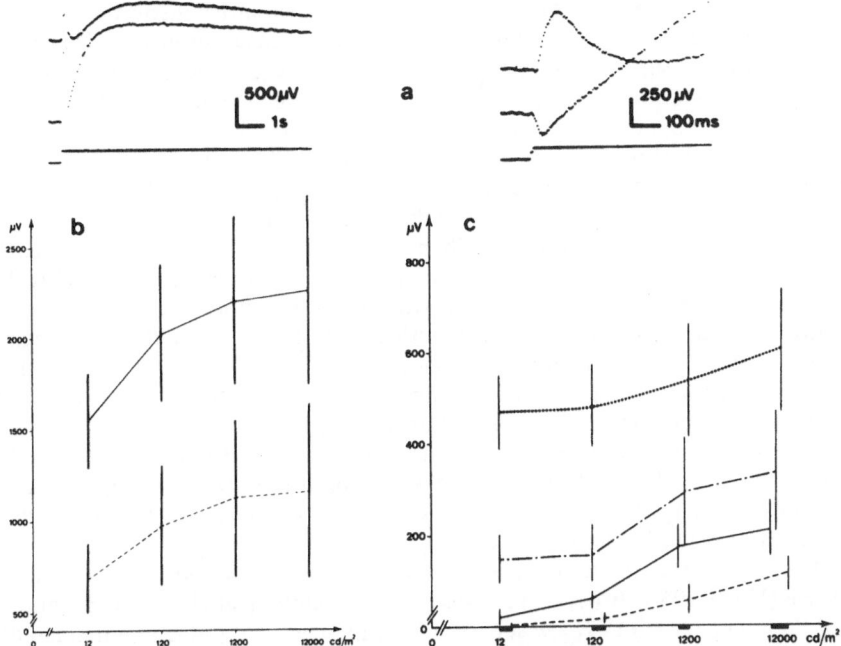

Fig. 1. (a) Characteristic ERG traces 13.5 h after injection of α-AAA into one eye (lower traces) and saline into the contralateral eye (upper traces). Expanded time scale in right part of the figure. Stimulus duration 10 s. Stimulus intensity 1200 cd/m². (b) Relation between *c*-wave amplitude and stimulus intensity 13.5–15 h after intravitreal injection of α-AAA into one eye (———) and saline into the fellow eye (- - - -). (c) Relation between *a*- and *b*-wave amplitudes and stimulus intensity 13.5–15 h after intravitreal injection of α-AAA into one eye (———, *a*-wave; –.–.–.–, *b*-wave) and saline into the fellow eye (– – – –, *a*-wave; . . . . ., *b*-wave). Means and standard errror of the means from four experiments.

One rabbit was reexamined after two weeks. The ERG of the eye injected with α-AAA was virtually extinguished, but that of the contralateral eye was still normal.

DISCUSSION

DL-α-aminoadipic acid is a selective antagonist of amino acid mediated synaptic excitation in the mammalina spinal cord (Biscoe et al., 1977). When injected intravitreally it acts as a gliotoxin, producing morphological changes in the Müller cells of rats (Lund Karlsen 1978; Pedersen and Lund Karlsen 1979), frogs and chicken (Bonaventure et al., 1980, personal communication). However, this cell injury could be reversible.

Previous electrophysiological investigations (Szamier et al., 1981) have demonstrated a profound suppression of the ERG *b*-wave in skate eyecup preparations superfused with a 50–100 mM solution of α-AAA. Histological examination revealed loss of electron density and extensive disruption of the plasma membranes in the Müller cells. However, after return to Ringer's solution the plasma membranes reformed and the b-wave could again be elicited. A reduction of the b-wave amplitude was also reported by Bonaventure et al., (1980, personal communication) and by Wachtmeister (1981).

The b-wave is thought to arise passively in the Müller cells as a consequence of potassium changes following neuronal activity (Faber 1969; Miller and Dowling 1970; Kline et al., 1978; Dick and Miller 1978; Newman 1979, 1980), but this view is not universally prevailing (Vogel 1980). In the present study the observed reduction of the b-wave amplitude after intravitreal injection of α-AAA is in accordance with previous reports (see above), and seems to support the Müller cell hypothesis on the origin of this potential. However, since α-AAA is a potent antagonist of amino acid medicated synaptic excitation (Biscoe et al., 1977) it cannot be excluded that the b-wave suppression might be due to this property of the drug.

The a-wave is mainly generated by the photoreceptors (Brown and Wiesel 1961; Faber 1969). The increased a-wave amplitude produced by α-AAA probably reflects the marked reduction of the b-wave, which allows the negative a-wave to be more fully developed.

The pigment epithelium generates the main positive component of the c-wave (Noell 1953; Brown and Wiesel 1961; Steinberg et al., 1970; Schmidt and Steinberg 1971) as the result of a light-induced and potassium mediated differential hyperpolarization of its apical and basal membranes (Oakley and Green 1976; Oakley et al., 1977; Oakley 1977). This positive pigment epithelial component is modified by negative potentials, such as slow PIII (Noel 1953; Faber 1969; Oakley 1977), which presumably originates in the Müller cells in response to a light-induced decrease in potassium concentration (Witkowsky et al., 1975; Oakley 1977; Lurie and Marmor 1980).

In the present study the c-wave amplitude was markedly increased 13.5 — 15 h after intravitreal injection of α-AAA. This ERG reaction supports the view that the Müller cells generate the negative slow PIII, since a reduction of this potential would allow the positive pigment epithelial component to become more or less unmasked, which can be seen as the increased c-wave amplitude.

The time interval between treatment with α-AAA and registration of the ERG was of importance. The increase of the c-wave and decrease of the b-wave amplitudes did not occur immediately after the injections but were deferred several hours. This observation was made in preliminary experiments, which also showed that a higher dose of α-AAA (3.2 mg) produced the ERG changes earlier than the lower dose (2.4 mg) used in the main investigation.

In conclusion, the present findings, which are discussed more fully by Welinder et al., 1982, support the view that the Müller cells are related to the generation of the b-wave and to the negative slow PIII-potential.

ACKNOWLEDGEMENT

This investigation was supported by grants from the Swedish Medical Research Council (Project No. 12X-734) and the Committee for Research and Development of Östergötlands läns Landsting.

REFERENCES

Biscoe, T. J., Evans, R. H., Francis, A. A., Martin, M. R. and Watkins, J. C.: D-α-amino-adipate as a selective antagonist of amino acid-induced and synaptic excitation of mammalian spinal neurones. Nature (Lond) 270: 743–745 (1977).

Brown, K. T. and Wiesel, T. N.: Localization of origins of electroretinogram components by intraretinal recording in the intact cat eye. J. Physiol. (Lond) 158: 257–280 (1961).

Dick, E. and Miller, R. F.: Light-evoked potassium activity in mudpuppy retina: its relationship to the b-wave of the electroretinogram. Brain Res. 154: 388–394 (1978).

Faber, D. S.: Analysis of the slow transretinal potentials in response to light. Ph.D. Thesis. State University of New York at Buffalo (1969).

Kline, R. P., Ripps, H. and Dowling, J. E.: Generation of b-wave currents in the skate retina. Proc. Natl. Acad. Sci. USA 75: 5727–5731 (1978).

Lund Karlsen, R.: The toxic effect of sodium glutamate and DL-α-aminoadipic acid on rat retina: changes in high affinity uptake of putative transmitters. J. Neurochem 31: 1055–1061 (1978).

Lurie, M. and Marmor, M. F.: Similarities between the c-wave and slow PIII in the rabbit eye. Invest. Ophthalmol. Vis. Sci. 19: 1113–1117 (1980).

Miller, R. F. and Dowling, J. E.: Intracellular responses of the Müller (glial) cells of mudpuppy retina: their relation to b-wave of the electroretinogram. J. Neurophysiol 33: 323–341 (1970).

Newman, E. A.: B-wave currents in the frog retina. Vision Res. 19: 227–234 (1979).

Newman, E. A.: Current source-density analysis of the b-wave of frog retina. J. Neurophysiol. 43: 1355–1366 (1980).

Nilsson, S. E. G. and Skoog, K.-O.: Covariation of the simultaneously recorded c-wave and standing potential of the human eye. Acta Ophthalmol (Kbh.) 53: 721–730 (1975).

Noell, W. K.: Studies on the electrophysiology and the metabolism of the retina. US Air Force, SAM Project 21-1201-0004. Randolph Field, Texas (1953).

Oakley, B. II: Potassium and the photoreceptor – dependent pigment epithelial hyper-polarization. J. Gen. Physiol. 70: 405–425 (1977).

Oakley, B. II and Green, D. G.: Correlation of light-induced changes in retinal extra-cellular potassium concentration with c-wave of the electroretinogram. J. Neurophysiol. 39: 1117–1133 (1976).

Oakley, B. II, Steinberg, R. H., Miller, S. S. and Nilsson, S. E. G.: The in vitro frog pigment epithelial cell hyperpolarization in response to light. Invest Ophthalmol. Vis. Sci. 16: 771–774 (1977).

Olney, J. W., Ho, O. L. and Rhee, V.: Cytotoxic effects of acidic and sulphur containing amino acids on the infant mouse central nervous system. Exp. Brain Res. 14: 61–76 (1971).

Pedersen, O. Ø. and Lund Karlsen, R.: Destruction of Müller cells in the adult rat by intravitreal injection of DL-α-aminoadipic acid. An electron microscopic study. Exp. Eye Res. 28: 569–575 (1979).

Schmidt, R. and Steinberg, R. H.: Rod-dependent intracellular responses to light recorded from the pigment epithelium of the cat retina. J. Physiol. (Lond) 217: 71–91 (1971).

Skoog, K.-O.: The directly recorded standing potential of the human eye. Acta Ophthalmol. (Kbh.) 53: 120–132 (1975).

Skoog, K.-O. and Nilsson, S. E. G.: The c-wave of the human d.c. registered ERG. I. A study of the relationship between c-wave amplitude quantitative and stimulus intensity. Acta Ophthalmol (Kbh.) 52: 759–773 (1974a).

Skoog, K.-O. and Nilsson, S. E. G.: The c-wave of the human d.c. registered ERG. II. Cyclic variations of the c-wave amplitude. Acta Opthalmol. (Kbh.) 52: 904–912 (1974b).

Steinberg, R. H., Schmidt, R. and Brown, K. T.: Intracellular responses to light from cat pigment epithelium: origin of the electroretinogram c-wave. Nature (Lond) 227: 728–730 (1970).

Szamier, R. B., Ripps, H. and Chappell, R. L.: Changes in ERG b-wave and Müller cell structure induced by α-aminoadipic acid. Neurosci. letters 21: 307–312 (1981).

55

Textorius, O., Nilsson, S. E. G. and Skoog, K.-O.: Studies on acute and late stages of experimental central retinal artery occlusion in the Cynomolgus monkey. I. Intensity-amplitude relations of the d.c. recorded ERG with special reference to the c-wave. Acta Ophthalmol. (Kbh.) 56: 648−664 (1978).

Textorius, O. and Welinder, E.: Early effects of sodium iodate on the directly recorded standing potential of the eye and on the c-wave of the DC registered electroretinogram in albino rabbits. Acta Ophthalmol. (Kbh.) 59: 359−368 (1981).

Vogel, D. A.: Potassium release and ERG b-wave current flow in the frog retina. Dissertation (Bioengineering), University of Michigan (1980).

Wachtmeister, L.: Further studies of the chemical sensitivity of the oscillatory potentials of the electroretinogram (ERG). II. Glutamate- aspartate- and dopamine antagonists. Acta Ophthalmol. (Kbh.) 59: 247−258 (1981).

Welinder, E., Textorius, O. and Nilsson, S. E. G.: Effects of intravitreally injected DL-α-aminoadipic acid on the c-wave of the D.C.-recorded electroretinogram in albino rabbits. Invest. Opthalmol. Vis. Sci. 23: 240−245 (1982).

Witkovsky, P., Dudek, F. E. and Ripps, H.: Slow PIII component of the carp electroretinogram. J. Gen. Physiol. 65: 119−134 (1975).

Mailing address:
Department of Ophthalmology
University Hospital, University of Linköping
S-581 85 Linköping,
Sweden

THE CANINE c-WAVE: BREED AND ANESTHETIC-DEPENDENT VARIATIONS

W. W. DAWSON, A. I. WEBB, R. PARMER and D. ARMSTRONG

(Gainesville, Florida, U.S.A.)

ABSTRACT

Understanding of the mammalian c-wave is enhanced by recent clarification of the role of the cells of the pigment epithelium. Profound between and within human variability is reported by Hock and Marmor (1982), while the classical literature exhibits a confusing number of citations to species variation for c-wave amplitude and latency. Among others, the canine eye has been reported to have no c-wave (Rodieck, 1973). We report here that this view is incorrect although DC-recorded canine c-waves are highly breed dependent and exhibit sensitivity to both inhalation and parenteral anesthetics. For example, in the pure breed beagle, normally large c-waves were eliminated by end-tidal halothane concentrations of 2%. More sensitive English setters lost 70% of c-wave amplitude with end-tidal halothane concentrations of 0.1%. Setters also show significant c-wave reductions with graded pento-barbital concentrations up to 10 mg/kg. One mixed breed dog showed poten-tiation of the c-wave in the presence of 2% halothane. An overview of per-formance across breeds disclosed moderate or mild a-, b-wave sensitivities, while c-wave reductions up to 100% were recorded. Species, breed, anesthetic and general physiological state probably account for the varied results in the classical c-wave literature.

INTRODUCTION

The ion gradients that contribute to the intraretinally recorded mammalian c-wave have been explained with great clarity by Steinberg and Miller (1979). This lucid account leaves the casual reader with a feeling of in-depth under-standing and with the assumption that there is little work of great importance left to be done in the area. The clinical electrophysiologist and the compara-tive physiologist are left with a less secure feeling after reviewing related literature pertaining to c-waves recorded from the corneal surface. Rodieck (1973) reviewed literature showing that rat, owl monkey and dog have no c-wave. While Marmor and Laurie (1979) report large variations in c-wave characteristics between rats, rabbits, cats and humans. Similar compelling indications of variation in c-wave characteristics from human subjects were

Doc. Ophthal. Proc. Series, Vol. 37, ed. by H. E. J. W. Kolder
©1983 Dr W. Junk Publishers, The Hague/Boston: Lancaster

described by Hock and Marmor (1982). In this paper we examine further the breed and anesthetic-dependent variations in the canine c-wave.

METHODS

Animal material for these experiments was provided by the kennels of the College of Veterinary Medicine and consisted of 2 pure bred Beagles and 4 English setters. Mixed breed dogs were represented by a Labrador retriever-like animal and a malamute-like animal. Methods of restraint and recording were adopted to maximize the physiological state of the animal and to provide for careful control of the inhalation and parenteral agents. Maintenance procedures were monitored by a veterinary anesthesiologist. Careful attention to consistent protocol was maintained across animals and experiments. Because of circulatory changes in long muscle relaxation, experiments were designed to require less than 2 hours of paralysis. But on one occasion it was necessary to adjust blood pressure with dopamine. In each case, the dogs were maintained in an environment at approximately 0 log foot lamberts (fl) for one hour prior to the experiment. Sodium thioamylal was used as an ultra short acting anesthetic for intubation, starting an I.V. drip and inducing muscle relaxation with pancuronium bromide. Cardiac and vascular signs were monitored with a Doppler ultrasonic device or by electrocardiography. Ventilation was assisted manually or mechanically and end-tidal CO_2 was maintained between 4.2 and 4.8%. Temperature was maintained by a heat-exchanger mattress. End-tidal halothane concentration was measured by a Beckman LB-2 gas analyzer.

Intubation and preparation were done at an adaptation level of about 1 log fl. The right pupil was dilated with neosynephrine and a topical anesthetic was applied. A molded plastic contact lens fitted with a recessed electrically reversible conductor was attached to the dilated right eye over a film of saline and methylcellulose. An electrically reversible disc electrode was attached with EEG paste to the right outer canthus approximately 3 cm from the eye. A tangent screen which subtended approximately 140 degrees of visual angle was positioned 15 cm in front of the right eye and could be illuminated uniformaly by adaptation lights. The xenon arc stimulus also illuminated the tangent screen uniformly and provided a fixed 0.51 log fl-sec flash lasting 25 μsec.

Following preparation the eye was adapted to darkness for 15 minutes and then brought to −2 log fl. All experiments began following at least 4 minutes of adaptation at that level. Signals from the corneal electrode were amplified (2000 ×) with a passband of DC to 1 kHz. Signals were recorded for 1 second before the stimulus flash and for 20 subsequent seconds. Ten second segments will be presented. Data were simultaneously digitized for storage on magnetic disc and recorded by FM tape. Digital resolution for the 20 second records was insufficient for high accuracy b-wave measurements which were reacquired from FM tape.

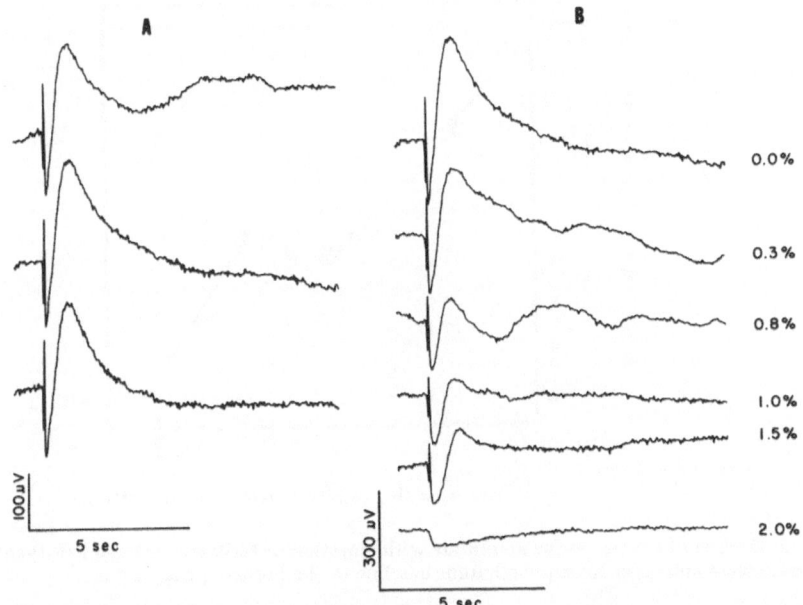

Fig. 1. Beagle c-waves. (A) Records taken at 3 minute intervals following 4 minutes at −2 log fl. (B) Progressive effects of halothane anesthesia measured as end-tidal percent. Stimuli were presented one second after the beginning of the records.

RESULTS

All results were generated by the same protocol. Following light adaptation to −2 log fl for 4 minutes stimuli were presented at 3 minute intervals to establish response stability. Subsequent inhalation or parenteral agents were manipulated in graded series and responses recorded. Responses from a typical Beagle are shown in Fig. 1A before graded halothane delivery, Fig. 1B. Stimulus delivery was just prior to the a-, b-wave complex which occurs at 1 second. C-wave latency was 895 msec. As circulating halothane concentration was built (Fig. 1B) stimuli were delivered at 3 minute or longer periods. C-wave amplitude and latency changed linearly. Diastolic pressure was maintained above 60 mm of Hg until the 2% level was reached. There pressure dropped to 40 but control was regained with the addition of dopamine. Fig. 2 graphically describes the relationship between the Beagle c-wave amplitude (measured from the pre-stimulus reference level to the positive peak) and end-tidal halothane. End-tidal halothane is a good estimate of the arterial halothane level and is approximately 1% below the haloethane content of the inspired mixture. The loss of c-wave at 2% may be a consequence of transiently lowered blood pressure.

Figure 3A describes the repeatability of the c-wave response in the English setter for comparison to the Beagle. Signals after adaptation to −2 log fl and for the ensuing 12 minute period show little variation in b-wave but a relatively delayed c-wave which peaked at 3.5 to 5 seconds. In this breed sensitivity to

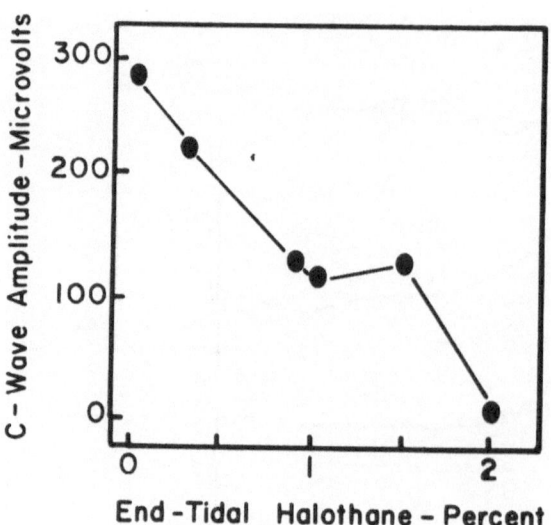

Fig. 2. Decline of beagle c-wave amplitude with elevation of estimated arterial halothane. C-waves were measured from pre-stimulus baseline to the positive peak.

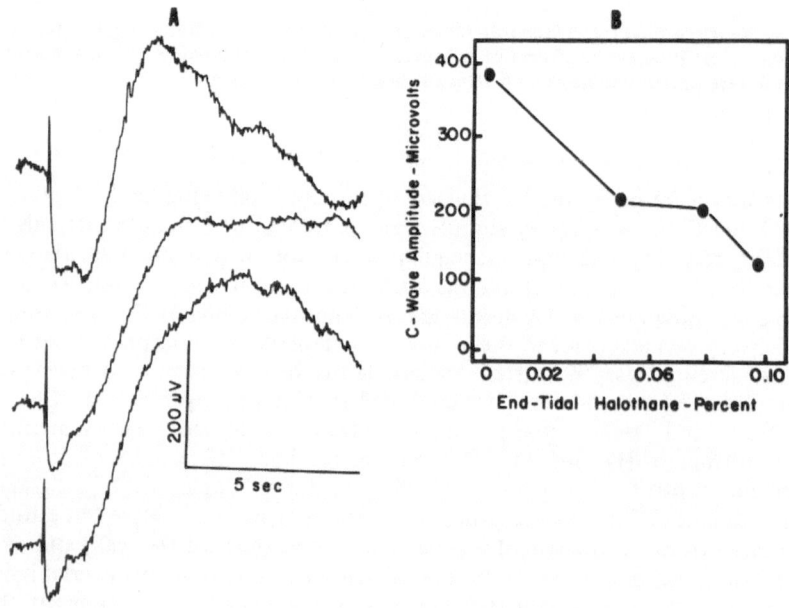

Fig. 3. English setter c-waves. (A) As Fig. 1. (B) Halothane effects as Fig. 2.

halothane is greater than in Beagles. Fig. 3B shows that setter c-wave amplitudes are reduced by 70% when the end-tidal halothane increased to only 0.1%. More halothane (Fig. 4) appears to eliminate the c-wave in this breed. However, recovery from halothane at these levels is rapid (Fig. 4). For records A and B

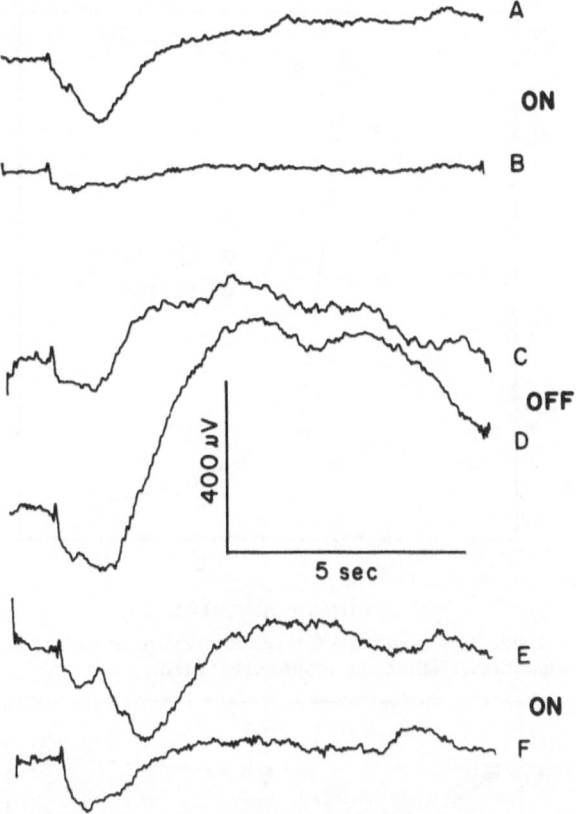

Fig. 4. English setter c-wave. Reversibility of halothane effects A–B, following the inhalation of halothane, end-tidal concentrations 0.08 and 0.12 percent respectively. C–D, halothane off, end-tidal concentration 0.05 percent (C) and 0.00 percent after 15 and 30 minutes respectively. E–F, halothane on, end-tidal concentration 0.06 and 0.12 percent respectively.

halothane was turned on briefly and reached 0.08% (A) and 0.12% (B). At that point the gas was turned off and after 15 minutes 0.05% was measured (C) and at 30 minutes 0.00% was measured (D). Then the gas was turned on once more with 0.06% registered for record E and 0.12% registered for record F. Similar results were given by the mixed breed retriever which was used in April of 1982. Subsequently this animal was retested with a graded halothane series but the results were reversed. That is, the maximum c-wave was recorded with 2% inspired halothane where c-wave decreased after halothane was discontinued and b-wave increased (Fig. 5).

Another English setter was used to generate the data summarized by Fig. 6. Graded doses of Na pentobarbital were delivered via the I.V. drip. The usual criterion for c-wave measurement (prestimulus baseline to positive peak) was abandoned for this set of records. In this case c-wave was measured from the negative trough (post b-wave) to the following positive peak. The usual canine anesthetic dose is 20–35 mg/kg. Fig. 6 shows that with the gradual

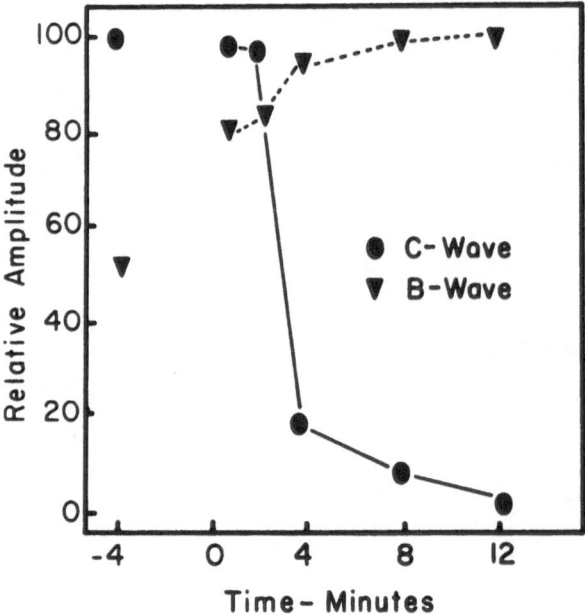

Fig. 5. Relative c- and b-wave amplitudes from a retriever (mixed breed) during recovery from two percent halothane. Halothane stopped at zero time.

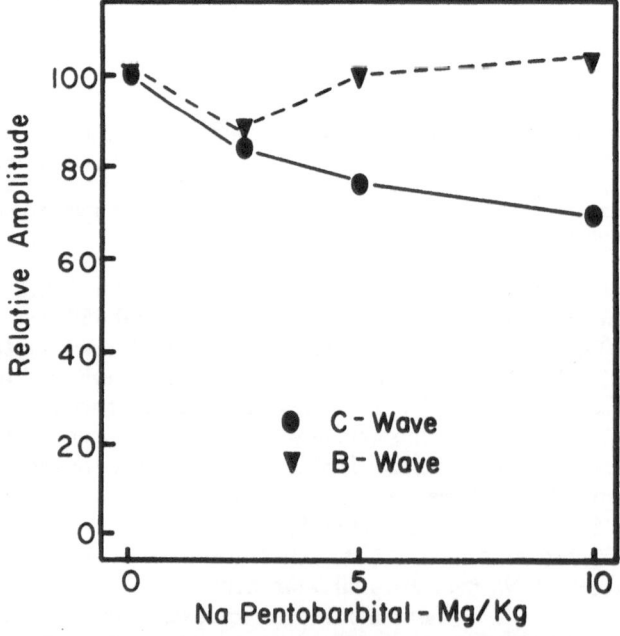

Fig. 6. Comparison of c- and b-wave amplitudes from an English setter before and at three minute intervals following increments of intravenous Na pentobarbital. C-wave amplitudes were measured from the positive peak to the preceeding negative trough.

62

increase of circulating pentobarbital over a 12 minute period, concentrations of 10 mg/kg. reduced the c-wave by 30%. The reduction would be 100% if the (Fig. 2) c-wave convention were applied. The b-wave was minimally affected.

DISCUSSION

The procedure was designed to minimize departures from the normal physiological state, chemical artifacts, animal discomfort and large, rapid changes in light level or extended periods of dark adaptation for an animal whose dark adaptation process has not been described. The stability of the a-, b- and c-waves recorded prior to the use of inhalation of parenteral compounds indicates little contamination by concomitantly changing standing potentials such as described by Welinder (1981) and by Nilsson and Skoog (1975). Their data suggests that large standing potential changes would register as varied c-wave amplitudes. Apparently either the protocol was sufficient to eliminate large standing potential changes or the relationship in the dog eye is different from that in humans and monkeys. But it no longer seems likely that the relationship between the standing potential and the c-wave is simple or direct. Steinberg and Niemeyer (1981) have demonstrated a large degree of independence, decoupling the standing potential light peak from the intraretinal K^+ concentration, which is so important to the c-wave.

The data presented show that popular anesthetics have c-wave effects which are usually (but not always, depending upon individual) predictable. Compounds which effect the c-wave do not necessarily have b-wave effects. Further, the c-wave and its sensitivity to anesthetics appears to vary between canine breeds and even for the same dog at different times of the year.

Failure to control or standardize physiological conditions, c-wave criteria and anesthetic artifacts may account for a significant amount of the supposed 'species' variation mentioned in the older literature. However, real species effects and breed effects do indeed exist. While the interacting influences of species, breed and anesthetics may be perplexing today, the understanding of their basis and interactions will provide for significant future research and a better understanding of retinal-pigment epithelium function.

ACKNOWLEDGEMENT

Assisted by National Science Foundation grant BNS-7914129, National Eye Institute grants EY-4083 and EY-0236, the Children's Brain Disease Foundation and in part by an unrestricted departmental grant from Research to Prevent Blindness, Inc., New York.

REFERENCES

Hock, P. and Marmor, M. (1982). Variability of the normal human c-wave. Invest. Ophthalmol. Visual Sci. (Suppl.) 22, 138.

Marmor, M. and Laurie, M. (1979). Light-induced electrical responses of the retinal pigment epithelium. In: K. Zinn and M. Marmor (eds.) The Retinal Pigment Epithelium, Cambridge, Harvard University Press, 226–244.

Nilsson, S. and Skoog, K.O. (1975). Covariation of the simultaneously recorded c-wave and standing potential of the humen eye. Acta Ophthalmol. 53, 721–730.

Rodieck, R. W. (1973). The Vertebrate Retina, San Francisco, W. H. Freeman, 546.

Steinberg, R. and Miller, S. (1979). Transport and membrane properties of the retinal pigment epithelium. In: K. Zinn and M. Marmor (eds.) The Retinal Pigment Epithelium, Cambridge, Harvard University Press, 205–225.

Steinberg, R. and Niemeyer, G. (1981). Light peak of cat DC electroretinogram: not generated by a change in $[K^+]_0$. Invest. Ophthalmol. Visual Sci. 20, 414–417.

Welinder, E. (1981). Cyclic amplitude variations of a slow ERG off-effect, the h-wave in the cynomolgus monkey. Vision Res. 21, 1159–1163.

Mailing address:
Department of Ophthalmology
University of Florida
Box J-284, JHMHC
Gainesville, Florida 32610,
U.S.A.

ELECTRORETINOGRAM BELOW b-WAVE THRESHOLD IN THE CAT: STUDIES OF RETINAL DEVELOPMENT AND RETINAL DEGENERATION

S. G. JACOBSON and H. IKEDA

(London, U.K.).

ABSTRACT

The cornea negative ERG below b-wave threshold was recorded in dark adapted cats. Retinal arterial occlusion resulted in a loss of the negative potential. During postnatal development of the cat, amplitude of the negativity was found to be adult-like at 4—6 weeks of age; it became greater than that of adults between 6 and 14 weeks of age; and thereafter decreased again to adult levels. The negativity was also recorded in adult cats with retinal degeneration caused by taurine deficiency. The amplitude of the negative potential decreased with increasing severity of the retinal degeneration, eventually becoming non-detectable.

INTRODUCTION

In the fully dark adapted eye, a very weak light stimulus evokes a cornea negative electroretinogram (ERG). This negativity below b-wave threshold has been described in man and in experimental animals (Finkelstein et al., 1968; Knave et al., 1972). The exact origin of this negative response is not known but it is of interest because it represents an objective indicator of the lowest level of scotopic retinal function and is though to be closer to psychophysical absolute threshold than the smallest detectable b-wave (Finkelstein et al., 1968).

Although it is a recognised ERG phenomenon, the negative potential has not been previously used to monitor changes in retinal function. We therefore developed techniques to elicit and record the negative potential serially and reliably in cats and then applied these techniques to the study of two groups of cats known to be undergoing changes in retinal structure and function. The results of our investigations of the negative ERG in normal adult cats, in kittens during postnatal development and in cats with a nutritionally-induced retinal degeneration are reported herein.

Doc. Ophthal. Proc. Series, Vol. 37, ed. by H. E. J. W. Kolder
©1983 Dr W. Junk Publishers, The Hague/Boston: Lancaster

METHODS

Cats in this study were from a specific pathogen free colony. ERGs were recorded under anaesthesia using alphaxalone alphadolone acetate (14.5 mg/ kg/hr). Details of our methods for recording the ERG of the cat have been published elsewhere (Jacobson and Ikeda, in press). Cats were dark adapted for at least 2 hours before ERG recording began. The contact lens electrode used was similar in principle to a Burian-Allen double contact lens electrode but had a 7 mm diameter artificial pupil and a diffuser in front of the aperture to provide ganzfeld stimulation. Amplification (bandpass 0.08–320 Hz) and computer averaging were performed with a Medelec AA-DAV6.

The stimulus was a xenon-filled gas discharge tube stroboscope (Devices Photostimulator 3180) with a short wavelength filter (Wratten 47). Intensity of the stimulus could be varied over 7 log units using a neutral density wedge. ERGs were elicited first with stimuli of the lowest intensity (7 log units below maximum) and then in 0.2 to 0.3 log unit steps of increasing intensity. At each step, 20 responses were elicited and summed by computer. A higher stimulus intensity (see Fig. 1, last response) was achieved with the same stroboscopic light source in a matt white dome, but neither the short wavelength filter nor the contact lens diffuser; peak luminance in the dome was 3.8 log cd/m^2. This stimulus was about 2 log units more intense than the maximum intensity possible with the other stimulus (as determined by comparing b-wave amplitude versus log intensity functions of the 2 stimuli). The ERGs of kittens were corrected for known changes in the axial length of the eye with age.

RESULTS

Figure 1A shows dark adapted ERGs from the left eye of an adult cat elicited with progressively increasing stimulus intensity over a 5–6 log unit range. The lowest intensities evoke no response while at higher intensities a cornea negative response can be recorded. In 8 adult cats the threshold of this negative potential, i.e. the first measurable response, was between 2.3 and 2.8 log units (mean, 2.55) above the 'zero' log relative intensity. For comparison, the threshold of a dark adapted human observer was tested psychophysically using the same apparatus (ganzfeld stimulation, natural pupil) and was found to be 1.25 log units of relative intensity.

With increasing stimulus intensity, the negative potential increases in amplitude. Maximum amplitude of the negativity in 8 adult cats ranged from 2.0 to 6.4 μV (mean, 4.0 μV). The latency (time to first negative deflection) of the response was between 65 and 85 msec after stimulus onset, while the implicit time (time to maximum amplitude) varied between 125 and 175 msec after the stimulus. In adult cats the negative response usually did not return to baseline during the recording period of 700 msec that followed each stimulus.

Between 1 and 2 log units above the threshold of the negative potential, the cornea positive b-wave is recorded. An apparent interaction between the

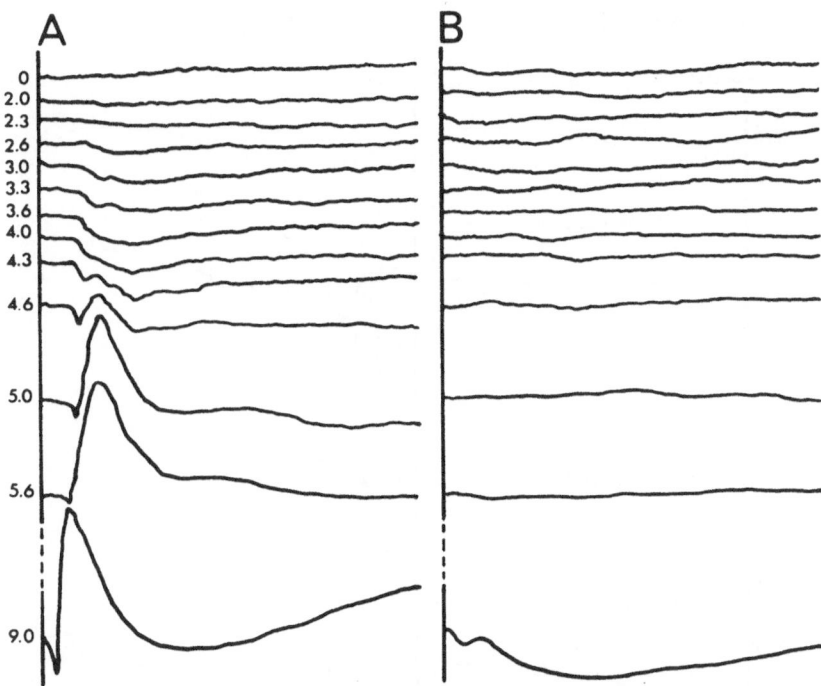

Fig. 1. ERGs from an adult cat, elicited with logarithmically increasing stimulus intensity, before (A) and after (B) retinal arterial occlusion. Calibration symbol is vertically 8 μV for log stimulus intensities 0–5.0; 20 μV for 5.6; and 100 μV for 9.0 Horizontally, the calibration symbol represents 100 msec.

b-wave and the negativity occurs and at higher intensity levels, the negative response is no longer identifiable. The last response in Figure 1A is at much higher intensity and demonstrates the typical ERG of the cat with both a- and b-wave components.

In Figure 1B are dark adapted ERGs recorded from the left eye of the same cat 4 hours later, after xenon photocoagulation of the retinal vessels at the margin of the optic disc. Occlusion of the retinal circulation is a technique that has been used previously to isolate the response of receptors at the expense of the inner retinal layers (Brown and Watanabe 1962). A comparison of the responses before and after arterial occlusion in this cat reveals that both the negative potential and the b-wave have been abolished by the procedure, at least for the 6 log units of intensity above zero. At the highest stimulus intensity in Figure 1B (lowest trace), however, a prominent a-wave and a residual small b-wave can be recorded.

We determined the postnatal development of the negative potential in kittens between the ages of 4 and 20 weeks. Representative ERGs from kittens of different ages are shown in Figure 2. Figure 2A displays negative potentials recorded from a 44 day old kitten; the maximum aplitude of these responses was like that of adult cats. Some kittens beyond the age of 6–7 weeks had amplitudes of the negative potential that were even greater than those of

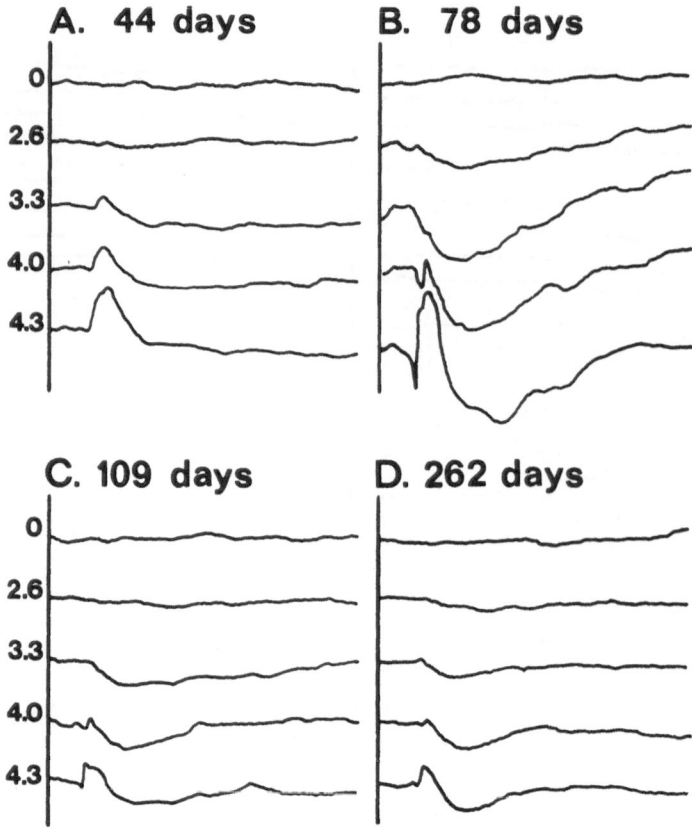

A. 44 days

0
2.6
3.3
4.0
4.3

B. 78 days

C. 109 days

0
2.6
3.3
4.0
4.3

D. 262 days

Fig. 2. ERGs from kittens of different ages elicited with logarithmically increasing stimulus intensity. The responses in C and D are from the same cat at two different ages. Calibration symbol is 10 μV vertically and 100 msec horizontally.

adult cats. In Figure 2B are examples of such large amplitude negative responses from a kitten of 78 days of age. After about 14 weeks of age, however, the amplitude of the negativity decreased and became adult-like again. The recordings in Figure 2C and 2D are from the same cat recorded at 109 days and then again at 262 days of age. It is evident that responses at the two sessions, separated by nearly 22 weeks, are very similar.

Certain other features of the responses shown in Figure 2 are worthy of mention. It has been reported that kittens between the ages of 6 and 14 weeks of age can have lower rod ERG thresholds than adult cats and supra-threshold rod ERG b-wave amplitudes greater than adults (Ikeda and Jacobson, 1982; Faulkner et al., in press). The b-wave thresholds of the 44 and 78 day old kittens are certainly lower than those of the kitten recorded at 109 and 262 days of age. Furthermore, the rod ERGs to the higher intensity stimulus (lowest trace in each series) had greater b-wave amplitude in the kittens of 44 and 78 days of age than at the later ages depicted.

Figure 3 shows ERGs from cats before and after being fed a diet with

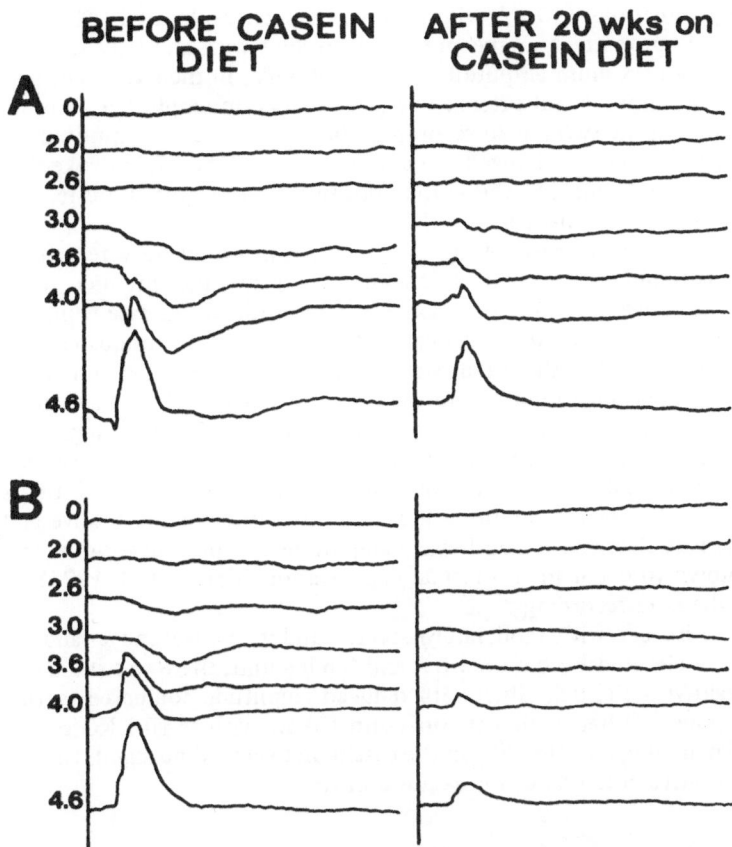

Fig. 3. ERGs from 2 adult cats before and 20 weeks after being fed a casein diet that produced retinal taurine deficiency. A. Cat with mild fundus lesions; B. Cat with severe fundus lesions. Vertical axis is log relative intensity. Calibration symbol is 5 μV vertically for intensities 0–4.0, and 10 μV for intensity 4.6; horizontally, 100 msec.

casein as the sole source of protein. The retinal degeneration that results from this diet has been shown to be due to a deficiency in retinal taurine (Schmidt et al., 1976). We tested 3 adult cats before they were placed on the diet and all had a well-defined negative potential below b-wave threshold. After about 20 weeks on the diet, the cats showed fundus lesions in the area centralis typical of this nutritionally-induced retinal degeneration. The degree of severity of the lesions, however, differed in the 3 cats. The lesions ranged from mild hyperpigmentation and granularity in the area centralis to a large elongate hyperreflective central 'scar'. The ERGs in the cats also differed in degree of change from pre-diet recordings.

Figure 3A shows ERGs recorded before and after 20 weeks on the diet in the cat with the least fundus change. Rod b-wave thresholds, measured in two ways (see Faulkner et al., in press), became elevated by about 0.3 log unit after 20 weeks on the diet. The a-wave threshold determined from amplitude-intensity functions (10 μV criterion) was similarly elevated. The negative potential is prominent in the pre-diet recording with an easily recognisable onset and a maximum amplitude of about 4.5 μV. In the later recording, the negative potential is still present but it is reduced in amplitude. It is evident by comparing the two sets of recordings that the decrease in amplitude of the negative potential has changed the configuration of the ERGs evoked by low intensity stimuli, making the cornea positive components more readily discernible at lower intensities.

Figure 3B shows ERGs from a cat with a more severe effect from the nutritionally-induced retinal degeneration. Again, the pre-diet recording shows a negative potential, the maximum amplitude in this case being 3.2 μV. After 20 weeks on the diet, this cat had the most severe fundus change and had a rod b-wave threshold that was elevated by about 0.7 log unit compared to the threshold measured before the diet was started. The a-wave threshold was also elevated to at least this level. In contrast to the recordings in Figure 3A, the recordings after 20 weeks on the diet in Figure 3B show no detectable negative potential. The last response in the vertical sequence of ERGs for each cat in Figure 3 is at suprathreshold intensities for the b-wave and the characteristic decrease in rod b-wave amplitude and prolongation of implicit time known to occur in this retinal degeneration (Rabin et al. 1973) can be seen in the later recordings.

In a third cat with moderately severe fundus change and a- and b-wave thresholds elevated by between 0.5 and 0.6 log unit, there was still a measurable negative potential, albeit with reduced amplitude compared to the pre-diet response. Other adult cats on normal diets with serial ERG recordings at similar intervals to the cats on the casein diet showed no significant change in the negative potential or the a- and b-waves.

DISCUSSION

In the present study, we recorded ERGs using very low intensity stimuli in the fully dark adapted eyes of cats. The first detectable response was a cornea negative potential followed at higher intensities by the cornea positive b-wave. The sequence of changes in the cat ERG with increasing stimulus intensity was similar to what has been previously described when such recordings have been made in other animals (Knave et al., 1972) or in man (Finkelstein et al., 1968). With the present technique of eliciting and recording the negative potential there was little variability in the responses on serial testing of normal adult cats (see, for example, Figures 2C and 2D). Furthermore, although the negative potential is of relatively small amplitude, every normal adult cat tested had an easily identifiable and measurable response. The negative waveform therefore has the prerequisites for being a useful additional ERG parameter for assessing retinal function. The exact origin of the negative potential, however, is not known, but there has been speculation that it may represent the 'receptor potential' (Finkelstein et al., 1968; Knave et al., 1972). The results of our recordings in a cat before and after retinal arterial occlusion (see Figure 1) suggest that the negative potential in the cat is more likely to be a post-receptoral electrical phenomenon.

70

A value of recording the negative potential is that it could provide an electrophysiological and hence objective estimate of the absolute threshold. In humans, the threshold of the negative potential was only about 0.6 log unit higher than the psychophysically-determined value (Finkelstein et al., 1968). Previous attempts at defining the absolute threshold in the cat using electrophysiological recordings (e.g. ERG b-waves and retinal ganglion cell responses) have found that the estimates were much higher than any behaviourally-determined values (see Berkley 1976). Our finding that the threshold of the negative potential as recorded at the cornea is between 1 and 2 log units lower than b-wave threshold suggests that the behavioural absolute threshold in the cat might, like the human, be better correlated with the negative potential threshold than with other physiological measures. A formal comparison of this electrophysiological threshold using similar stimuli and, preferably the same animals, is necessary to clarify this issue.

Dramatic changes in the negative potential were found during postnatal development in the cat. A negative potential similar in amplitude to that of adult cats was already present in 4 to 6 week old kittens. During the next 6 to 8 weeks of life, the negativity increased in amplitude and then decreased again to adult levels. Other studies of the ERG during development in the cat (Ikeda and Jacobson, 1982; Faulkner et al., in press) have described a similar period of increased excitability between about 6 and 14 weeks of age. A form of hyperexcitability has also been observed in recordings from retinal ganglion cells of kittens (Rusoff and Dubin, 1977; Ikeda, personal communication). An exact mechanism for this phenomenon is not yet known but existing morphological evidence confirms that retinal maturation continues until 4–5 months of age in the cat and that considerable retinal differentiation occurs between the first and fifth months of life (Vogel, 1978).

In another series of experiments we recorded the negative potential in adult cats before and after they developed a nutritionally-induced retinal degeneration. It has been proven that a diet such as these cats were fed causes a retinal taurine deficiency which leads eventually to photoreceptor cell death (Hayes et al., 1975). Both a- and b-waves of the ERG become progressively diminished with increasing severity of this lesion but the early receptor potential is preserved until late in the condition (Berson et al., 1981). The negative potential was found to be sensitive to the effects of taurine deficiency. A reduction in amplitude of the negativity occurred in a relatively mildly affected cat and it became non-detectable in a cat that was more severely affected. Whether such changes in the negative potential occur exclusively in the retinal degeneration of taurine deficiency will only be determined by further studies of these responses in other experimental retinal degenerations and in retinitis pigmentosa in man.

ACKNOWLEDGEMENT

We thank the Retinitis Pigmentosa Foundation (Baltimore, Maryland, U.S.A.) and St. Thomas' Hospital for their support. We appreciate Dr K. Ruddock's expert advice and Professor R. Fletcher's help with the design and construction

71

of the contact lens electrodes. This work was performed at the Vision Research Unit of the Sherrington School, The Rayne Institute, St. Thomas' Hospital, London, U.K.

REFERENCES

Berkley, M. A. : Cat visual psychophysics: neural correlates and comparisons with man. In: Progress in Psychobiology and Physiological Psychology. 61–119, Academic Press, New York, 1976.

Berson, E. L., Watson, G., Grasse, K. L. and Szamier, R. B.: Retinal degeneration in cats fed casein: IV. The early receptor potential. Invest. Ophthalmol. Vis. Sci. 21: 345–350, 1981.

Brown, K. T. and Watanabe, K.: Isolation and identification of a receptor potential from the pure cone fovea of the monkey retina. Nature. 193: 958–960, 1962.

Faulkner, D. J., Ikeda, Hisako, Jacobson, S. G. and Kemp, C. M.: Rhodopsin levels and rod electroretinogram thresholds during development in the cat. J. Physiol. (in press).

Finkelstein, D., Gouras, P. and Hoff, M.: Human electroretinogram near the absolute threshold of vision. Invest. Ophthalmol. 7: 214–218, 1968.

Hayes, K. C., Rabin, A. R. and Berson, E. L.: An ultrastructural study of nutritionally induced and reversed retinal degeneration in cats. Am. J. Pathol. 78: 505–516, 1975.

Ikeda, Hisako and Jacobson, S. G.: Cone and rod electroretinograms during development in the cat. J. Physiol. 329: 21–22P, 1982.

Jacobson, S. G. and Ikeda, H.: Rod and cone electroretinograms in the cat. In: Proceedings of an International Workshop on Problems of Normal and Genetically Abnormal Retinas. Academic Press (in press).

Knave, B., Moller, A. and Persson, H. E.: A component analysis of the electroretinogram. Vision Res. 12: 1669–1684, 1972.

Rabin, A. R., Hayes, K. C. and Berson, E. L.: Cone and rod responses in nutritionally induced retinal degeneration in the cat. Invest. Ophthalmol. 12: 694–704, 1973.

Rusoff, A. C. and Dubin, M. W.: Development of receptive-field properties of retinal ganglion cells in kittens. J. Neurophysiol. 40: 1188–1198, 1977.

Schmidt, S. Y., Berson, E. L. and Hayes, K. C.: Retinal degeneration in cats fed casein: I. Taurine deficiency. Invest. Ophthalmol. 15: 47–52, 1976.

Vogel, M.: Postnatal development of the cat's retina. Advances in Anatomy, Embryology and Cell Biology. 54: 1–66, 1978.

Mailing address:
Dr. S. G. Jacobson
Massachusetts Eye and Ear Infirmary
243 Charles Street
Boston, Massachusetts 02114,
U.S.A.

ORIGIN OF THE FAST OSCILLATION IN THE MACAQUE

D. VAN NORREN and H. G. M. HEYNEN
*Institute for Perception TNO, Kampweg 5,
Soesterberg, The Netherlands*

The fast oscillation is a damped oscillatory wave with a period time of 2.5 min. It generally appears superimposed on the slow oscillation which has a period time of 25 min. Microelectrode recordings across the retinal pigment epithelium in intact eyes of macaca speciosa showed that both fast and slow oscillation are generated in this structure. The neural retina yields no contribution to these components. A similar conclusion was recently reached by Griff and Steinberg for an isolated preparation of the gecko retina (ARVO, 1982). Despite extensive manipulation of the stimulus parameters the fast oscillation always had a much smaller amplitude than the slow oscillation. In fact no more than one negative and one positive deflection could be discerned.

Doc. Ophthal. Proc. Series, Vol. 37, ed. by H. E. J. W. Kolder
©1983 Dr W. Junk Publishers, The Hague/Boston: Lancaster

INCREMENT THRESHOLD FUNCTION OF THE LIGHT-INDUCED SLOW OSCILLATION OF THE EOG

C. J. KRÜGER AND M. BAIER

(Frankfurt/Bad Nauheim and Hannover, F.R.G.)

ABSTRACT

Using Ganzfeld illumination the criterion threshold for a light rise of the standing potential of 30 per cent was determined in the electrooculogram at increasing levels of adaptive illumination. The amplitudes of the first positive peak of the slow oscillation were measured and the increment threshold was determined by the linear regression of amplitude vs. log test light illumination at various levels of adaptive illumination. Plots of the test light luminance necessary for the criterion amplitude vs. adaptive illumination revealed a curve, which can best be described by two separate e-functions probably representing the scotopic and photopic increment threshold functions of the human electrooculogram.

INTRODUCTION

As shown by microelectrode recordings the standing potential of the eye is built up along Bruch's membrane (for recent results see van Norren, 1982). In order to determine the retinal structure producing this potential the effect of brightness, duration and colour of the adaptation and test light (Kolder, 1959; Arden and Kelsey, 1962; McCord, 1963; Elenius and Karo, 1966; Täumer et al., 1976; Hache et al., 1976) as well as the size and localization of the stimulated area (Hochgesand and Schicketanz, 1975; Aschoff, 1981; Krüger, 1981) was investigated by measuring the amplitude of the light-induced slow oscillation of the standing potential in the human electrooculogram. Both the photopic and the scotopic system were shown to contribute to the light rise with a major contribution of the scotopic system. In order to evaluate more precisely the contribution of the photopic system to the light rise of the electrooculogram, we used the measurement of the increment threshold introduced into electroretinography at Dodt et al. (1960). For this purpose we measured the test light luminance, necessary for a constant amplitude of the slow oscillation of the standing potential at increasing levels of adaptive illumination. It was found that the increment threshold can best be described by a curve of two e-functions separating at an adaptive illumination of approx. 1 cd/m^2.

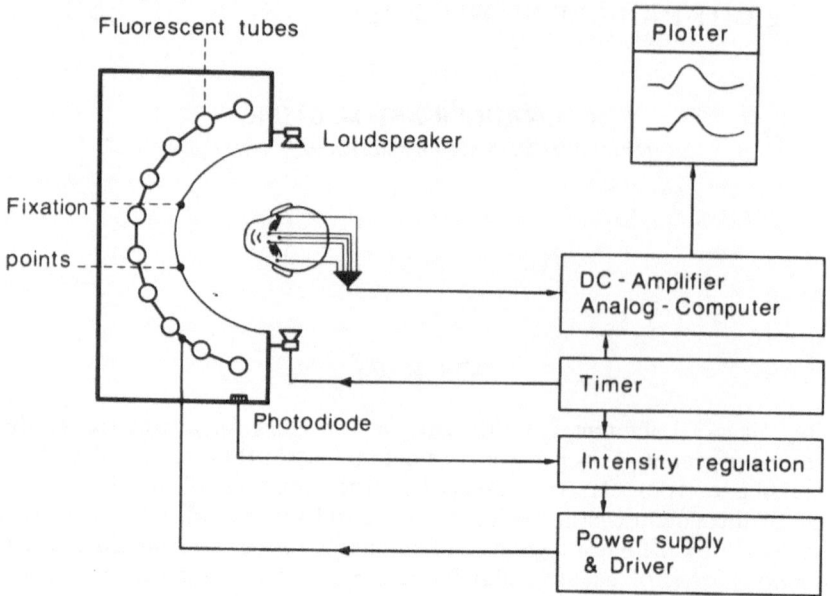

Fig. 1. Schematic diagram of the stimulus and recording procedure. The lights used for adaptation and testing are presented in a Ganzfeld mode of stimulation by means of the half-cylindrical frosted acryl screen homogenously illuminated from the backside by ten fluorescent tubes (5500° K), DC-driven and of adjustable luminance within 3 log units by feedback control. Additional light attenuation of 3 log units was obtained by inserting another neutral grey screen. A timer controlled the duration of the time periods used for adaptation and testing and prompted the eye movements by acustical signals at the right and left ear of the subject. The fixation points marked the extend of the eye movements (40° of visual angle). The standing potential was picked up by Ag-AgCl skin-electrode at the canthi of the eyes, the grounding electrode was attached to the forehead. The electrical potentials induced by the eye movements were DC-amplified and calculated by an analog-computer, averaged for each minute, and plotted on an Y-T recorder.

METHOD

Six healthy subjects took part in the experiment. All of them had normal visual fields and a visual acuity of 1.0 or better.

The stimulus set up and the recording procedure are shown in Figure 1. The light used for adaptation (0.001 to 40 cd/m²) and testing (0.02 to 980 cd/m²) was provided by fluorescent tubes on a back-illuminated screen. The standing potential was indirectly recorded by measuring the amplitude of the electrooculogram led off by two pairs of electrodes at the canthi of each eye. After an adaptation period to constant illumination of at least one hour, eye movements of 40° between the fixation points were performed for 30 min at intervals of 1 s at the beginning of each minute, monitored by an acustic signal. Light stimulation did not start until the standing potential was constant. All subjects received Mydriaticum Roche® for dilatation of the pupil to at least 8 mm. From the electrooculogram amplitude the light-induced

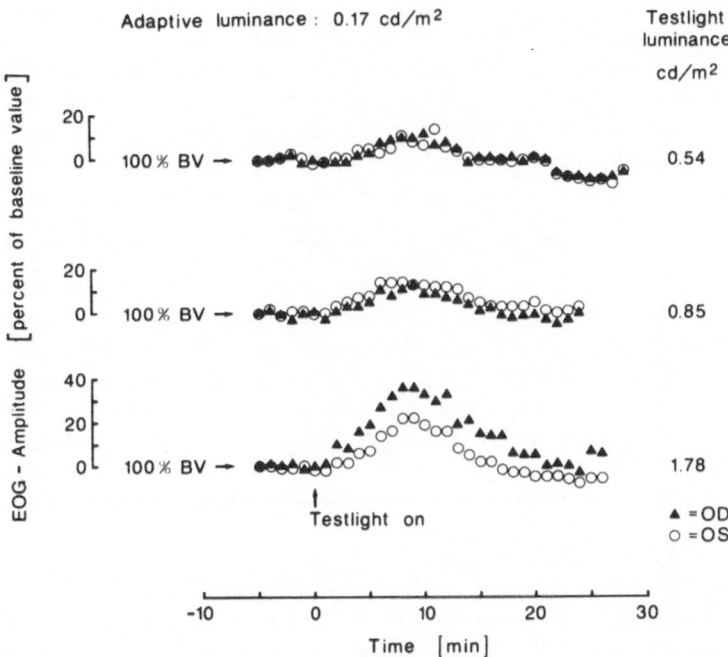

Fig. 2. Subject H.K. Plots of the light-induced slow oscillation of the standing potential in response to Ganzfeld-stimuli of different luminance during the exposure to a constant adaptation light (0.17 cd/m²). Change of potential of the right (OD) and left (OS) eye indicated by different symbols. Prior to the test light the subject was exposed to the adapting light for at least one hour. Measurements began when the standing potential had become constant. Baseline value 100 per cent determined by the last five measurements at the end of the adaptation period.

slow oscillation of the standing potential was calculated by an analog computer at one minute intervals and plotted on an Y-T recorder (Rhode et al., 1976). The amplitudes of the last five measurements before light stimulation were averaged and determined as the baseline value of 100 per cent. For test lights of various luminance the amplitude of the first positive peak of the slow oscillation was expressed in per cent of the baseline value (Figure 2). In consecutive sessions the experiment was repeated at different levels of adaptive illumination.

RESULTS

From the measurement illustrated in Figure 2 plots of the light rise of the standing potential (averaged for both eyes) vs. log test light luminance were drawn. Figure 3 shows such plots including the regresssion lines of three subjects at different levels of adaptive illumination.

In order to obtain the increment threshold of the standing potential a criterion amplitude of 30 per cent light rise (Figure 3, dashed lines) was

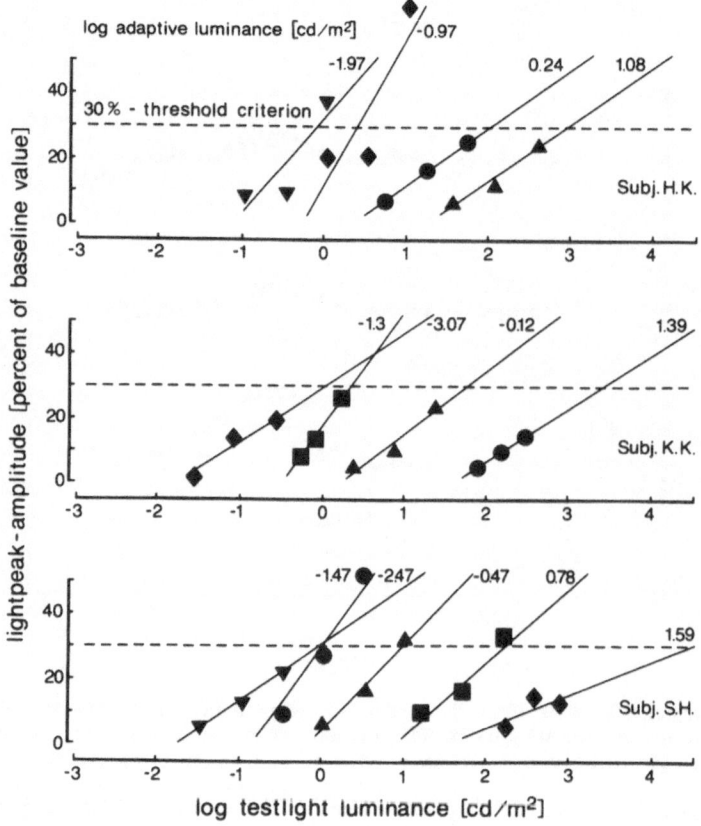

Fig. 3. Plots of the amplitude of the light rise vs. log test light luminance at different levels of adaptive illumination (indicated besides the regression lines in log cd/m^2). Averaged results of the right and the left eye of three subjects (H.K., K.K. and S.H.). The amplitudes of the light peaks are given in per cent of the baseline value. Amplitude criterion (30 per cent) indicated by the dotted line.

chosen and the corresponding test light luminance was plotted against adaptive illumination. The results of all subjects investigated, plotted on a log/log scale, are depicted in Figure 4. The data can be described by two e-functions, indicated in Figure 4 by solid line, in a way that the standard deviation of the individual data attains a minimal value. No better fitting was obtained by using a single e-function or by computing a family regression program.

DISCUSSION

The increment threshold function of the light-induced slow oscillation of the standing potential as measured by the electrooculogram indicates the presence of two systems of different light sensitivity, operating at different levels of

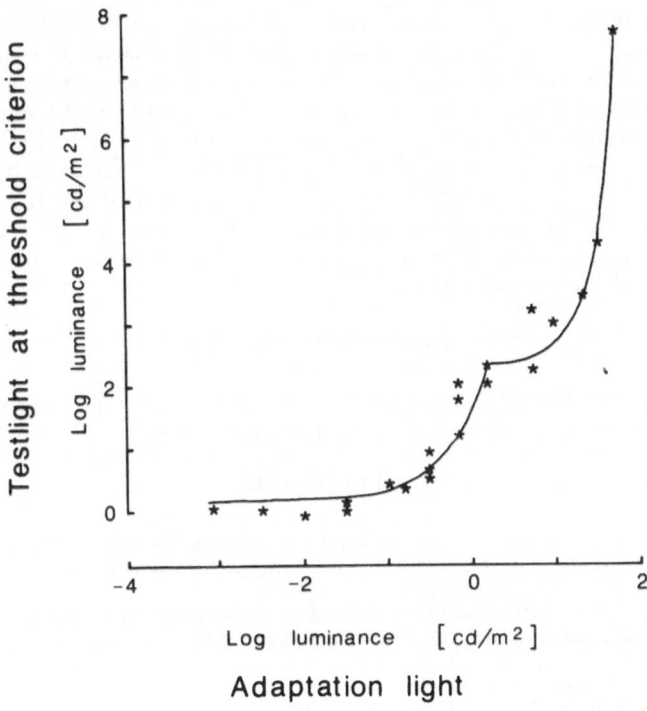

Fig. 4. Increment threshold function of the light-induced slow oscillation of the standing potential using Ganzfeld illumination.
Ordinate: Log test light luminance required for a light peak amplitude of 30 per cent above the baseline value.
Abscissa: Log adaptive luminance. Averaged values of the right and the left eye. Six subjects.
The solid line represents two calculated e-functions of least square deviations of the individual data. The two functions point to two generators of different relative sensitivity under scotopic and photopic conditions.

adaptive illumination. The adaptive luminance where the two systems cross over is at $1.0 \, cd/m^2$ which closely corresponds to Stiles' (1959) psychophysical measurements of increment threshold of the parafoveal human retina determined with small test fields. This implies that the slow light-induced oscillation of the standing potential in man exhibits different sensitivities under scotopic and photopic conditions.

The amplitude criterion of 30 per cent light rise was selected since with a lower (15%) or higher (50%) criterion the separation of the two e-functions was less evident in the graphical display. Further, the 15 per cent amplitude criterion lies close to the lowermost amplitude of the light rise of 8 per cent that could be resolved from background noise by the recording procedure presently used, whereas the luminance for the 50 per cent amplitude criterion is far from the electrooculogram threshold of the dark adapted eye.

The lines of regression of the amplitude vs. test light luminance function

79

under photopic conditions exhibited a smaller increment than those recorded at low luminance levels of adaptation. This can best be explained by the low number of retinal elements responding at high luminance levels of adaptation. Unfortunately the test light available under photopic conditions did not permit measurements at higher criterion values. However, the separation of the two branches of the increment threshold function at 1 cd/m² adaptive luminance for all criteria between 15 and 50 per cent led us to believe that the data presented indicate the relative contribution of the rod and cone system to the light rise of the standing potential. The results are in agreement with previous studies showing a reasonable contribution of the photopic system to the electrooculogram.

ACKNOWLEDGEMENT

We are greateful to Dr. Zrenner for stimulating the study and to Prof. E. Dodt for supporting and monitoring the project in all phases.

REFERENCES

Arden, G. B., Kelsey, J. H.: Some observations on the relationship between the standing potential of the human eye and the bleaching and regeneration of visual purple. J. Physiol. 161: 205–226 (1962).

Aschoff, U.: Skotopische und photopische Anteile der Hell- und Dunkelschwingung im Elektrookulogramm. Dev. Ophthal. 4: 149–166 (1981).

Dodt, E., Echte, K., Jessen, K. H.: Elektroretinographische Messung der Unterschieds-schwelle (increment threshold) bei Steigerung der adaptiven Beleuchtung. Ber. Dtsch. Ophthalmol. Ges. 63, 319–322 (1960).

Elenius, V., Karo, T.: Cone activity in the light-induced response of the human electro-oculogram. Pflügers Arch. 291: 241–248 (1966).

Hache, J. C., Francois, P., Geominne, P.: Macular electrooculography. Docum. Ophthal. Proc. Ser. 10: 37–47 (1976).

Hochgesand, P., Schicketanz, K. H.: Das Elektro-Okulogramm der zentralen Retina. Ber. Dtsch. Ophthal. Ges. 73: 115–126 (1975).

Kolder, H.: Spontane und experimentelle Änderungen des Bestandpotentials des mensch-lichen Auges. Pflügers Arch. 268: 258–272 (1959).

Krüger, C. J.: Der Anteil zentraler und peripherer Netzhautbezirke an der langsamen Hellschwingung im Electrookulogramm (EOG). Ber. Dtsch. Ophthalmol. Ges. 78: 741–749 (1981).

McCord, C. D.: The corneo fundal potential, the effect of monochromatic light. Thesis. Emory University, Atlanta, Ga. 1963.

Rhode, N., Täumer, R., Braas, F.: An EOG computer and stimulator for the investi-gation of the slow retinal potential. In: Täumer, R. (ed.). Electro-oculography – its clinical importance. Bibl. Ophthal. 85: 75–83 (1976).

Stiles, W. S.: Colour vision: the approach theory increment threshold sensitivity. Proc. Nat. Acad. Sci. USA 45: 100–114 (1959).

Täumer, R., Rohde, N., Pernice, D.: The slow oscillation of the retinal potential, a bio-chemical feedback stimulated by the activity of rods and cones. In: Täumer, R. (ed.). Electro-oculography – its clinical importance. Bibl. Ophthal. 85: 40–56 (1976).

van Norren, D., Valeton, J. M.: Relation between the EOG, corneal-, and in the retinal slow potentials. Docum. Ophthal. Proc. Ser. 31: 104 (1982).

Mailing address:
Mellendorferstr. 3
3000 Hannover 61
West Germany

CORNEORETINAL POTENTIALS IN HUMAN INFANTS

R. M. HANSEN AND A. B. FULTON

(Boston, Massachusetts, U.S.A.)

ABSTRACT

Vestibularly induced horizontal eye movements were recorded to investigate the corneoretial potential of 23 infants ages 4 to 48 weeks. Infants were tested for 15 minutes in the dark, and 15 minutes in room light (85 ft. Lamberts). Under these conditions, the EOG did not change systematically with age. Also, the amplitude of this potential at the dark trough (mean = $230\,\mu$V; SD = $77\,\mu$V), amplitude at the light peak (mean = $492\,\mu$V; SD = $165\,\mu$V), time to dark trough (mean = 7.7 minutes; SD = 1.0 minute) and time to light peak (mean = 7.6 minutes; SD = 1.1 minute) were not significantly different from those obtained with adults. Thus, the present results suggest that retinal structures and processes responsible for the corneoretinal potential mature early.

INTRODUCTION

In the postnatal period, there are significant developmental changes in the human visual system that may affect the corneoretinal potential by changing the eye's electrical properties. For example, the diameter of the globe (Larsen, 1971) and retinal surface area (Robb, 1982a) increase 25 to 30 percent during infancy; this change in eye size should increase the eye's electric dipole moment, and thereby, change the standing potential. In addition, the total number of pigment epithelial and neural retinal cells remains relatively constant during this period of rapid growth (Mund, Rodrigues and Fine, 1972; Robb, 1982b) leading to a change in the eye's charge distribution. This factor could also affect the corneoretinal potential. Finally, distal retinal function matures postnatally. The sensitivity, latency and amplitude of retinal responses to diffuse, flashed stimuli (assessed by the ERG b-wave) undergo developmental changes (Fulton and Hansen, 1982). Since the corneoretinal potential is thought to depend upon the function of the retinal epithelium and cells of the neural retina (Berson, 1981), changes in distal retinal function may also affect the corneoretinal potential. The interaction of these factors in determining the corneoretinal potential is not understood. Previous investigators (Henkes and Legein, 1969; Trimble, Ernest and Newell, 1977) have tested infants and children, but did not consider very young babies during the period of rapid developmental change. The present study concentrates on this group to determine whether there are developmental changes in the corneoretinal potential.

METHODS

The electrooculograph (EOG) was recorded using skin electrodes placed near the right and left outer canthi, and a ground electrode placed over the mastoid. Potentials were amplified (A-C coupled, gain = 1000, 0.5 to 1000 Hz bandwidth) and displayed on an oscilloscope and chart recorder. Eye movements were elicited using the method of Trimble *et al.*, (1977). Briefly, the mother sat in a rocking chair with the infant lying across her lap, while the chair was rocked gently back and forth. Stops beneath the chair's rockers restricted chair rotation to about 45°. Illuminated toys were used to attract the baby's attention. Vestibularly induced compensatory eye movements drove the eye horizontally through 30° to 50° of visual angle. An adult watched the infant throughout testing to ensure that the baby remained alert and continued attending to the fixation target. Testing stopped when the baby became fussy or fell asleep.

Following pre-adaptation in a bright, uniformly illuminated room (85 ft. Lamberts producing a retinal illumination of about + 3.0 log photopic trolands) for 15 minutes, the EOG was recorded for at least 15 minutes in the dark, and then for an additional 15 minutes with the room lights on (85 ft. Lamberts).

Thirty-one infants ages 4 to 48 weeks were tested; twenty-three infants successfully completed the test (median age = 12 weeks). The eight infants who did not complete the test were either sleepy or fussy; their data were not included in the analysis. All infants had been born within seven days of term. Thorough ophthalmic examination revealed no ocular abnormalities. Cycloplegic retinoscopy revealed no significant refractive errors. The mean right eye spherical equivalent for 23 subjects was + 1.89 diopters (SD = 1.20 diopters; Range: 0 to + 5.0 diopters). Five adults were also tested using the same apparatus and procedure to provide normative data.

RESULTS

Sample horizontal eye movement records from a 12 week old infant, and an adult control subject are presented in Figure 1. Qualitatively, the eye movement records from infants and adults appeared similar consisting of smooth compensatory movements and occasional saccades. Records such as these were measured to determined the average peak-to-peak amplitude of the EOG during each minute of testing. This approach was chosen to reduce variability in estimating the amplitude of the EOG with records contaminated by inappropriate eye movements or poor attention to the fixation target.

82

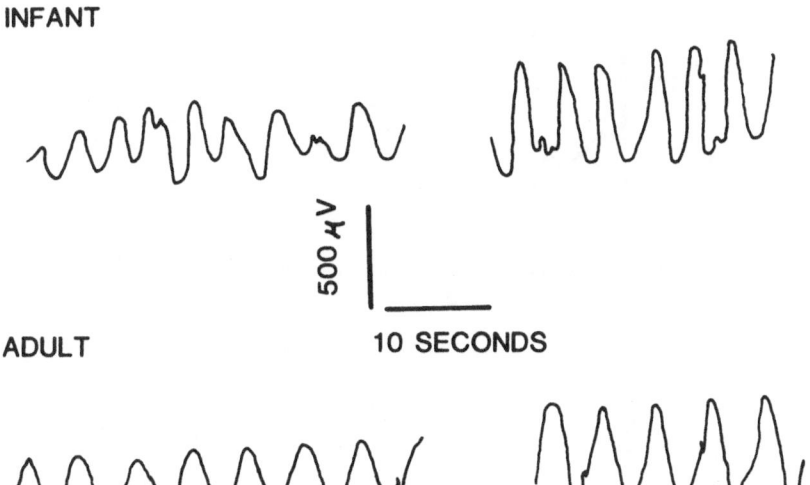

Fig. 1. Sample eye movement records from a 12 week old infant and an adult subject. The potential difference produced by horizontal eye movements is plotted as a function of time. These samples were selected from times near the dark trough and light peak. The horizontal bar represents 10 seconds, and the vertical bar represents 500 μVolts.

For each subject, the amplitude of the EOG was plotted as a function of time to determine the minimum value of the potential in the dark (*dark trough*), the maximum value of the potential in the light (light peak), and the times when these events occurred. Figure 2 presents a sample graph of this potential as a function of time for a 12 week old infant, and an adult control. Figure 2 shows that, under these testing conditions, light induced changes in the EOG are comparable in infants and adults.

Figure 3 summarizes individual results obtained from 23 infants and 5 adult subjects. In this figure, the amplitude of the EOG at the dark trough and light peak, and the times of the dark trough and light peak are plotted as a function of age. There were no clear age related changes in any of these measures. In fact, analysis of variance indicated that no systematic age related changes in the amplitude of the EOG at the dark trough ($F = 1.17$, $df = 5,22$; n.s.), amplitude at the light peak ($F = 0.76$, $df = 5,22$; n.s.), the time of the dark trough ($F = 1.20$, $df = 5,22$; n.s.), or the time of the light peak ($F = 1.22$, $df = 5,22$; n.s.) occurred. Table 1 summarizes all of these results, including the Arden ratio.

DISCUSSION

The present results showed that the EOG did not change systematically with age; results from 4 to 16 week old infants were not reliably different from

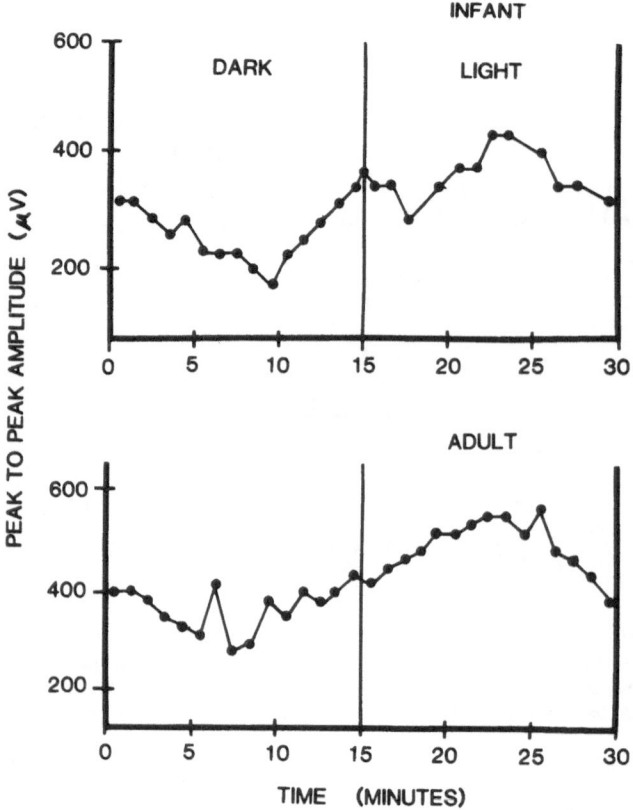

Fig. 2. Peak-to-peak EOG amplitude as a function of time for a 12 week old infant and an adult subject. The amplitudes represent the average value of the EOG during each minute of testing. *Dark* refers to testing with the room lights out; *Light* refers to testing with normal room illumination (85 ft. Lamberts).

those obtained with adults. This finding suggested that the corneoretinal potential does not change significantly during a period of rapid growth of the eye (Larsen, 1971) and maturation of distal retinal function (Fulton and Hansen, 1982).

Our results are consistent with those of other investigators who have used the EOG to study the corneoretinal potential. For example, the Arden ratios derived from the infants' data (mean = 2.17; SD = 0.19; Range: 1.68 to 2.53) agree with those reported by Adams (1973) for older (10 to 69 years) subjects. EOG amplitudes from our subjects are consistent with those reported by Trimble *et al.*, (1977) for 5 to 21 month old subjects. They are, however, somewhat lower than reported previously for adults (for example, see Krogh, 1976). Electrode placement may explain this difference with earlier reports; Shackel (1960) reported comparable initial EOG amplitudes for 30° eye movements using a similar electrode placement.

The retinal pigment epithelium and cells of the neural retina are thought

84

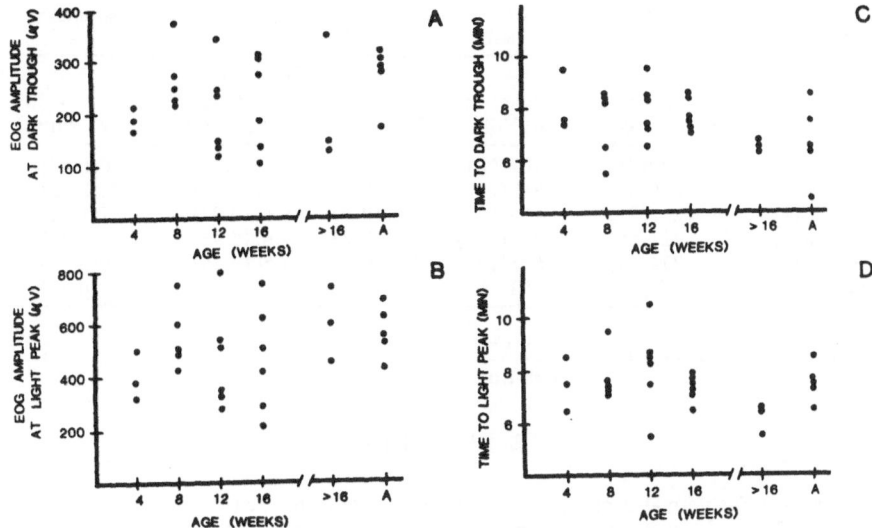

Fig. 3. Summary of results from infants and adults. *A*. The amplitude of the EOG at its minimum value in the dark (*dark trough*) is plotted as a function of age in weeks. Each point represents results from one subject. Adult results are shown at one age point, labelled *A*. *B*. The amplitude of the EOG at its maximum value in the light (*light peak*) as a function of age. *C*. Time from the start of testing to the minimum amplitude in the dark as a function of age. *D*. Time from turning room lights on to the maximum amplitude as a function of age. All other features of *B*, *C*, and *D* are similar to those in part *A*.

to be the generators of the eye's standing potential, and to be involved in producing the light induced rise in the EOG (Gouras and Carr, 1965; Marmor and Lurie, 1979; Noell, 1954). One implication of the present results is that these generators are operative and possibly mature soon after birth. Since the total number of cells of the retinal epithelium and neural retina appears to remain constant during this period (Robb, 1982b), our results suggest that these cells must adjust their electrical activity to maintain a constant standing potential.

In summary, our results revealed no significant age related changes in the EOG suggesting that the corneoretinal potential is adult-like soon after birth. These results can be used as norms for the testing of young patients with retinal diseases.

ACKNOWLEDGEMENT

We thank Susan Harris and Deborah Clark for their assistance. This research was supported by Research Grant EYHD 3211 from the National Institutes of Health.

Table 1. Summary of EOG results from infant and adult subjects. For each parameter, the mean and standard deviation (in parentheses) are given.

Age	N	Amplitudes dark trough (μ Volts)	light peak (μ Volts)	Arden Ratio[*]	Latencies time to dark trough (min)	time to light peak (min)
4 weeks	3	188(21)	402(48)	2.10(0.18)	8.17(1.00)	7.50(0.87)
8 weeks	5	270(57)	543(122)	2.01(0.13)	6.82(2.51)	7.90(0.82)
12 weeks	6	202(81)	466(179)	2.25(0.17)	8.00(0.97)	8.17(1.51)
16 weeks	6	221(85)	468(189)	2.11(0.23)	7.83(0.48)	7.33(0.38)
> 16 weeks	3	274(57)	595(121)	2.13(0.13)	6.50(0.24)	6.50(0.87)
Adults	5	272(55)	561(89)	2.12(0.25)	6.75(1.36)	7.50(0.65)

[*]The Arden Ratio is defined as $\dfrac{\text{Light peak}}{\text{Dark trough}}$

REFERENCES

Adams, A.: The normal electro-oculogram (EOG). Acta Ophth., 51, 551–561, 1973.

Berson, E. L.: Electrical phenomena in the retina. In Adler's physiology of the eye. Seventh edition. R. A. Moses, editor. St. Louis, 1981, The C. V. Mosby Company, Chapter 17.

Fulton, A. B. and Hansen, R. M.: Background adaptation in human infants: Analysis of b-wave response. Docum. Ophthal. Proc. Series, 31, 191–197, 1982.

Gouras, P. and Carr, R. E.: Light induced DC responses of monkey retina before and after central retinal artery interruption. Invest. Ophthalmol. Vis. Sci., 4: 310–317, 1965.

Henkes, H. E. and Legein, C. P.: Electrodiagnostic procedures in the blind and partially sighted young child. Int. Ophthalmol. Clin., 9: 921–934, 1969.

Krogh, E.: Normal values in clinical electrooculography. II. Analysis of potential and time parameters and their relation to other variables. Acta Ophtha., 54: 389–398, 1976.

Larsen, J.: The sagittal growth of the eye. Ultrasonic measurements of the axial length of the eye from birth to puberty. Acta Ophthal., 49: 873–886, 1971.

thelium. In: The retinal pigment epithelium, K. M. Zinn and M. F. Marmor, editors. Cambridge, MA, 1979, Harvard University Press, Chapter 13.

Mund, M. L., Rodrigues, M. M. and Fine, B. S.: Light and electron microscopic observations on the pigmented layers of the developing human eye. Am. J. Ophthalmol., 73: 167–182, 1972.

Noell, W. K.: The origin of the electroretinogram. Am. J. Ophthalmol., 38: 78–90, 1954.

Robb, R. M.: Increase in retinal surface area during infancy and childhood. J. Pediatr. Ophthalmol. Strabis., 19: 16–20, 1982a.

Robb, R. M.: Personal communication, 1982b.

Shackel, B.: Pilot study in electro-oculography. Brit. J. Ophthalmol., 44: 89–113, 1960.

Trimble, J. L., Ernest, J. T. and Newell, F. B.: Electrooculography in infants. Invest. Ophthalmol. Vis. Sci., 16: 668–670, 1977.

Mailing address:
Department of Ophthalmology
Children's Hospital Medical Center & Harvard Medical School
300 Longwood Avenue
Boston, Massachusetts, 02115, U.S.A.

EOG DRIVEN BY THE CONTRALATERAL READING EYE

L. RONCHI AND A. SERRA

(Florence, Italy and Cagliari, Italy)

ABSTRACT

The present report deals with the comparison of monocular EOG responses recorded while reading printed material. The amplitudes of monocular tracings are measured at 40 ms intervals. We neglect the return sweep at the end of every line, so that our digitization is confined to the complex of jumps and fixation pauses across the line. Next, we estimate the correlation coefficient (r) between the two sets of 30 data points. Two experimental conditions are considered: a) both eyes are reading simultaneously; b) one eye is reading, the contralateral one is screened out. The EOG recorded from the latter represents a driven movement. In normals, r is higher in case a) than in b), and differs according to whether the right or the left eye is screened out. The correlation with ocular dominance is sought for. Also people with binocular imbalances, and diabetic people are examined.

INTRODUCTION

The present report is part of a research program which is being developed in two different Labs (at Florence and at Caglairi). Briefly, we are recording simultaneously EOG responses from either eye (in the horizontal plane), while reading printed material, and we compare the monocular tracings. The literature is rich of reports on factors influencing eye movements, partly observer-related, partly stimulus-related (Rayner et al., 1976).

A fundamental property of *large* eye movements is their binocular coordination, and normal eyes 'nearly' always move synchronously together (Alpern, 1972). the problem is more complicated for eye micromovements, where some controversies are still open (Krauskopf, 1960).

The pattern of eye movements while reading has been widely investigated, but, as far as we know, the inter-ocular feedback timing operations of the two eyes deserves further attention (Smith et al., 1971; Gruber, 1962).

In a previous experiment (Ronchi et al., 1982), we noted that binocular coordination is 'good' (according to our criterion, the evaluation of the correlation coefficient, for a set of pairs of monocular amplitudes of tracing,

Doc. Ophthal. Proc. Series, Vol 37, ed. by H.E.J.W. Kolder
© 1983 Dr W. Junk Publishers, The Hague/Boston:Lancaster

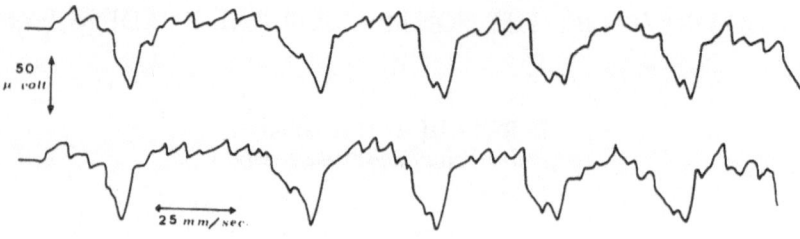

Fig. 1. An example of tracings, when reading binocularly.

digitized at the same time), when target contrast does not drop below a given value (three times above threshold), and when transient adaptational effects are avoided.

In the present experiment we wonder to what extent one eye (not reading, being screened out), is 'driven' by the contralateral reading one. It seems to us that approach is a promising source of information, in addition to the observation of eye movement and static eye position in various situations, the classical basis for the diagnosis and treatment of some ocular anomalies (Ciuffreda et al., 1976; Smith et al., 1970; Adler Grindberg et al., 1978).

MATERIALS AND METHOD

The observer was seated in a screened booth. His eyes were well adapted to the average luminance of the target (which produced 0.33 lux at the eye).

The target to be read (silently) consisted of a printed, well contrasted, typewritten material, placed vertically, at a viewing distance of 60 cm, being 7 cm wide, 10 cm long, letter size being 2 x 3 mm. The content of the text changed from trial to trial. No perceptual difficulties were met, since the material was taken from a book on great explorers.

To record eye movements we made use of the EOG technique. Silver chloride skin electrodes were placed close to the canthi of each eye, the reference electrode being pasted on the forehead. The signal from the electrodes was amplified by AC techniques with 0.1 sec time constant.

We did not adopt the classical technique of data analysis, consisting in counting the shifts of fixation, the fixations pauses, the regressions, etc. We digitized the amplitude of the tracing (Figure 1) after having traced an arbitrary baseline, at 40 ms intervals, by neglecting the return sweep at the end of each line. Thus, for each read line (or a portion of it), we gathered two sets of 30 data, one for the right eye, the other for the left eye. Next we calculated the correlation coefficient r, being:

$$r = \frac{n\,Sxy - Sx \cdot Sy}{\sqrt{[n\,Sx^2 - (Sx)^2]\,[n\,Sy^2 - (Sy)^2]}}$$

for n = 30, by considering pairs of 'monocular' readings, x, and y respectively, at 30 different points in time.

In this way we compare the overall shapes of monocular tracings.

In some trials both eyes are reading, and we wonder whether r is high enough to consider as 'good' the binocular coordination. In other trials one eye is reading while the other is screened out (but left free to move). We assume that when r is high, the occluded eye, driven by the reading one, follows it quite synchronously. This is no longer the case when r is low.

Subjects

We tested 13 subjects, described in Table 1.

Table 1

Subject	age	binoc. vision	(after correction) Visual acuity R.E	LE	Notes
ME	26	normal	10/10	10/10	
DC	56	normal	10/10	10/10	
SC	28	exophoric	10/10	10/10	well corrected myopia (9D for either eye)
LP	18	normal	10/10	10/10	
RM	40	normal	10/10	10/10	
PA	22	esophoric (5°)	10/10	10/10	
RV	39	(L.E.)aphakic	10/10	8/10	left eye's refraction corrected after cataract surgery
PV	37	normal	10/10	10/10	diabetic (without ocular involvement
OR	22	(L.E.)exotropic	10/10	4/50	amblyopia ex anisometropia
FO	30	anisometropia	10/10	10/10	
TO	29	(L.E.)esotropic	10/10	2/10	squint
MA	17	alternating esotropia	5/10	10/10	L.E. dominant
MC	36	hyperphoria	10/10	10/10	

Experimental Findings

An overview of our data is shown in Figure 2. On the axis of the ordinates, the correlation coefficient r is displayed. The significance level is $r = 0.35$, for $df = 30,2$, at $P < 0.05$. We assume that when r exceeds 0.35, the two eyes move in a fairly synchronous manner, while reading. When r is less than 0.35 the two monocular patterns differ in shape (let us recall that we neglect the return sweep at the end of each line by considering only the set of jumps and fixation pauses across the line).

Subjects are subdivided into four groups, a) through d).

To group a) belong subjects who exhibit r values above the significance level both when both eyes are reading or when one eye reads and other is 'driven', being screened out.

To group b) belong two subjects for which r is above the significance level both when both eyes are reading and when one of the eyes is screened out (but not when, instead, the other eye is screened out).

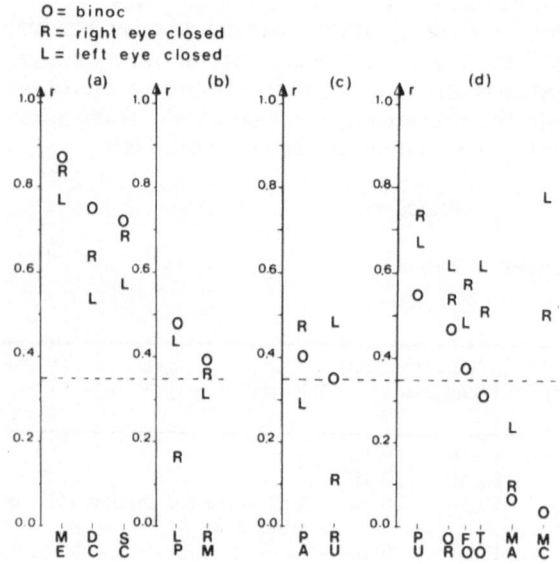

O = binoc
R = right eye closed
L = left eye closed

Fig. 2. Ordinates: correlation coefficient r.
Abscissae: label denoting the subject.
Each data point represents the average of ten r values, obtained by reading ten different lines.
Open circles: both eyes are simultaneously reading.
R, right eye is occluded; L, left eye is occluded.

To group c) belong people for whom the r value for binocular vision lies between those for monocular reading, respectively.

The most interesting subjects seem to be those belonging to group d). For them, the r value for binocular vision is lower than those for monocular reading. It is as if the two eyes were mutually disturbing one another, when working together.

Possibly, records of the kind described in the present experiment can provide a quantitative measurements of the transition from ocular dominance to sub-clinical binocular imbalance. However it is imperative to ascertain to what extent a small r value represents an impairment rather than a different way of acquiring information through differential monocular inputs.

REFERENCES

Adler Grinberg, D. and Stark, L.: Eye movements and dislexia. Amer. J. Optom., 55, 557–570, 1978.
Alpern, M.: Eye movements. In- Handbook of Sensory Physiology, Vol. VII/4, Visual Psychophysics, Jameson, D. and Hurvich Eds. Springer Verlag, Berlin, pp. 303–330, Ch. 12, 1972.
Ciuffreda, K. J., Terry Bahill, A., Kenyon, R. V. and Stark, L.: Eye movements during reading: case reports. Amer. J. Optom., 53, 385–389, 1976.

90

Gruber, E.: Reading ability, binocular coordination and the ophthalmograph. Amer. J. Ophthal., 67, 34–42, 1962.

Krauskopf, J., Cornsweet, T. N. and Riggs, L. A.: Analysis of eye movements during monocular and binocular fixation. J. Opt. Soc. Am., 50, 572–578, 1960.

Rayner, K., and McConkie, G. W.: What guides a reader's eye movements? Vision Res., 16, 829–837, 1976.

Ronchi, L., Stefanacci, S. and Macii, R.: Interocular comparison of EOG Tracings recorded while reading under various viewing conditions. Doc. Ophth. Proc. Ser., 31, 106–107, 1982.

Smith, K. U., Schmidt, J. and Putz, V.: Binocular coordination, feedback of synchronization of eye movements in space perception. Amer. J. Optom., 47, 679–689, 1970.

Smith, K. U., Schremser, R. and Putz, V.: Binocular coordination in reading. J. Appl. Psychol., 55, 251–255, 1971.

Mailing address:
National Institute of Optics
Arcetri
Florence, Italy

THE ELECTROOCULOGRAM IN 'VITELLIFORM' MACULAR LESIONS

R. SABATES, R. C. PRUETT AND T. HIROSE

(Kansas City, Missouri and Boston, Massachusetts, U.S.A.)

ABSTRACT

Fifty seven patients originally referred with the tentative diagnosis of Best's vitelliform dystrophy were examined. With the aid of electrooculography the cases could be clearly divided into three groups: Best's vitelliform dystrophy (BVD), (12 cases); Pseudovitelliform macular degeneration (PMD), (42 cases); and Pigment epithelium detachment (PED), (3 cases). All cases of BVD had abnormal EOG's with an average L_p to D_t ratio of 1.38. Cases with PMD had normal or only slightly abnormal EOG's with an average L_p to D_t ratio of 2.16. The three cases with PED had normal EOG's.

INTRODUCTION

The term 'vitelliform' (egg yolk-like) is used to describe the yellow macular lesions which are frequently seen in Best's disease. When a patient present with bilateral 'vitelliform' macular lesions the presumptive diagnosis of Best's vitelliform dystrophy (BVD) is considered. The light peak to dark trough ratio of the electrooculogram has been found to be abnormally depressed in BVD (Krill, Morse, Potts and Klien, 1966; François, DeRouck and Fernandez-Sasso, 1966). A number of other disorders may present with morphologically similar 'vitelliform' macular lesions. In this study we evaluate the role of electrooculography in the differential diagnosis of 'vitelliform' macular lesions.

MATERIALS AND METHODS

Fifty seven patients originally referred with the tentative diagnosis of Best's vitelliform dystrophy were examined. All patients had complete ocular examinations which included fundus photography and in most cases fluorescein angiography. In one hundred and one eyes of 51 patients the electrooculogram (EOG) was recorded by the method of Arden and others (Arden, Barrada and Kelsey, 1962). Detailed description of our recording method is described elsewhere (Hirose, Wolf and Hara, 1976). A family history was obtained in all cases and family members examined when possible. The cases have been followed for periods ranging from one to eleven years.

RESULTS

The cases in this study could be clearly classified into three groups: Best's vitelliform dystrophy (12 cases), Pseudovitelliform macular degeneration (42 cases) and Pigment epithelium detachment (3 cases).

Best's Vitelliform Dystrophy (BVD)

The twelve patients in this group ranged in age from 6 to 32 years at the time of initial diagnosis. There were five (5) females and seven (7) males with a median age of 15 years. Ten eyes in seven patients presented with the classic 'egg-yolk' macular lesion (Figure 1a, b). The others presented in more advanced vitelliruptive stages (Figure 2a, b). The electrooculogram was abnormal in all cases. The average L_p and D_t ratio was 1.38 (Table 1). A documented family history with autosomal dominant transmission was present in all cases.

Pseudovitelliform Macular Degeneration (PMD)

There were 31 females and 11 males in this group ranging in age from 16 to 75 years. The median age for the females at initial diagnosis was 48 years, and 61 years for the males. The most common presenting complaint was a gradual blurring of vision in one or both eyes over a period of several months. The presenting visual acuity was typically good, in most cases ranging from 20/20 to 20/50. The macular lesions presented at the level of the retinal pigment epithelium (RPE) as a slightly raised yellow lesion approximately ¼ to ½ disc diameter in size. They were round or oval in shape and had sharply demarcated borders. At this stage of the disease the lesions always blocked fluorescence during angiography (Figure 3a–d). Two cases presented with unilateral lesions, but during the follow-up period both developed bilateral disease.

Progression occurred slowly over several years and was characterized by dispersion of the yellow material, which resulted in an angiographic RPE window defect. Eventually all the yellow material absorbed leaving a well circumscribed area of atrophy with an occasional pigment clump centrally (Figure 4a, b). The electrooculogram was recorded in 71 eyes and was normal or only slightly subnormal in all cases. (Average L_p to D_t ratio of 2.16) (Table 1). Long-term follow-up in ten cases (5 to 11 years) showed that useful vision (20/50 or better) is retained in at least one eye. (These patients also underwent other electrophysiologic and psychophysical studies which are described in detail elsewhere (Sabates, Pruett and Hirose, 1982)). Except for two siblings in the group, a positive family history could not be elicited in any of the cases. Multiple family members including all living relatives of two patients (16 members) were examined and macular lesions could not be found.

94

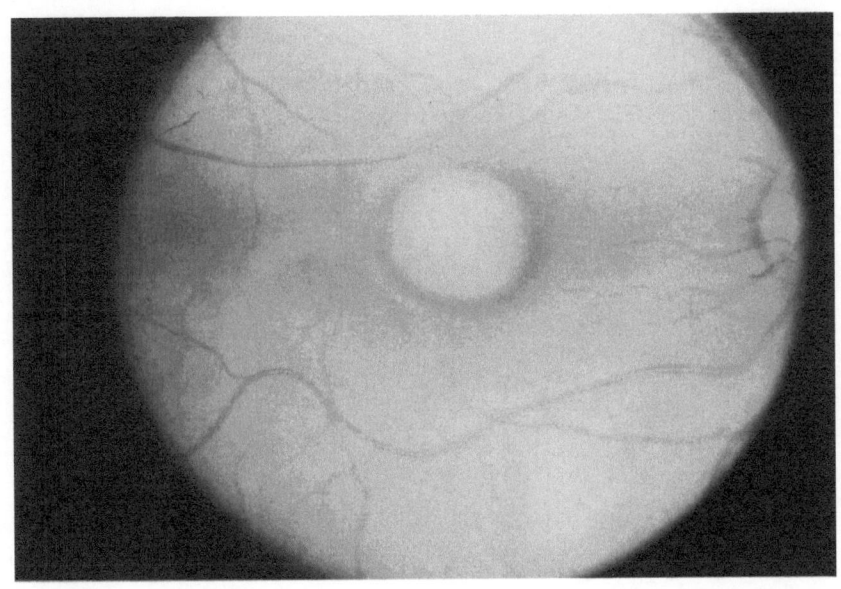

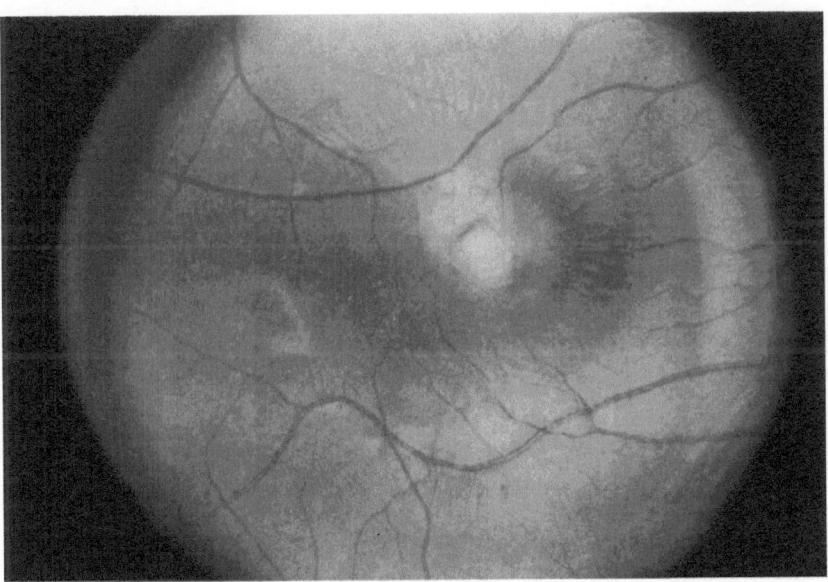

Fig. 1. (a) Fundus of a ten year old with BVD showing a classic 'vitelliform' lesion. The EOG was markedly abnormal. (b) The same fundus four years later shows the resorption of the yellow material and the development of a hypertropic scar.

95

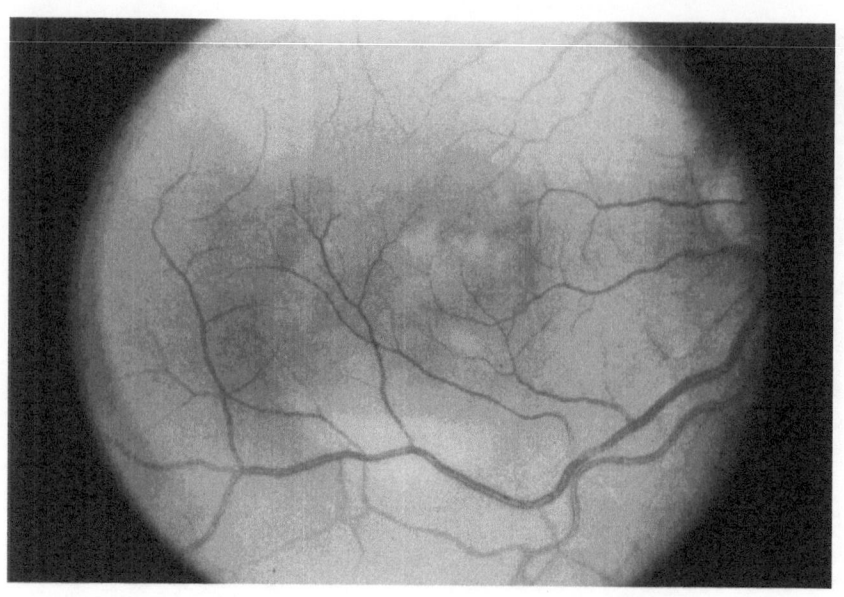

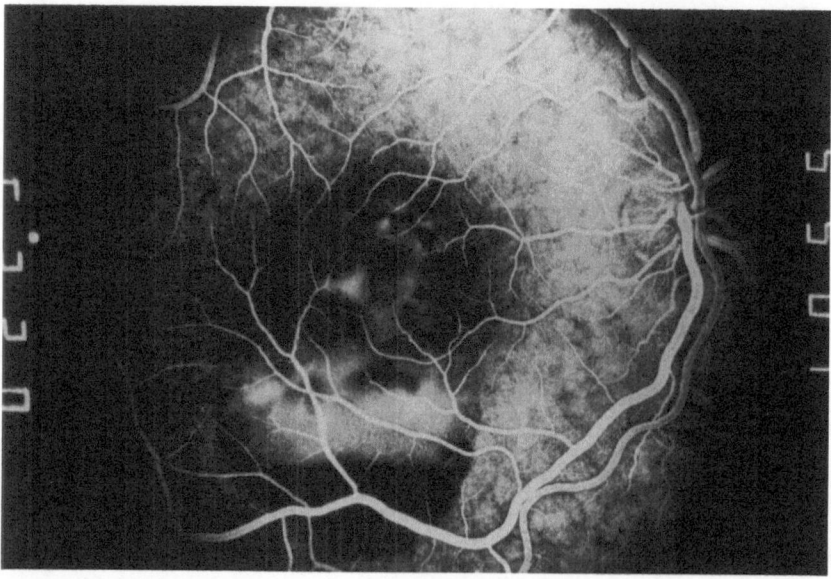

Fig. 2. (a) Fundus of a 20 year old male with BVD demonstrating a pseudohypopyon lesion. (b) Fluorescein angiography clearly shows a fluid level with blockage of fluoroescence by the turbid subretinal material.

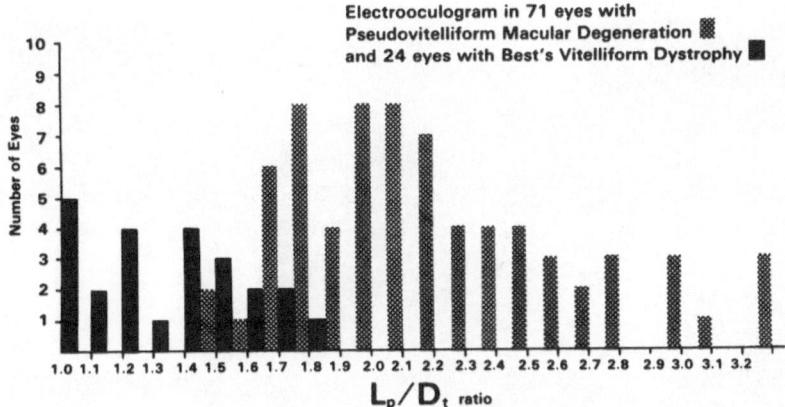

Table 1. Electrooculogram responses in 71 eyes with pseudovitelliform macular degeneration and 24 eyes with Best's vitelliform dystrophy.

Pigment Epithelium Detachment (PED)

The three patients in this group were 48, 55 and 60 years of age. Two were males and one female. All had normal electrooculograms. (Average L_p and D_t ratio of 2.4). All had bilateral dome shaped macular or paramacular lesions. Fluorescein angiography was most useful for the diagnosis (Figure 5a–d).

COMMENT

Best's vitelliform dystrophy (BVD) has been thoroughly studied and its natural history is well documented (Krill, Morse, Potts and Klien, 1965; François, DeRouck and Fernandez-Sasso, 1966; Deutman, 1969; Mohler and Fine, 1981). Pseudovitelliform macular degeneration (PMD) is a less well recognized entity which may bear a clear morphologic resemblance to BVD. It has been referred to as a peculiar foveomacular dystrophy (Gass, 1974), pseudovitelliform macular degeneration (Fishman, Trimble, Rabb and Fishman, 1977) vitelliform macular degeneration (Kingham and Lochen, 1977), adult vitelliform macular degeneration (Epstein and Rabb, 1980) and adult-onset foveomacular pigment epithelial dystrophy (Vine and Schatz, 1980).

Vitelliform macular degeneration is the most descriptive term because the early lesions are 'vitelliform' and the disease appears to be a degenerative process, but perhaps the term 'pseudovitelliform' would be more appropriate so as not to be mistaken for vitelliform dystrophy.

PMD is a distinct entity which can be clearly differentiated from BVD as well as other degenerative or dystrophic processes. There are five main differentiating features: age of onset, EOG responses, family history, evolution of the lesion and late stage complications.

97

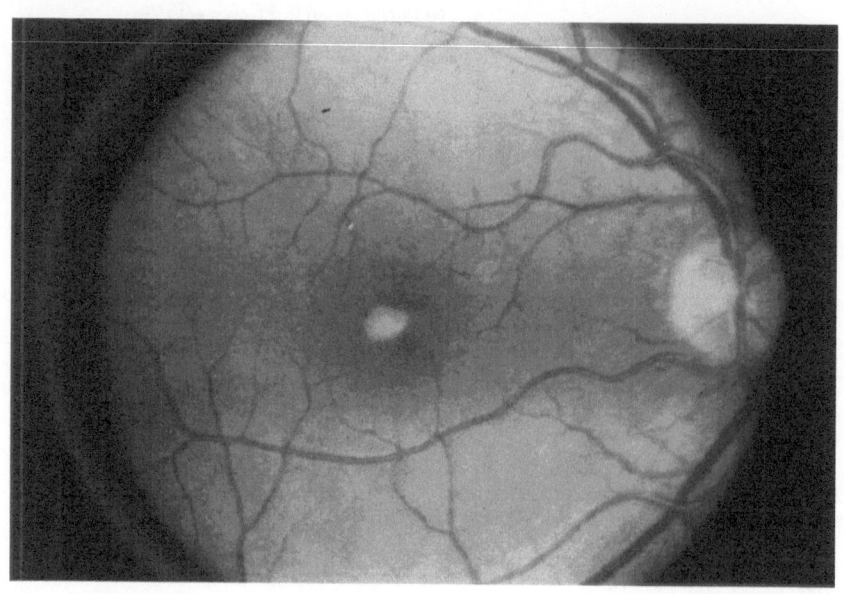

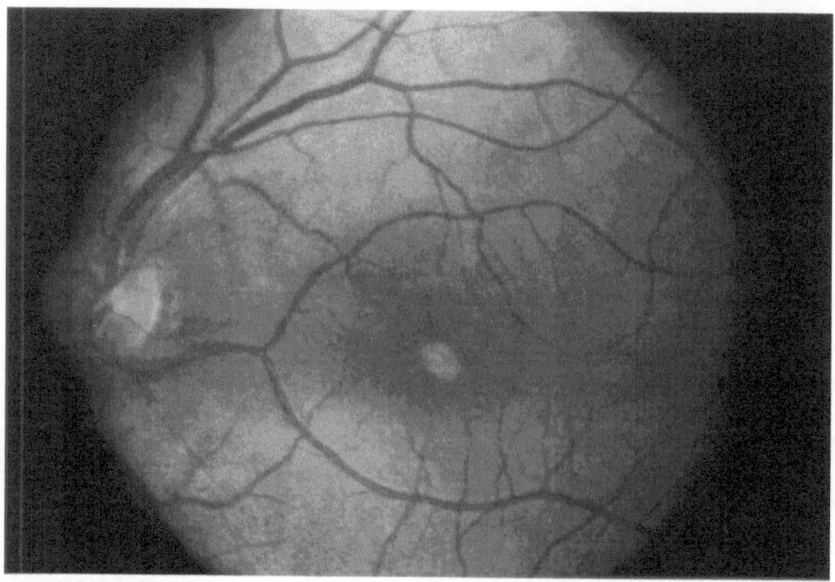

Fig. 3. (a, b) Fundus photographs of a 40 year old female with pseudovitelliform macular degeneration. The lesions are at the level of the RPE. The EOG was normal in both eyes.

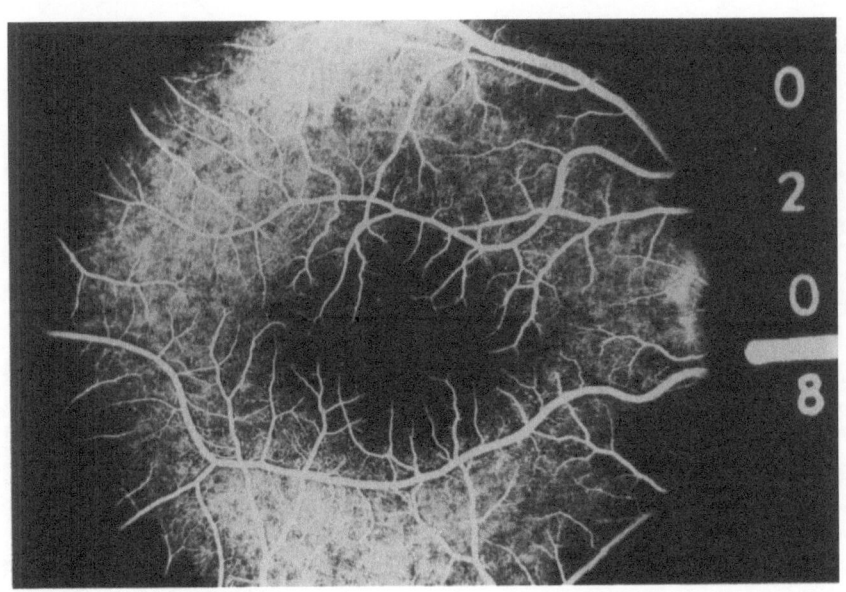

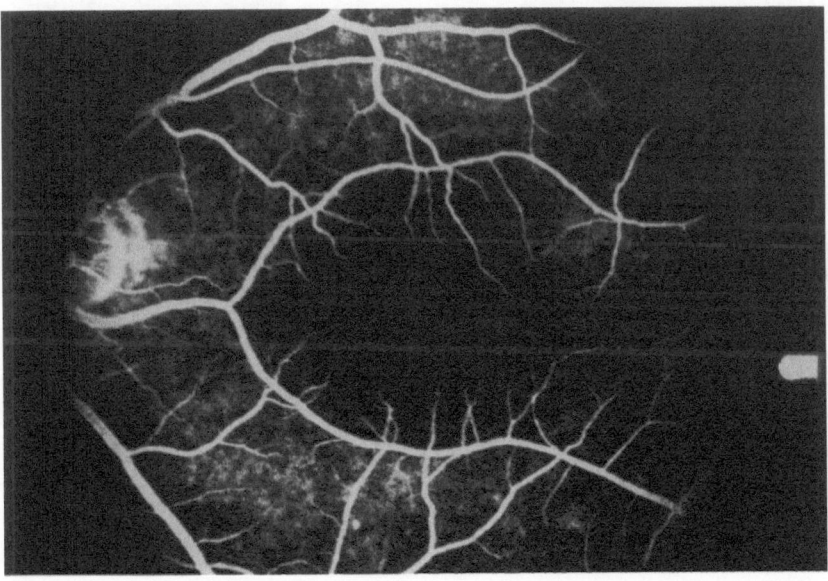

Fig. 3. (c, d) Fluorescein angiography shows blocked fluorescence by the yellow material.

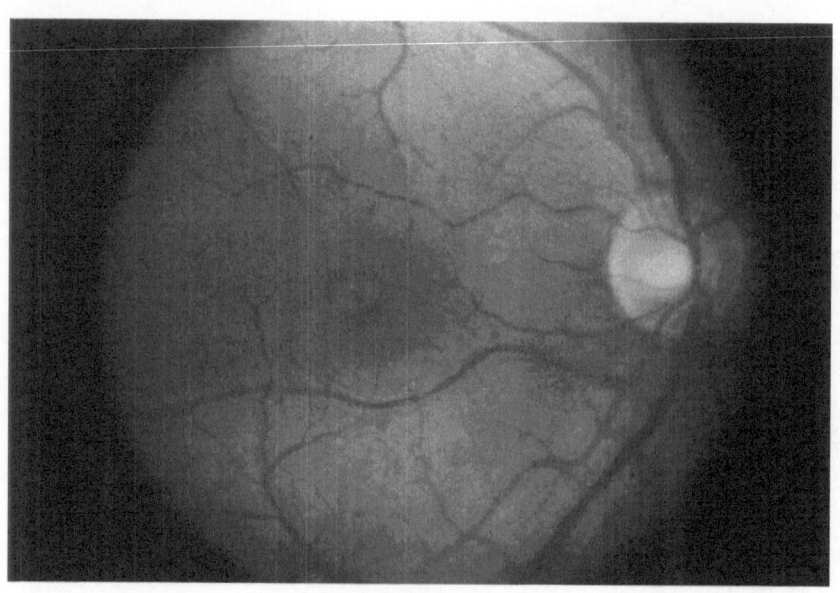

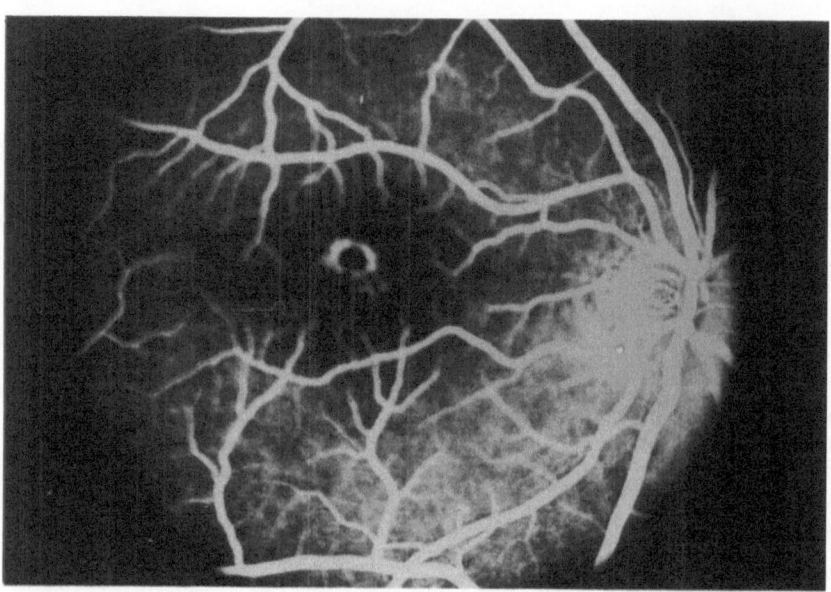

Fig. 4. (a) Endstage lesion of pseudovitelliform macular degeneration showing atrophy of the RPE with a central pigment clump. (b) Fluorescein angiography demonstrates a window defect with blockage of fluorescence by the pigment.

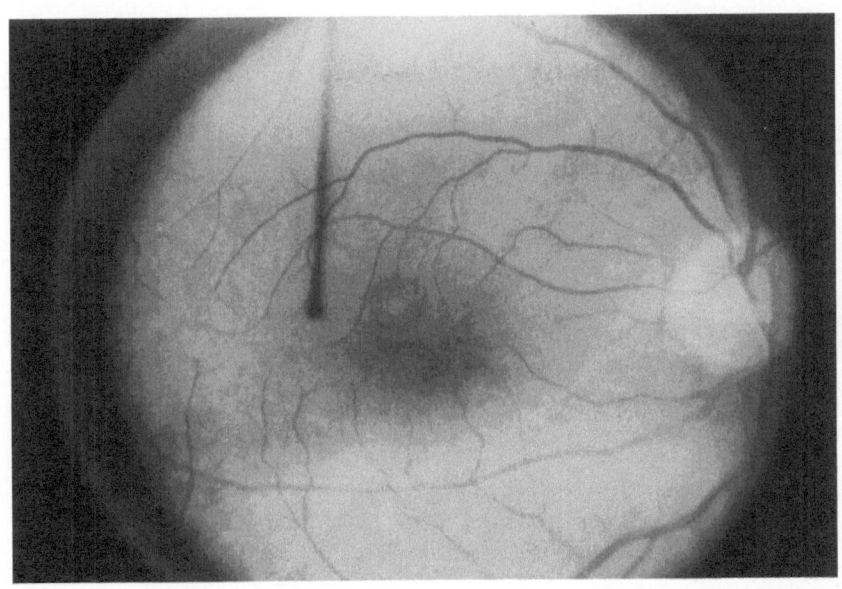

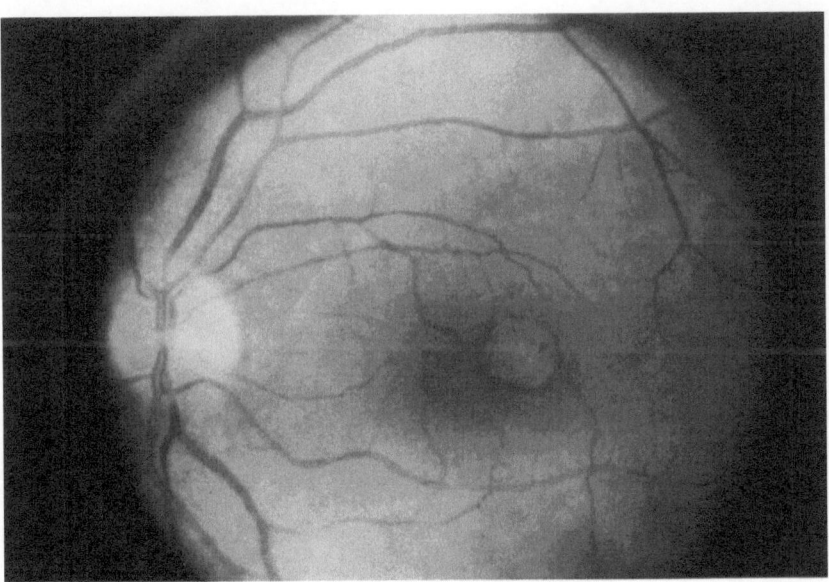

Fig. 5. (a) Right fundus of a 55 year old male with normal EOG showing two small dome shaped parmacular lesions. (b) The left fundus shows a central lesion.

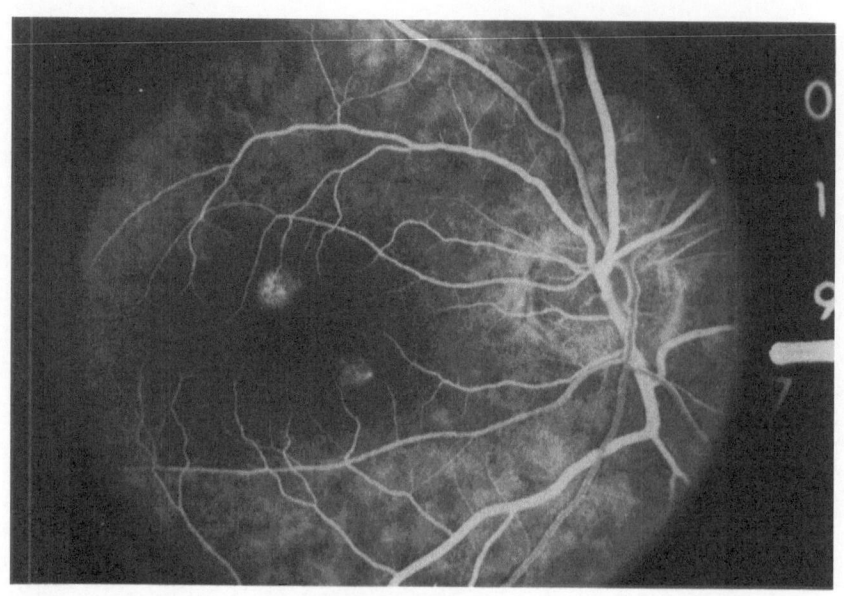

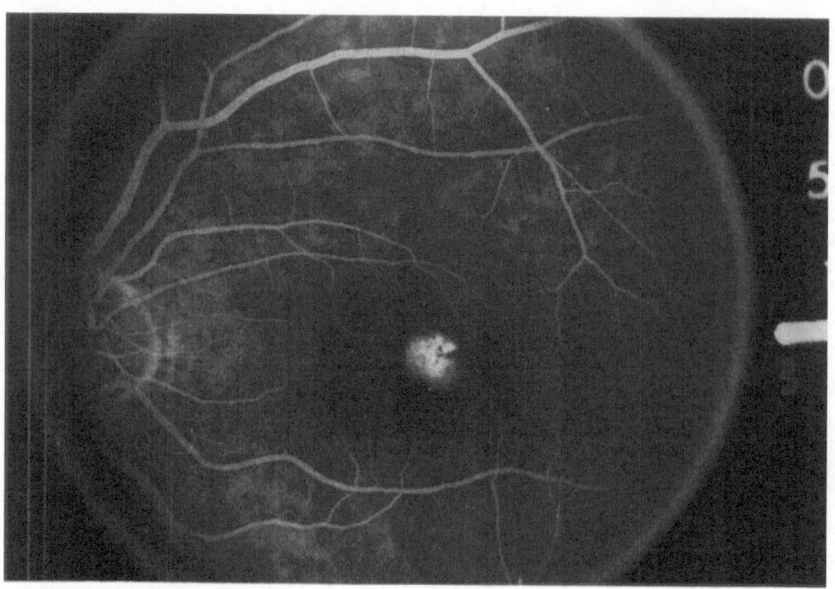

Fig. 5. (c, d) The fluorescein angiogram shows transmission of fluorescence typical of a retinal pigment epithelium detachment.

In PMD the disease usually presents in middle age from apparently normal retina. The lesions progress slowly over several years to form a discrete area of atrophy. Family history is negative and the EOG is normal or only slightly subnormal. On the other hand, BVD is usually diagnosed at a young age and is clearly transmitted as an autosomal dominant disease. The EOG is abnormal in all cases and a significant number of cases form hypertrophic scars in the late stages (Figure 1b).

The cause of PMD is unknown. Psychophysical and electrophysiologic studies suggest a pathologic process limited to the central retina. (Sabates, Pruett and Hirose, 1982). The blockage of fluorescence during angiography by the yellow material, further suggests an intracellular deposition in the RPE. Although the lesion is first clinically visible in the RPE an initial patho-logic process of the photoreceptors cannot be rules out.

REFERENCES

1. Arden, G. B., Barrada, A., Kelsey, J. H.: New clinical test of retinal function based upon standing potential of the eye. Brit. J. Ophthal. 46: 449–467, 1962.
2. Deutman, A. F.: Electrooculography in families with vitelliform dystrophy of the fovea. Arch. Ophthalmol., 81: 305, 1969.
3. Epstein, G. A., Rabb, M. F.: Adult vitelliform macular degeneration: Diagnosis and natural history. Brit. J. Ophthalmol., 64: 733–740, 1980.
4. Fishman, G. A., Trimble, S., Rabb, M. F., Fishman, M.: Pseudovitelliform macular degeneration. Arch. Ophthalmol., 95: 73–76, 1977.
5. François, J., DeRouck, A., Fernandez-Sasso, D.: L'electrooculographic dans les degenerescences vitelliformes de la macula. Bull. Soc. Belge. Ophthalmol., 143: 545–552, 1966.
6. Gass, J. D. M., A clinicopathologic study of a peculiar fovemacular dystrophy. Trans. Am. Ophthalmol. Soc., 72: 139–155, 1974.
7. Hirose, T., Wolf, E., Hara, A.: Electrophysiologic and psychophysical studies in congenital retinoschisis of x-linked recessive inheritance. Doc. Ophthalmol. Proceedings Series 13: 173–184, 1976.
8. Kingham, J. D., Lochen, G.P.: Vitelliform macular degeneration. Am. J. Ophthalmol. 84: 526–531, 1977.
9. Krill, A. E., Morse, P. A., Potts, A. M., Klien, B. A.: Hereditary vitelliruptive macular degeneration. Am. J. Ophthalmol., 61, 1405–1415, 1966.
10. Mohler, C. W., Fine, S. L.: Long-term evaluation of patients with Best's vitelliform dystrophy. Ophthalmology., 88: 688–692, 1981.
11. Sabates, R., Pruett, R., Hirose, T.: Pseudovitelliform macular degeneration. Retina 2: 197–205, 1982.

Mailing address:
Department of Ophthalmology
University of Missouri-Kansas City
23rd and Holmes
Kansas City, Missouri 64108, U.S.A.

EOG CHANGES IN DOMINANTLY INHERITED DRUSEN
(MALATTIA LEVENTINESE)

F. HESS AND G. NIEMEYER
(Zürich, Switzerland)

ABSTRACT

Dominant drusen typically lead to decrease in visual acuity at age 40–60 years and to low-normal or reduced cone and rod b-waves in the ERG. To assess electrophysiologically changes in the pigment epithelium we used the extended EOG ramp test (Rohde et al., 1981), which provides stimulation for the fast oscillation during dark adaptation of 30 min prior to a light step of 4 log units. From 14 control subjects we obtained the following data:

Control EOGs (n = 28 eyes)	mean	SD
Light peak (% of basic level)	198	15
Latency of light peak (min)	9.4	1.0
Fast oscillation (μV)	143	57.9
Fast oscillation, period (min)	2.5	0.2

14 patients (28 eyes tested), all members of affected families, exhibited drusen at the posterior pole, with or without visual loss. The fast oscillation of their EOGs revealed normal amplitudes ($157 \pm 28 \, \mu$V) and period length of 2.4 ± 0.2 min. The light peak revealed a mean of 208; i.e., 26% above the dark adapted basic level, with 2 eyes presenting ratios of less than 2 SD below mean control. The latency of the light peak-maximum was increased (10.5 ± 1.7 min), with 6 eyes presenting a delay of more than 2 SD from mean control. The data provide electrophysiologic evidence for pathology in the retinal pigment epithelium as reflected in the changes in the ratio and the frequent delay of the EOG light peak.

INTRODUCTION

Dominantly inherited drusen of the posterior pole are associated with progressive degeneration of the central retina. The synonymous term 'Malattia leventinese', used for this disease by Swiss and German authors, refers to the geographic location of several involved families in the Leventina valley of southern Switzerland.

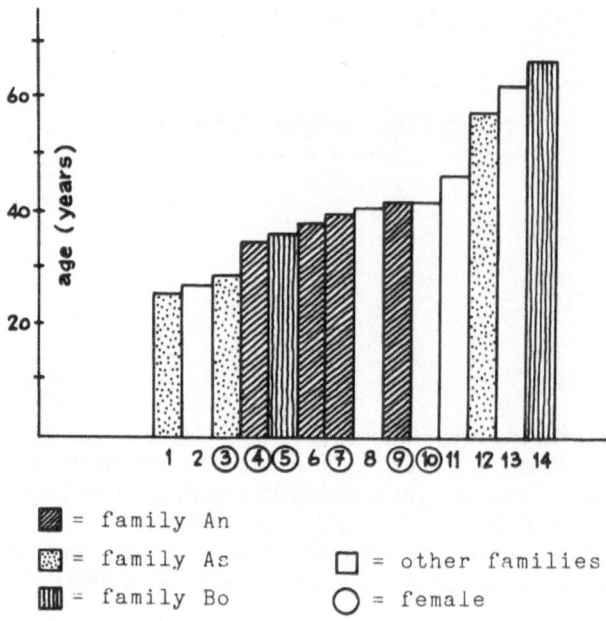

Fig. 1. Age, sex and kinship of the patients with dominantly inherited drusen.

This rare disease is characterized by the presence of drusen in the region of the macula and/or the optic disc. The drusen appear between the ages of 12 and 20 (Wagner and Klainguti, 1943; Forni and Babel, 1962) leading to a reduction in visual acuity in the fourth to sixth decades of life. At this stage electroretinograph (ERG) shows low-normal to subnormal b-wave amplitudes of both the rod and cone systems (Niemeyer, 1977; Scarpatetti et al., 1978). Since light- and electron-microscopic studies have demonstrated the marked involvement of the retinal pigment epithelium in this disease (Farkas et al., 1971; Dusek et al., 1982), we looked for corresponding changes in the electrooculogram (EOG).

MATERIAL

We examined 14 patients (Figure 1), all with an established diagnosis of dominant drusen and a typical fundus appearance. All patients examined belonged to families with several members involved. Most of the patients have been known to and examined by authors of previous publications (Forni, 1957; Forni and Babel, 1962; Niemeyer, 1977; Scarpatetti et al., 1978). The distribution of age, sex and kinship is graphically presented in Figure 1. Beside a complete history and examination of each patient, fundus photography, ERG and EOG were performed. The EOG parameters of the patients were compared to those of a normal control group, consisting of 10 women and 4 men. The results of these control EOGs are listed in Table I.

Means and standard deviations of the normal control group (n = 28 eyes)		$\bar{x}$	s
fast oscillation	amplitude (uV)	143	58
	time (min.)	2.5	0.2
light peak (slow oscillation)	standing potential (uV) (= basic level)	576	142
	amplitude (uV)	1176	289
	% of basic level	198	15
	peak time	9.5	1.0

Table 1. EOG parameter values from a control group.

METHODS

ERG recording: The ERG was recorded by the method of Gouras (1970) and Gunkel et al. (1976), i.e. using a Ganzfeld stimulator under two conditions of adaptation: with dark adaptation a blue and a red filter, matched for the rods, was used, and with light adaptation, a blue-green and an orange filter, matched for the cones, was used. The ERG was recorded with low-vacuum Henkes electrodes, amplified by a Tektronix preamplifier Type 122 at a bandpass of 0.2–1000 Hz and displayed on a Tektronix oscillostrope Type 502A (Niemeyer, 1976, 1979). Subnormal amplitudes of b-waves were defined as two standard deviations below the normal mean value.

EOG recording: The microprocessor-assisted EOG test, 'extended EOG ramp test' (Rohde et al., 1976; Rohde et al., 1977; Rohde, 1979; Rohde et al., 1981; Täumer, 1976), schematically shown in Figure 2, begins with the recording of the 'fast oscillation' (FO): starting at room light of about 100 lux the illumination is gradually decreased to 0.1 lux within 30 min. During this period the light decrease is sinusoidally modulated for 8 min with an amplitude of 3 log and a cycle of 2.5 min. Subsequently, the light peak ('slow oscillation') is induced. At 31 min the illumination is suddenly increased to 1000 lux and maintained at this level until the end of the 60 min test, while the subject continues alternating the fixation. For recording, Beckmann Ag-AgCl skin electrodes were placed close to the inner and outer canthi, nasally and temporally of each eye. An X-Y recorder (type HP 7005B) was used for the display of averaged EOG amplitudes.

EOG evaluation: The amplitude of the FO is determined by a line perpendicular to two parallel lines running through the light peaks and the dark

107

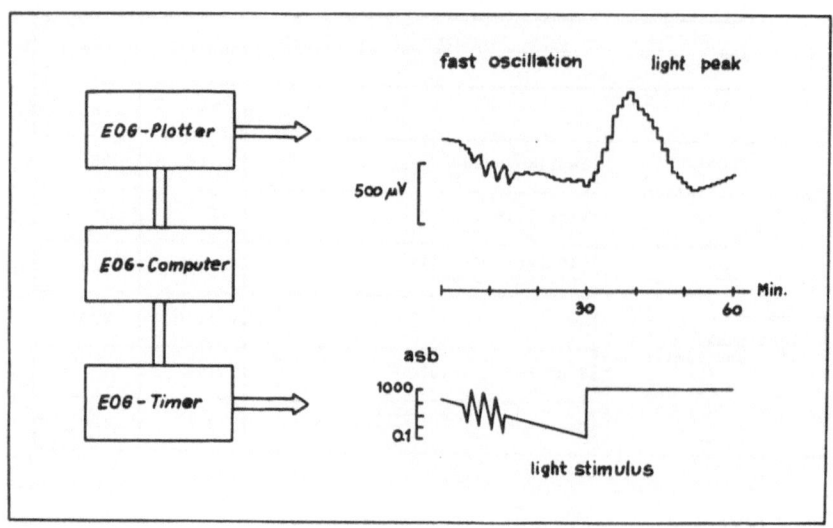

Fig. 2. Schematic of the set-up for recording of the EOG.

troughs, respectively. The basic level in dark adaptation is determined at 30 min of the test. The amplitude and the latency (onset of light step to maximum of response) of the light peak are then measured. The relative amplitude of the light peak is calculated according to Rohde (Rohde et al., 1977; Rohde, 1979; Rohde et al., 1981) and expressed in percent of the basic level.

RESULTS

Ophthalmoscopy: All the patients exhibited typical fundus changes, i.e. drusen around the macula and, in 9 out of 14 cases, nasal to the optic disc. Later changes included confluence of the drusen and fine granularity of the pigment. In agreement with previous reports (Wagner and Klainguti, 1943; Forni, 1957; Forni and Babel, 1962; Niemeyer, 1977; Scarpatetti et al., 1978) decrease in visual function was found in older patients (the youngest was 46 year old) and was associated with pronounced changes in the fundus, such as heavily pigmented or atrophic macular degeneration.

ERG: We recorded rod- and cone ERGs with *low-normal b-wave* amplitudes in most patients with drusen; about one third of them exhibited subnormal b-waves (Niemeyer, 1977; Scarpatetti et al., 1978). In the present study the youngest patient with marked ERG changes was a 35 year old female (Table 2), who had subnormal cone responses in one eye. Two patients exhibited *low normal* cone-, and two other patients exhibited *low normal* rod-b-wave amplitudes. A total of 7 eyes in 4 patients had *subnormal* cone ERGs (Table 2). None of the 12 ERGs (24 eyes) showed subnormal rod responses or increased peak times.

108

Table 2. Data from patients with dominantly inherited drusen

Age		25	26	28	34	35	37	39	40	41	41	46	57	62	66
Visual acuity	right	1.0	1.0	1.0	0.9	1.0	1.0	1.0	1.0	1.0	1.0	0.1	0.1	0.3	0.1
	left	1.0	1.0	1.0	0.9	1.0	1.0	1.0	1.0	1.0	1.0	1.0	0.8	0.6	FC
ERG	Rods	no	no	no	no	no	no	no	no	no	no	no	no	no	no
	Cones	no	no	no	no	subn	no	no	no	no	no	subn	no	no	subn
EOG	FO	no	no	no	no	no	no	no	no	no	no	no	no	no	no
	L.p. in % of BL	no	no	no	no	160*	no	no	no	165*	no	no	no	no	no
	Peak time right	no	no	no	no	no	no	no	no	14.7	no	no	no	no	13.5
	Peak time left	no	no	no	no	12.9	no	12.1	no	12.5	no	no	no	no	13.5

Data pooled from 14 patients. Pathological values are thickly framed. Empty spaces represent values that could not be measured. Peak time is given in minutes. Symbols and abbreviations: M = surrounding the macular region; O = surrounding the optic disc; C = confluent drusen; pat = patchy pigmentation; hyp = hyperpigmentation; FC = finger counting; no = normal; sub = subnormal; BL = basic level; * = pathological value in one eye, fellow eye normal

EOG: Normal values

The control group comprised 28 eyes of 14 subjects aged 18–47 years. All control data are listed in Table 1. The normal range of the basic level (standing potential in dark adaptation), of the light peak and of its latency is graphically shown by the dotted area in Figure 3.

EOG in dominant drusen

In all the examined patients the 'fast oscillation' remained normal regarding both, amplitude and latency (Table 2). The basic level of the standing potential was normal in all the patients. High-normal amplitudes of the light peak were found in 9 cases. Pathological ratios, i.e. light peak in percent of basic level, were seen in only 2 patients (2 eyes) (Table 2 and Figure 4) and border-line (2 SD above the mean) in 2 patients (2 eyes). Latency was increased in 4 patients (6 eyes) and borderline in 3 patients (5 eyes), as shown in Figures 3 and 4 and in Table 2. It is striking that these borderline or pathologically long latencies are seen in patients at a relatively advanced age, and thus in a late stage of the condition.

DISCUSSION

In our attempt to assess electrophysiologically functional defects in the pigment epithelium of patients with dominant drusen we found moderate changes in the EOG. This was surprising since the rod- and cone-ERG revealed comparatively more pathology of the retina in dominant drusen (Niemeyer, 1977).

Fast oscillation

Compared to the normal values (Table I) the fast oscillation in our patients was not significantly changed in amplitude or time course. This finding was a

109

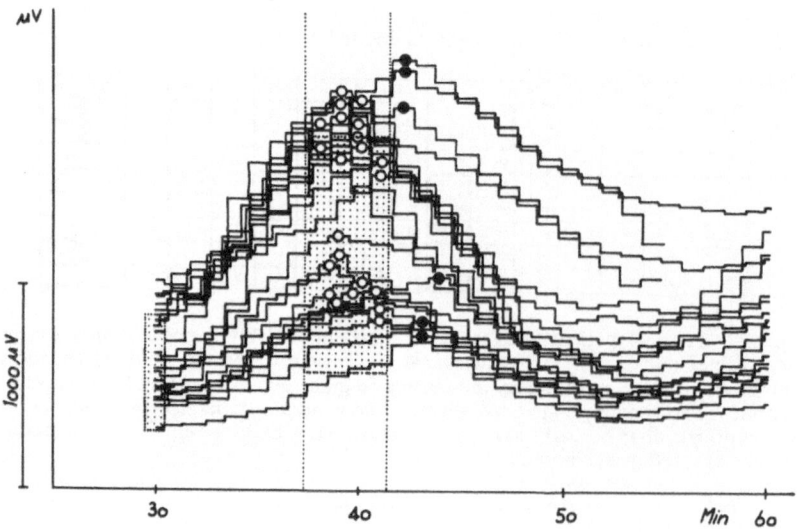

Fig. 3. 28 light peaks of patients are plotted against time. The normal ranges of the basic level, of the light peak and of its latency are indicated by the dotted areas. The empty circles represent the normal amplitudes and latencies of the light peaks. The full circles represent the pathological values.

surprise in the light of distinct ophthalmoscopic changes and occasionally severe functional defects (Niemeyer, 1977; Scarpatetti et al., 1978). We conclude that the fast oscillation is not a sensitive test in retinal degenerations that are primarily characterized by drusen, although it can be informative in other pathologic conditions of the retina (Rohde et al., 1981). Experiments on the cat retina in vitro revealed a particular resistance of the fast oscillation to hypoxia as well as to acidosis (Niemeyer, 1982).

Light peak

In contrast to only two pathological 'light peak' amplitudes (patients no. 5 and 9), there were 6 pathologically increased latencies (Table 2). The latency therefore appears to be a more sensitive EOG parameter than the amplitude. This is best seen when the light peak in percent of the basic level is plotted against latency (Figure 4). If we add the 6 eyes with pathologically increased latency and the 5 eyes with borderline-prolonged latency, 11 out of 28 eyes show *noticeable change* in this parameter.

A possible cause of the increased latency of the light peak could be a pH change, or some other metabolic effect. Niemeyer and Steinberg (1981) showed that a pH change from 7.4 to 7.1 (HCl acidosis) can cause an increase in latency of the light peak in the isolated perfused cat eye.

Subnormal light peak amplituded could be due to a widespread functional defect in the RPE. To resolve mechanisms underlying these changes is, however, outside the range of this work. Recent publications correlated the normal function of the retinal pigment epithelium with electrophysiology

110

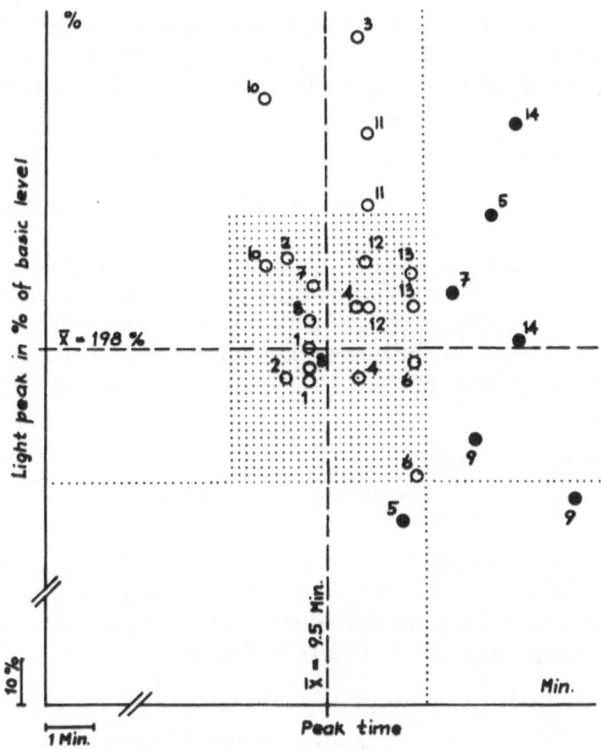

Fig. 4. Light peak in percent of basic level plotted against peak time. Normal range is indicated by the dotted area. Empty circles represent the normal, full circles the pathological values.

(for review see Zinn and Marmor, 1979), excluded changes in extracellular retinal potassium as a mechanism involved in the light peak (Steinberg and Niemeyer, 1981) and located the generation of the light peak at the basal membrane of the pigment epithelium (Linsenmeier and Steinberg, 1981; Griff and Steinberg, 1981; Griff and Steinberg, 1982).

Correlation of ophthalmoscopic findings with ERG and EOG

Table 2 shows that there is no obvious relationship between the ophthalmo-scopic changes and the ERG or EOG. As regards the ERG, this has been pointed out in the previous studies of this disease (Niemeyer, 1977; Scarpatetti et al., 1978). The finding is not surprising in view of the fact that anatomical structures probably responsible for the generation of the ERG b-wave are not primarily involved in dominant drusen. On the other hand, the lack of correlation with EOG is surprising, because the retina-RPE complex responsible for the generation of the EOG is the tissue predominantly affected by dominant drusen in the first place (Deutmann, 1970; Farkas et al., Streicher, 1982; Dusek et al., 1982). Thus, extension of drusen and their

111

confluence would have been expected to be reflected in the EOG. Furthermore, increased latency of the light peak often precedes a decrease in visual acuity, as seen in Table 2, especially if patients aged 35, 37, 52 years with border-line latency are included.

CONCLUSION

The 'fast oscillation' of the EOG is normal in dominantly inherited drusen. Destruction of the RPE is reflected mainly by the increase in latency, rarely by a subnormal amplitude of the light peak. The increase in latency could be related to progression of the disease. EOG changes often appear before visual function decreases, and they are less marked than the changes in the rod- and cone-ERG.

ACKNOWLEDGEMENT

We thank Dr. S. Forni, Bellinzona, for discussions and his help in chosing the patients whom he has been following for many years. Dr. E. Demant contributed valuable suggestions during the preparation of the manuscript. We appreciated the secretarial help of Mrs. V. Szabo.

REFERENCES

Deutmann, A. F., Jansen, L. M. A.: Dominantly inherited drusen of Bruch's membrane. Brit. J. Ophthal., 54: 373-382, 1970.
Dusek, J., Streicher, T., Schmidt, K.: Hereditäre Drusen der Bruch'schen Membran. II. Untersuchung von Semidünnschnitten und elektronenmikroskopischen Ergebnissen. Klin. Mbl. Augenheilk. 181: 79–83, 1982.
Farkas, T. G., Sylvester, V., Archer, D.: The ultrastructure of drusen. Amer. J. Ophthal. 71: 1196–1205, 1971.
Forni, S.: Nouvel arbre généalogique de dégénérescence tapétorétinienne de la région maculaire et péripapillaire, type 'Malattia leventinese'. Probl. act. Ophthal., Vol. 1: 570–575, 1957, S. Karger, Basel/New York.
Forni, S. and Babel, J.: Etude clinique et histologique de la malattia leventinese. Ophthalmologica (Basel), 143: 313–322, 1962.
Gouras, P.: Electroretinography: some basic principles. Invest. Ophthal. 9: 557–569, 1970.
Griff, E. R., Steinberg, R. H.: The origin of the light peak: in vitro study of gekko gekko. Invest. Ophthalmol. Vis. Sci. 20, Suppl. ARVO: 43, 1981.
Griff, E. R., Steinberg, R. H.: Light evokes retinal pigment epithelium basal membrane hyperpolarisation. Invest. Ophthalmol. Vis. Sci. 22, Suppl. ARVO: 280, 1982.
Gunkel, R. D., Bergsma, D. R., Gouras, P.: A Ganzfeld stimulator for electroretinography. Arch. Ophthal. 94: 669–670, 1976.
Linsenmeier, R. A., Steinberg, R. H.: Origin and sensitivity of the light peak of the intact cat eye. Invest Ophthalmol. Vis. Sci. 20, Suppl. ARVO: 43, 1981.
Niemeyer, G.: Stäbchen- und Zapfenaktivität im klinischen Elektroretinogramm. Ophthalmologica (Basel), 172: 175–180, 1976.
Niemeyer, G.: Rod- and cone-function in Malattia leventinese and in retinitis pigmentosa. Docum. Ophthal. Proc. Series, Vol. 17, 1977.

Niemeyer, G.: Information von der Netzhaut durch Elektroretinografie. A.v. Graefes Arch. klin. exp. Ophthal., 211: 129–137, 1979.

Niemeyer, G., Steinberg, R. H.: Effects of low pH and high CO_2 on the b-wave and light peak of the DC ERG in the perfused cat eye. Invest. Ophthalmol. Vis. Sci. 20, Suppl. ARVO: 43, 1981.

Niemeyer, G.: Light modulation of the standing potential in the perfused cat eye characteristics and responses to acidosis. 20th ISCEV Symposium, Iowa, 1982 (in press, this volume).

Rohde, N., Täumer, R., Pernice, D.: Vorschlag eines verbesserten klinischen EOG-Testes. Sonderdruck aus Bericht über die 74. Zusammenkunft der Deutschen Ophthalmol. Gesellschaft 1975. J. F. Bergmann-Verlag, München, 1977.

Rohde, N., Täumer, R., Braas, F.: An EOG Computer and Stimulator for the Investigation of the Slow Retinal Potential, Electro-Oculography – Its Clinical Importance. R. Täumer, ed., Bibliotheca ophthal., S. Karger, Basel, No. 85: 75–83, 1976.

Rohde, N.: Eine Bemerkung zur Interpretation pathologischer EOG-Veränderungen. Ber. Dtsch. Ophthalmol. Ges. 76: 437–440, 1979. J. F. Bergmann Verlag, München, 1979.

Rohde, N., Täumer, R., Bleckmann, H.: Examination of the fast oscillation of the corneoretinal potential under clinical conditions. A.v. Graefes Arch. klin. Ophthalmol. 217: 79–90, 1981.

Scarpatetti, A., Forni, S., Niemeyer, G.: Die Netzhautfunktion bei Malattia leventinese (dominant drusen). Klin. Mbl. Augenheilk. 172: 590–597, 1978.

Streicher, T., Schmidt, K., Dusek, J.: Hereditäre Drusen der Bruch'schen Membran. I. Klinische und lichtmikroskopische Beobachtungen. Klin. Mbl. Augenheilk, 181: 27–31, 1982.

Täumer, R.: Electro-oculography – its clinical importance. Bibliotheca ophthal. No. 85, S. Karger, Basel, 1976.

Wagner, H. and Kleinguti, R.: Weitere Untersuchungen über die Malattia leventinese. Ophthalmologica (Basel), 105: 225–228, 1943.

Zinn, K. M., Marmor, M. F.; The retinal pigment epithelium. Harvard University Press, 1979.

Mailing address:
Department of Ophthalmology
Universitätsspital, CH-8091
Zürich, Switzerland

EOG APPLICATION FOR STARGARDT'S DISEASE AND X-LINKED JUVENILE RETINOSCHISIS

D. YONEMURA, K. KAWASAKI, K. WAKABAYASHI AND J. TANABE

(Kanazawa, Japan)

ABSTRACT

A case of Stargardt's disease and a case of X-linked juvenile retinoschisis were studied by our electrophysiological tests for the cone receptor cell and the retinal pigment epithelium (RPE). The cone activity was evaluated by the electroretinographic rapid off-response which is mainly composed of the decay of the late receptor potential of cones. The RPE activity was assessed by the susceptibility of the ocular standing potential to hyperosmolarity and to Diamox with the EOG method (hyperosmolarity response and Diamox response respectively).

In a case of Stargardt's disease the EOG L/D and the Diamox response in both eyes and the hyperosmolarity response in the left eye were within normal limits. The hyperosmolarity response in the right eye, however, was subnormal, indicating pigment epitheliopathy. In a case of X-linked juvenile retinoschisis the EOG L/D, the hyperosmolarity response and the Diamox response all remained normal. The spectral sensitivity of the rapid off-response was within normal limits in both cases.

INTRODUCTION

A recent histological study on a well-documented case of fundus flavimaculatus with atrophic macular degeneration (Eagle et al., 1980) revealed widespread abnormalities in the retinal pigment epithelium (RPE). We reported the retinal pigment epitheliopathy in a case of fundus flavimaculatus by our new electrophysiological tests; the hyperosmolarity response and the Diamox response (Yonemura et al., 1982). Juvenile retinoschisis is a X-linked recessive inherited disorder and the schisis is seen histologically as a splitting within the nerve fiber layer (Yanoff et al., 1968).

In the present study we analyzed a case of Stargardt's disease, the basic defect of which might reside in the RPE, and a case of juvenile retinoschisis, the basic disorder of which might be at the level of the nerve fiber and ganglion cell layers, by our new methods of testing the cone receptor cell and the RPE.

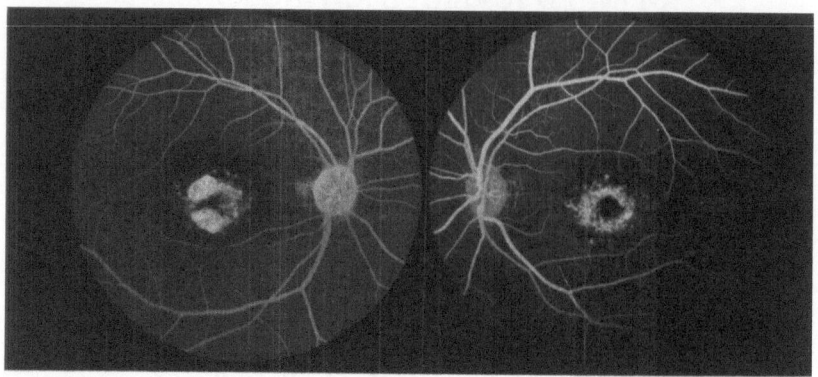

Fig. 1. Fluorescein angiograph of a case of Stargardt's disease. The transmitted hyperfluorescence was seen corresponding to the atrophic macular area and some perifoveal flecks.

METHODS

The detailed methods have been described elsewhere (Yonemura et al., 1979). The off-response of the ERG was evoked by rectangular monochromatic stimuli having equal quantal content. The stimulus light subtended about 30 degrees of visual angle. Responses were amplified (time constant: 2 sec) and were led to a signal averager. The scotopic b-wave (b_s) was evoked by a full-field stimulation of 1.0×10^{-3} to 1.0 lux at the cornea. The pupil was fully dilated for the ERG recording.

The change of the standing potential of the eye by osmotic stress or Diamox was recorded with the EOG method (30 degree horizontal saccade). A hypertonic solution of Fructmanit (15% mannitol, 10% fructose, 1.4×10^3 mOsm, Taiho Co.) or acetazolamide (500 mg, Diamox®) was given intravenously after the standing potential had been stabilized (V_0) in the dark. The reduction of the standing potential is expressed in percentage, $(V_0 - V_{min}/V_0) \times 100\%$, where V_{min} is a minimal EOG amplitude after an intravenous injection of Fructmanit or Diamox. The conventional L/D ratio of the EOG was estimated, using a luminance of 1.1×10^3 candela m^{-2}. No mydriatic was used for the EOG recording.

RESULTS

Stargardt's disease: The patient was a 36 year-old female, who had noted bilateral gradual visual loss for the past three years. The corrected visual acuity was 20/200 in the right eye and 20/60 in the left eye on her first visit to our clinic. Both fundi showed 'beaten bronze' macular atropic lesions with perifoveal yellowish flecks in a garland fashion. Fluorescein angiography revealed the transmitted hyperfluorescence corresponding to the atrophic macular area seen on ophthalmoscopy (Figure 1). Some of the perifoveal flecks also showed the transmitted hyperfluorescence. These ophthalmo-scopical and fluorographic findings indicated some degree of choriocapillaris atrophy in addition to retinal pigment epithelial atrophy in the macula. The degree of choriocapillaris atrophy in the macula was thought to be more severe in the right eye than in the left. The fluorescein angiography character-istically showed a generalized abolished visibility of the normal background fluorescence, which has been termed the 'sign of choroidal silence'. This sign is thought to result from the massive accumulation of a lipofuscin-like sub-stance in the RPE. Visual field examination revealed a normal peripheral field and a mild decreased sensitivity in a central field. By routine color vision tests no significant color vision defect was found except the increase of the total error score of the 100-hue test in the right eye. The dark adaptation was slightly delayed for cones and the final rod threshold was normal. The b_s-wave (b_p), the oscillatory potential (OP) and the 30 Hz flicker ERG were all normal. The rapid off-response to monochromatic repetitive stimuli remained normal (Figure 2), and its spectral sensitivity was normal within the wave-length range tested. The EOG L/D and the diamox response in both eyes, and the hyperosmolarity response in the left eye were within the normal range. The hyperosmolarity response in the right eye was, however, subnormal, indicating pigment epitheliopathy.

   X-linked juvenile retinoschisis: An 8 year-old boy visited our clinic because of poor vision found by a local ophthalmologist. His refractive error was 2 diopters hypermetropia in both eyes. His corrected visual acuity was 20/30 in the right eye and 20/60 in the left. The macula showed bilaterally a micro-cystic appearance and fine lines radiated from the fovea. Silver-gray, glistening spotty areas somewhat reminiscent of Berlin's edema were scattered in the midperipheral retina. There were no signs of peripheral schisis. Fluorescein angiography revealed some irregularity of the foveal capillary network in the right eye and no transmitted defect in either eye. Peripheral and central visual fields were normal. No significant color vision defect was found by routine color vision tests. Delayed dark adaptation for both rods and cones with a mild elevation of the final rod threshold was found. The b_p-wave, the OP and the 30 Hz flicker ERG were within normal limits. The amplitude of the b_s-wave, elicited by a full field dim stimulation, was lower in the case of juvenile retinoschisis than in a normal control of the stimulus intensities tested (Figure 3). The diminution of the b_s-wave was more apparent at the lower stimulus intensities. The rapid off-response in the ERG and its spectral sensitivity were within normal limits. The EOG L/D, the hyperosmolarity response and the Diamox response were all within normal range.

DISCUSSION

X-linked juvenile retinoschisis is characterized by a splitting of the sensory retina in the nerve fiber layer. Deutman (1977) stated that a subnormal b-wave was invariably found and that the rod system appeared in general to be affected more severely than the cone system in juvenile retinoschisis. The present study may confirm the above description from a different viewpoint. The spectral sensitivity of the rapid off-response was normal while the

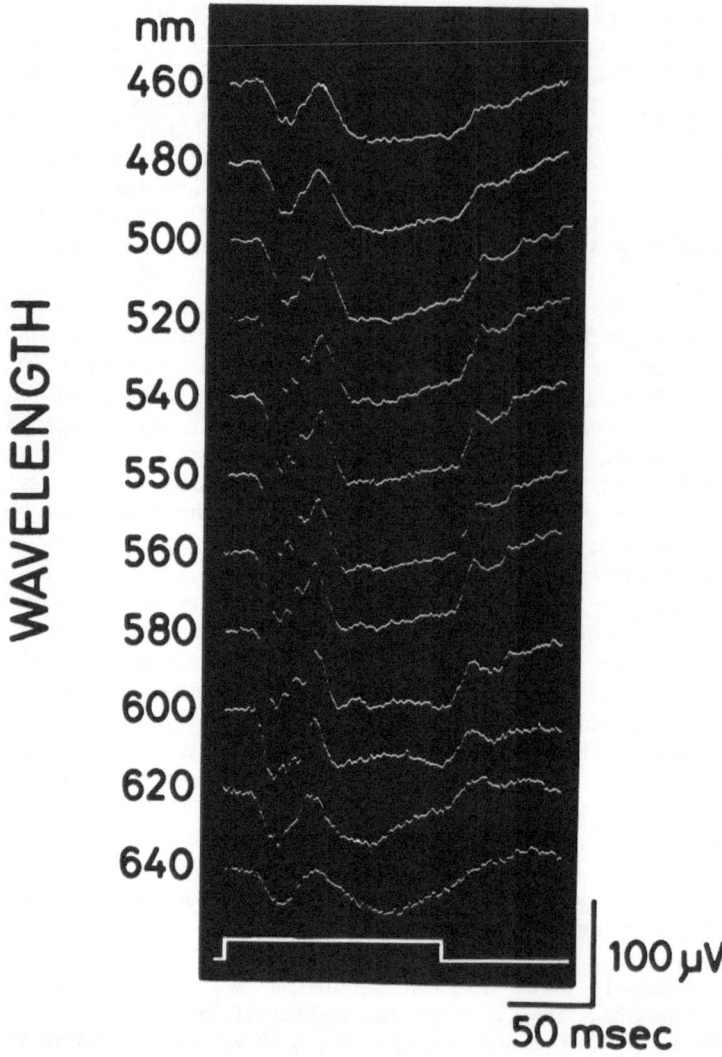

Fig.2. The ERG is Stargardt's disease by monochromatic rectangular stimuli having equal quantal content (3.0×10^{14} quanta $\cdot$ m^{-2} $\cdot$ sec^{-1} at the cornea). The stimulus of 125 msec duration was repeated at 4 Hz, 50 stimuli were averaged used. Upward deflection indicates cornea positive. The rapid off-response was of normal amplitude at all wavelengths tested.

amplitude of the b_s-wave was lower than normal especially at the lower stimulus intensities in our case of juvenile retinoschisis. The amplitude of the b_s-wave in this case was approximated by the equation $V = (I^n/I^n + \sigma^n)V_{max}$. where I, V_{max} and σ were respectively the stimulus intensity, the maximal amplitude of the b_s-wave and the stimulus intensity for eliciting the amplitude of $\frac{1}{2} V_{max}$. The sensitivity of the b_s-wave estimated by V_{max}/σ^n was only a half

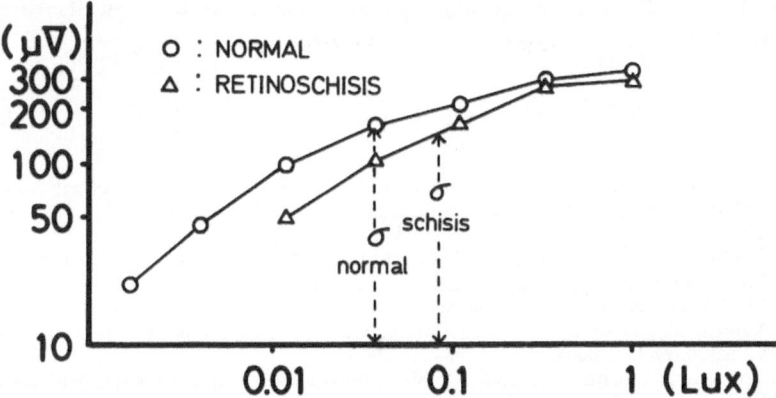

Fig. 3. The relationship between the stimulus intensity and the amplitude of the scotopic b-wave, elicited by a full field dim stimulation on a log-log plot. V_{max} and σ were respectively the maximal amplitude of the scotopic b-wave and the stimulus intensity for eliciting the amplitude of $\frac{1}{2} V_{max}$. The diminution of the scotopic b-wave in juvenile retinoschisis was more apparent at the lower stimulus intensities.

of that of the normal control in our case of juvenile retinoschisis. Deutman (1977) described that the EOG L/D might be normal or subnormal among patients with juvenile retinoschisis. The light rise depends on the photo-receptors as well as on the RPE. Further, retinal portions proximal to the receptors have to be normal to generate the normal light rise. One should be careful in evaluating the EOG L/D as a test for the RPE particularly in a patient with an affected ERG such as our case of juvenile retinoschisis. The normal results of the EOG L/D, the hyperosmolarity response and the Diamox response in our case of juvenile retinoschisis may indicate the integrity of the RPE.

A histological study by Eagle et al., (1980) revealed massive accumulation of a lipofuscin-like substance in the RPE in fundus flavimaculatus. They suggested that an altered lipopigment metabolism might play a major role in the pathogenesis of this retinal pigment epithelial disorder. In our case of Stargardt's disease the b_s-wave, the b_p-wave, the OP, the 30 Hz flicker ERG and the rapid off-response were normal, suggesting the integrity of the sensory retina. Although the EOG L/D was within the normal range bilaterally, the hyperosmolarity response was subnormal in the right eye and close to the lower limits of the normal range in the left eye, indicating retinal pigment epitheliopathy in our case of Stargardt's disease. The clinical and electrophysiological findings suggest that this patient corresponds to the cases of stage 2 by Fishman (1976). In our previous paper (Yonemura et al., 1982), we reported a patient with fundus albipunctatus showing a normal EOG L/D and a abnormal hyperosmolarity response and a patient with fundus flavi-maculatus showing a normal EOG L/D and an abnormal hyperosmolarity response. The elucidation whether this different result between the EOG L/D and the hyperosmolarity response may depend on a difference in sensitivity for detecting retinal pigment epitheliopathy or a characteristic difference

119

between the EOG L/D and the hyperosmolarity response awaits further investigations.

REFERENCES

1. Eagle, R. C., Lucier, A. C., Bernardino, V. B. and Yanoff, M.: Retinal pigment epithelial abnormalities in fundus flavimaculatus. Ophthalmology, 87: 1189–1200, 1980.
2. Deutman, A. F.: Vitreoretinal dystrophies. In Krill's Hereditary Retinal and Choroidal Diseases. pp. 1043–1108, Harper & Row, New York, 1977.
3. Fishman, G. A.: Fundus flavimaculatus. Arch Ophthalmol. 94: 2061–2067, 1976.
4. Yanoff, M. Rahn, E. K. and Zimmerman, L. E.: Histopathology of juvenile retino-schisis. Arch Ophthalmol., 79: 49–53, 1968.
5. Yonemura, D. and Kawasaki, K.: New approaches to ophthalmic electrodiagnosis by retinal oscillatory potential, drug-induced responses from retinal pigment epithelium and cone potential. Doc. Ophthalmol., 48: 163–222, 1979.
6. Yonemura, D., Kawasaki, K., Wakabayashi, K., Madachi-Yamamoto, S. and Kawaguchi, I.: New approach to electro-physiological analysis of flecked retina syndrome. Doc. Ophthalmol. Proc. Ser., 31: 165–175, 1982.

Mailing address:
Department of Ophthalmology, School of Medicine
Kanazawa University, 13–1, Takara-machi
Kanazawa, Japan

120

HYDROXYCHLOROQUINE AND RETINAL TOXICITY

R. INFANTE, D.A. MARTIN AND J.R. HECKENLIVELY

(Los Angeles, California, U.S.A.)

ABSTRACT

Fifty-eight patients on Plaquenil treatment were evaluated for retinal toxicity, using the electrooculogram (EOG), Farnsworth 100 hue test, and the Nagel anomaloscope. Ten patients showed supranormal values above 250% light/ dark ratios (L/D ratios), 13 had subnormal L/D ratios, while 28 patients had abnormal color vision tests either with normal or abnormal EOG. Interestingly the patients with the supranormal EOG L/D ratios, may represent a pretoxic state. In some patients color vision alterations were the first sign of retinal toxicity. We will discuss the value of the electrophysiological and psychophysical testing in terms of management of the drug to avoid retinal toxicity.

INTRODUCTION

Retinal toxicity produced by chloroquine and its derivatives such as hydroxychloroquine (HC), has been a well-recognized entity since the report by Cambiagi (1950). The affinity of the drug for the retinal pigment epithelium (RPE) and the resultant toxic effect have been reported to be associated with the total dosage (Shearer, 1967), the duration of the treatment (Nylander, 1966; Tobin, 1982; Viopio, 1966), and the age of the patient and individual susceptibility (Tobin, 1982), the last probably depending on the melanine content in the RPE and choroidal tissue (Nylander, 1966; Schmöger, 1978).

To date, there appears to be no ideal test for detecting early HC toxicity. Tests suggested by various authors (Table 1) have included the electroretinogram (ERG), electro-oculogram (EOG), visual field test, dark-adaptation test, color vision (CV) test, and fluorescein angiogram. These tests have been performed individually or in combination (Nylander, 1966; Shearer, 1967; Henkind, 1964). Early detection of toxicity is difficult because the majority of patients have normal visual acuity and are completely asymptomatic, yet on testing they may demonstrate toxic changes.

The reported long-term effects of HC usage have been variable, with some patients showing progression of retinal degeneration even after the drug has been discontinued (Schmöger, 1978), and others showing visual field

Table 1. Tests for chloroquine retinal toxicity

Author	Test Preference	Reference
Fishman, G. A.	Static perimetry; Foveal sensitivity	Contemp. Ophthalmol. (1980)
Gouras, P. et al.	ERG, EOG	Arch. Ophthalmol. (1963)
Henkind, P. et al.	ERG, EOG	Am. J. Ophthalmol. (1964)
Marmor & Zinn	None specific	Book, The Retinal Pigment Epithelium, (1979)
Kearns, T. P. et al.	Fluorescein angiogram	Arch. Ophthalmol. (1966)
Tobin, E. et al.	Visual fields	Arch. Ophthalmol. (1982)

constriction returning to pretreatment levels following discontinuation of HC (Tobin, 1982). Some patients who have atrophic macular retinal pigment epithelial loss give a history of chloroquine use 20 years previously, which suggests a toxic origin to the degeneration.

Because we had noted color vision defects in patients on HC, and because toxic effects are known to have been accentuated by red targets on visual field examination (Tobin, 1982), we evaluated the joint use of color vision testing and the EOG in detecting early signs of chloroquine toxicity.

MATERIALS AND METHODS

Forty-six patients receiving HC were evaluated in our laboratory with EOG and CV testing during the past six years. All patients had been referred by other physicians to rule out retinal toxicity secondary to HC. Five patients were tested before starting treatment and eleven patients had been taking the drug for two months or less at the time of the initial test.

Patients were studied with the Farnsworth Munsell 100-hue test (FM-100), the Nagel anomaloscope and the EOG. The FM-100 hue test was conducted in the standard manner using the Macbeth Easel lamp for illumination. Patients were retested on the boxes on which they made errors. The Nagel anomaloscope test was performed in a standard manner as described by Krill (1977) and Pokorny et al. (1979), with each eye tested separately for color and intensity matching.

The EOG was performed with the pupils dilated, and the test was started after the patients had been dark adapted for 45 minutes. After the skin was cleansed with alcohol, electrodes were placed nasally and temporally to each eye, and an inactive electrode was placed on the forehead. Patients were positioned 2 m from the test board, which has a dim central fixation and two end-point red test lights that subtend a 20° arc. Patients were tested at 3 min intervals for 25 min, the first half in the dark and the second half in the light. The peak light amplitude was divided by the lowest dark-adapted amplitude to calculate the light to dark (L/D) ratio. Supranormal L/D responses $\geqslant 250$ were noted. Table 2 shows our normal values on these tests.

Patients were placed into four groups for the purposes of analysing the results. Group I had normal color vision and EOG, Group II recorded abnormal color vision and normal EOG, Group III had abnormal EOG and normal color vision, and Group IV had both abnormal EOG and color vision.

Table 2. Color vision and EOG data for a normal control group

Test	Normal Value
FM-100 hue test	Error score $\leq$ 100, no axis
Nagel anomaloscope	Rayleigh equation 37–45
EOG	Arden's Light/Dark Ratio $\geq$ 175%

RESULTS

The period of treatment in all groups of patients varied from two weeks to as long as six years. The average daily dose was 200 mg/day with a maximum cumulative dose of 980 gm.

Group I: Normal color vision and electro-oculogram

Twenty-three out of 46 patients had normal color vision and EOG. The maximum duration of treatment was three years, the average age 42 years, and the maximum cumulative dose was 980 gm. Some of the patients were tested several times and had small variations between the tests, but each time values were within normal limits. The average error score for the FM-100 hue test was 47 for the right eye and 49 for the left eye. The average midpoint for the Nagel anomaloscope was 40.3 scale units for the right eye and 42.8 for the left eye. The average value for the EOG was 212% for the right eye and 208% for the left eye. Three out of 23 (13%) patients had L/D ratios $\geq$ 250 in at least one eye.

Group II: Abnormal color vision and normal electro-oculogram

Fourteen patients had abnormal color vision but normal EOG results. All fourteen patients had Fansworth error scores greater than or equal to 100, which is abnormal for our laboratory. The L/D ratio varied from 175% to 339% (mean 212%) for the right eye and from 176% to 378% (mean 218) for the left eye. Five of 13 patients (36%) had supranormal L/D ratios $\geq$ 250. A history was available for 13 of 14 patients and the mean duration of the drug use was 16.5 months at the time of testing. The average age was 48 years. Only 3 of 9 patients who had the Nagel anomaloscope had abnormally wide Rayleigh equations.

The color vision test findings in three patients in this group are particularly interesting, and are presented in detail. Patient 4 (Table III) had an elevated error score for the FM-100 hue test of 113 for the right eye and 149 for the left eye. She was taking 400 mg/day of HC for 76 months with a total dose of approximately 5,000 gm during this period. On the basis of these results, her dose was reduced to 200 mg/day. The FM-100 was repeated five months later and had a markedly improved score of 66 in both eyes.

Similarly patient 10 (Table III) who was initially tested 1.5 months after starting 800 mg/day of HC, had an error score of 86 for the right eye and 64 for the left eye. She was tested four months later on a dose of 600 mg/day.

123

Table 3. Color vision and EOG data for four patients on hydroxychloroquine medication and examined more than once.

Patient number	Date	Dose (mg/day)	EOG		FM-100	
			OD	OS	OD	OS
4	10/81	400	275	225	113	140
	3/82	200	252	214	66	66
10	7/79	800	182	284	86	64
	11/79	600	178	176	128	103
	6/80	200	175	175	58	39
6	1/77	400	186	228	–	–
	9/77	400	171	162	57	46
	3/78	400*	188	176	103	120
	10/78	none	209	200	52	63
	6/79	200	233	225	63	56
	1/80	200	243	217	27	47
	12/81	unknown	150	159	16	36
	9/82	100	217	200	56	60

*drug discontinued 3/78

Her error scores were 128 for the right eye and 103 for the left eye. Her dose was reduced to 200 mg/day and seven months later she was retested. The F-100 error score was 58 in the right eye and 39 in the left eye. The Nagel anomaloscope remained normal.

Patient 6 (Table III) has been tested in our laboratory for HC toxicity since 1976. Before 1978 this patient had FM-100 values for 57 for the right eye and 46 for the left eye. When evaluated again in 1978 after taking the drug for three years, the patient had an abnormal error score of 103 in the right eye and 120 in the left eye. The drug was discontinued and six months later the patient was retested. The FM-100 values returned to a normal of 52 and 63 respectively. On two occasions the EOG became abnormal. In 1977, after the patient had been taking the drug for two years, the L/D ratio dropped from 186% in the right eye and 228% in the left eye to 171% and 162% respectively. The dose was reduced and the L/D ratio slowly increased to normal values of 243% in the right eye and 217% in the left eye. Two years after the drug was reinstituted, the EOG again was abnormal (150% right eye, 169% left eye). On both occasions the values returned to normal after the patient was taken off the drug for six months.

Group III: Abnormal electo-oculogram and normal color vision tests

Six patients developed abnormal EOG with normal color vision tests. The periods they took the drug ranged from eight months to three years. The mean values for the L/D ratio were 155% in the right eye and 127% in the left eye. The average age was 34 years. Four patients in this group had abnormal EOG at the first testing and had been on the drug for an average period of 2.5 years with total dosage of approximately 240 g. One of these four, patient 23, improved his L/D ratio when the dose was decreased from 600 to 400 mg/day (Table III).

Table 4. Color vision and EOG data for three patients on hydroxychloroquine medication and tested only once.

Pt. no.	Age	Date	EOG %		FM-100	
			OD	OS	OD	OS
11	65	8/79	168	173	123	142
37	66	12/80	150	167	170	140
34	58	11/80	171	171	80	138

Group IV: Abnormal electro-oculogram and abnormal color vision tests

Only three patients in our study had both abnormal EOG and abnormal color vision tests. The average age was 63 years. The EOG and color vision test results are shown in Table IV. Only patient 37 had an abnormal ERG. Of note in this group is the short duration of treatment, no longer than three months when first tested, and the older average age of the patient.

DISCUSSION

Numerous tests have been tried searching for the ideal way to detect early chloroquine/hydroxychloroquine retinal toxicity before irreversible damage takes place. No tests have been shown to be completely effective, and opinion varies as to which set of tests are most helpful in monitoring patients, with different investigators relying on different tests (Table I).

It is our impression that the ERG and the visual field test pick up chloroquine or HC toxicity at a stage in which irreversible damage usually has taken place. The EOG has been difficult to interpret, but clearly shows abnormalities in early stages of toxicity in some patients, and the test results improve when the drug is withdrawn. The data suggest that the EOG may be more helpful than the ERG and visual field test in monitoring patients before retinal damage occurs. In some cases of HC toxicity, the Farnsworth 100 hue test has become abnormal before the EOG changes.

One interesting phenomenon in this group has been the supranormal ($\geqslant 250\%$) Arden L/D ratio. In our laboratory, these values clearly are outside the two standard deviations, and our belief, although unproved at this point, is that this may represent a pretoxic state which needs to be followed closely. If the Arden ratio falls from this higher value while the patient is on the same or higher doses of chloroquine, or if the color vision becomes worse while the EOG is supranormal, we carefully consider reducing or stopping the drug.

The interval of follow-up testing is often difficult to judge, but we normally follow patients every four to six months depending on whether any of their scores are abnormal or if they are on a particularly high dosage. Undoubtedly, other risk factors that currently are not recognized may help us in the future to adjust testing intervals.

Multiple studies suggest that HC is a safer drug with less retinal toxicity than chloroquine in the treatment of systemic lupus erythematosus and rheumatoid arthritis (Tobin, 1982; Nylander, 1966; Shearer, 1967).

We conclude that the FM-100 hue test in association with the Nagel anomaloscope and EOG can be used effectively for the evaluation of HC toxicity. These results in addition to fundus findings and other tests will help in directing the management of these patients.

REFERENCES

Carr, R. E., Gouras, P., Gunkel, R. Chloroquine retinopathy. Arch. Ophthalmol. 75: 171–178 (1966).
Cambiagi, A. Unusual lesions in a case of systemic lupus erythematosus. Arch. Ophthalmol. 57: 451–453 (1957).
Fishman, G. A. Toxic retinopathies. Contemporary Ophthalmology 1: 1–5 (1980).
Gouras, P., Gunkel, R. D. The EOG in chloroquine and other retinopathies. Arch. Ophthalmol. 70: 629–639 (1963).
Henkind, P., Carr, R. E., Siegel, I. M. Early chloroquine retinopathy: clinical and functional findings. Arch. Ophthalmol. 71: 157–165 (1966).
Kearns, T. P., and Hollenhorst, R. W. Chloroquine retinpathy: evaluation by fluorescein angiography. Arch. Ophthalmol. 76: 378–384 (1966).
Krill, A. E. The Hereditary Retinal and Choroidal Diseases, Harper & Row, Publ. Hagerstown, 1977, vol. 1, p. 330.
Monahan, R. H., Horns, R. C. The pathology of chloroquine in the eye. Trans. Am. Acad. Ophthalmol. and Otolaryingol. 71: 49–54 (1964).
Nylander, U. L. F. Ocular damage in chloroquine therapy. Acta Ophthalmologica 44: 335–348 (1966).
Okun, E., Gouras, P., Bernstein, H., Von Sallmann, L. Chloroquine retinopathy. Arch. Ophthalmol. 69: 59–71 (1963).
Pokorny, J., Smith, V. C., Verriest, G., Pinckers, A. J. L. G. Congenital and Acquired Color Vision Defects, Grune and Stratton, Inc., Publ., New York, 1979.
Schmöger, E., Müller, W., Haase, E. Follow-up in a case of retinopathy more than 10 years after stopping chloroquine therapy. Doc. Ophthalmologica Proc. Series 15: 101–105 (1978).
Shearer, R. V., Dubois, E. L. Ocular changes induced by long-term hydroxychloroquine (Plaquenil) therapy. Am. J. Ophthalmol. 64: 245–252 (1967).
Tobin, D. R., Krohel, G. B. Ryners, R. I. Hydroxychloroquine: Seven years experience. Arch. Ophthalmol. 100: 81–83 (1982).
Viopio, H. Incidence of chloroquine retinopathy. Acta Ophthalmologica 44: 349–354 (1966).
Zinn, K. M., Greenseid, D. Z. Toxicology of the retinal pigment epithelium. Int. Ophthalmol. Clin. 4: 147–157 (1982).
Zinn, K. M., and Marmor, M. F. Toxicology of the human retinal pigment epithelium, in: Zinn, K. M. and Marmor, M. F. (eds). The Retinal Pigment Epithelium, Harvard University Press, Cambridge, Mass., 1979.

Mailing address:
John R. Heckenlively, M.D.
Deidre A. Martin, B.S.
Jules Stein Eye Institute
U.C.L.A. School of Medicine
Los Angeles, California 90024, U.S.A.

Ricardo Infante, M.D.
Apartado Aereo 19392
Bogota, Columbia

EOG CHANGES DUE TO SPONTANEOUS MACULAR PUCKER

M. H. FOERSTER, N. BORNFELD AND H. LAQUA

(Essen, West Germany)

ABSTRACT

In cases of spontaneous macular pucker operated by vitrectomy and micro-dissection as well as in other induced defects of the internal limiting membrane we were able to show reversible reductions of the EOG light-rise which were not attributable to the retinal pigment epithelium and the inner retinal layers. We suggest a short circuiting at the posterior pole to be responsible for this voltage drop of the ocular dipole, which in our cases was reversible contrary to situations like vitelliform dystrophy or in intraocular tumors without detachment.

INTRODUCTION

The standing potential of the clinical EOG and its light response is said to reflect mainly the activity of the retinal pigment epithelium. The contribution of the pigment epithelium to the standing potential is unquestioned. A contribution of cones and rods to the light response has been shown. The light rise of the ERG as well the c-wave however are compromised by a process in the inner retinal layers like interruption of the central retinal artery. The role of the inner retinal layers in influencing the light rise has been unclear and the clinical evaluation of the light rise had to be made by comparison with other electrophysiological data.

METHODS

We used the EOG according to the protocol of Täumer et al., where, after a preadaption of 30 minutes to continuously dimming light from 200 to 0.1 asb, a step increase in intensity to 1.000 asb. is applied. Seven EOG potentials from over an angle of 30° are averaged every minute for over 30 min.

The average light rise is 187% of the basic value in our laboratory with a standard deviation of ± 18%.

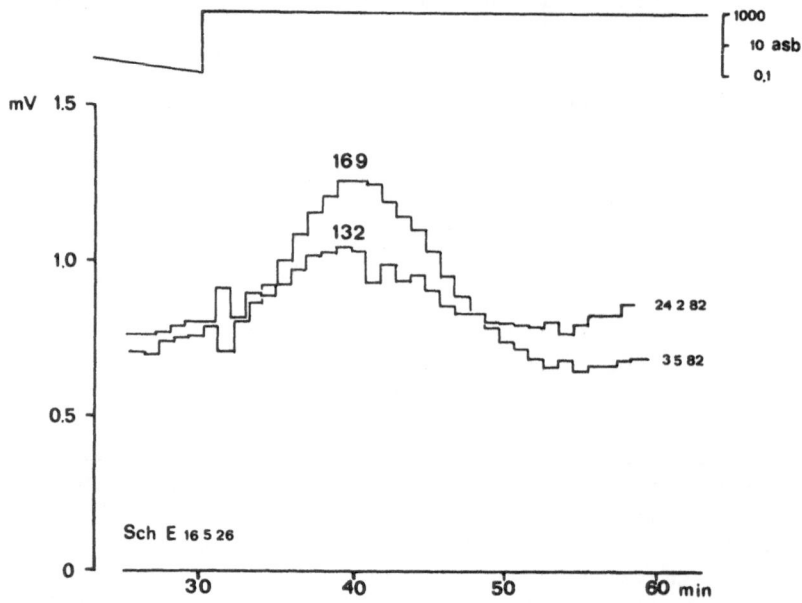

Fig. 1. EOG one week after vitrectomy and 9 weeks after vitrectomy respectively. The patient had a defect of the inner limiting membrane.

Before we examined patients with spontaneous macular pucker we studied 2 patients electrophysiologically prior to vitrectomy.

RESULTS

The first patient was a 56 year old railroad engineer who suffered from a preretinal hemorrhage in his left eye without any history of vascular disease. The amplitude intensity function of the ERG a- and b-waves was completely normal and a vitrectomy was performed, for occupational reasons, one week after the hemorrhage. In the course of the operation a defect of the internal limiting membrane developed and a bleeding retinal vessel was treated by endodiathermy. Fluoresceinangiography one week after the operation did not reveal any vascular abnormalities, but the light rise of the EOG was 132%. After 9 weeks the light rise was back to 169% which is in the lower normal range (Figure 1).

A second patient, 20 years old, had a macular pucker at the upper branch vein with a questionable history of contusion. His right eye showed, after vitrectomy, a preretinal hemorrhage indicating a defect of the internal limiting membrane. The histology of the membrane showed a collagenous material which did not contain any vessels. His EOG light rise one week postoperatively was 138%. It increased 7 months later to 157% being in the lowest normal range.

128

Since we saw these patients we have treated 4 patients with a spontaneous macular pucker. We would like to discuss our findings in a typical case. A 42 year old patient, who since 1977 noticed a decrease of visual acuity to 0.1 in his left emmetropic eye had no history of trauma and his medical record showed no other abnormalities. He complained about metamorphopsia in his left eye. Therefore a vitrectomy was performed in June of 1982. Indirect ophthalmoscopy showed a preretinal membrane with traction in the papillomacular bundle before the operation. The traction on the intraretinal vessels was relieved after the operation and the retina flattened. The metamorphopsia disappeared and the visual acuity improved. Fluorescein angiography before the operation revealed extensive vascular traction and 4 leakage sites at the posterior pole. Four weeks postoperatively the leakage of fluorscein was unchanged. There was no gross abnormality of the sensory retina. Light microscopy showed a wrinkled membrane which was different from the one of the second patient. The ultrathin sections demonstrated an epiretinal membrane mainly composed of a basement-membrane-like material which is morphologically identical with the inner limiting membrane described by Foos in human eyes. On the surface of this membrane, which is most likely the vitreal surface, a few longitudinally oriented cells were found similar to glial cells.

In some places glial cells interconnected different parts of the membrane with long cell processes. The other surface on the membrane was irregular with accumulation of cell debris. From the tentacle like processes of this side, which looked like remnants of Müller cells, we concluded, that it must be the retinal surface. The EOG was performed 3 times. Before the operation the light rise was 157% being in the lower normal range. One week after the operation the light rise had changed to 143% which is below our 2 standard deviation limit. Four weeks after operation it was back to 154% (Figure 2).

In conclusion we can state that 2 patients with defects of the inner limiting membrane and one patient with spontaneous macular pucker had a membrane peeling operation. All had a decrease in the light-rise in the EOG. A decrease of the light-rise in the EOG and the c-wave has been described before in central retinal artery occlusion. The mechanism by which it is induced remains unclear. Our patients with spontaneous macular pucker did not show any severe pigment epithelial abnormalities. It seems difficult to imagine that potassium changes are responsible for the reduction in light rise.

We would like to suggest a mechanism which is similar to the behaviour of the light rise in vitelliform dystrophy. The ocular dipole may be altered by short circuiting on both sides of the retina diminishing the vector of the dipole due to a small area exhibiting membrane pathology. In our cases with spontaneous repair of the internal limiting membrane the EOG light rise returned to the normal range after a certain time which seems to verify our hypothesis.

REFERENCES

Arden, S. B., Barrada, A. and Kelsey, I. M.: New clinical test of retinal function based upon the standing potential of the eye. Br. J. Ophthalmol. 46, 449–467, 1962.

129

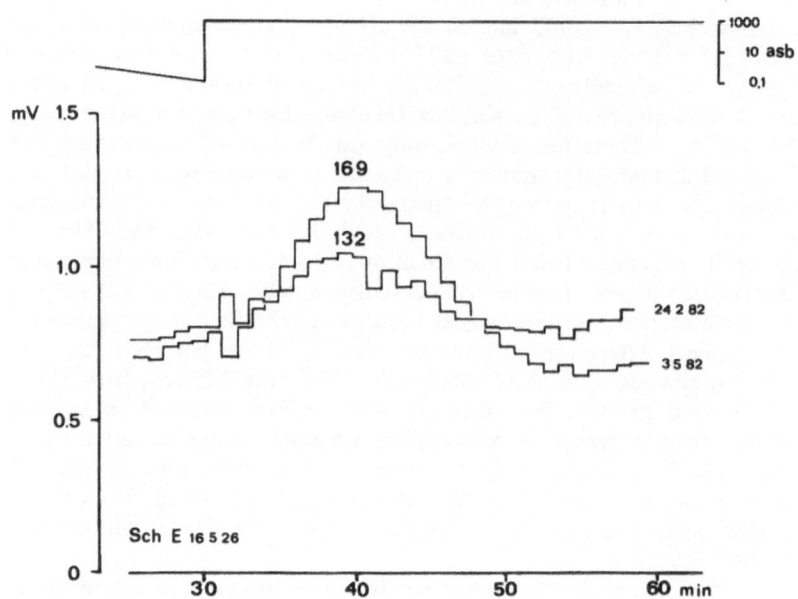

Fig. 2. EOG before and after a membrane peeling operation for spontaneous macular pucker. For details see text.

Gouras, P. and Carr, R. E.: Cone activity in the light induced DC-response of monkey retina. Invest. Ophthalmology 4, 318–324, 1965.

Gouras, P. and Carr, R. E.; Light induced DC-responses on monkey retina before and after central retinal artery interruption. Invest. Ophthalmology 4, 310–317, 1965.

Täumer, R., Rhode, N., Pernice, D. and Kohler, U.: EOG: light test and dark test Albrecht von Graefes Arch. klin. Ophthal. 199, 207–213, 1976.

Thaler, A. and Heilig, P.: EOG and ERG components in ischemic retinopathy Ophthal. Res. 9, 38–46, 1977.

Mailing address:
Universitäts-Augenklinik,
Hufelandstr. 55,
D-4300 Essen,
West Germany.

130

THE FAST OSCILLATION OF THE ELECTRO-OCULOGRAM, AMPLITUDES AND LATENCIES IN THE COURSE OF THE SLOW OSCILLATION

M. R. LESSEL, A. R. G. THALER AND P. HEILIG

(Vienna, Austria)

ABSTRACT

In 10 normal subjects the fast and slow oscillations of the electro-oculogram were elicited simultaneously by repetitive light stimuli. A slow oscillation evoked by continuous light of lower intensity was subtracted from the combined curve by use of a computer program. No influence of the slow oscillation on amplitudes and peak latencies of the fast oscillation could be proven.

INTRODUCTION

The fast oscillation (FO) of the electro-oculogram (EOG) was defined by Kolder and Brecher (1966). It can be recorded in the beginning of the light induced slow oscillation (SO) of the EOG. On-stimulation causes a cornea negative, off-stimulation a cornea positive deflection of the corneoretinal potential. The peak latencies of the FO range from 30 to 45 sec.

The following study was designed in order to determine whether the amplitudes and latencies of the FO are dependent on the time course of the SO.

METHODS

A series of 1 to 3 EOG-tests was performed in 10 ophthalmologically normal subjects. A total of 25 recordings was used for analysis. The recordings were performed in front of a 3/4 sphere of 35 cm diameter providing Ganzfeld-stimulation (Ulbricht sphere). Fluorescent tubes in connection with a stabilization circuity allowed continuously adjustable light intensities. 10 light emitting diodes were mounted equidistantly in the sphere and triggered sequentially serving as fixation aids. Repetitive horizontal eye movements over an angle of $30°$ were performed. A repetition rate of 2.5 sec was controlled by the computer digital output. Silver-silver-chloride electrodes (Beckman 39170) were fixed at the outer and inner canthi. The potentials were amplified $1:10^4$ and fed into a computer (PDP11E10) for further analysis. A return to zero correction was performed at each left-position of the eyes.

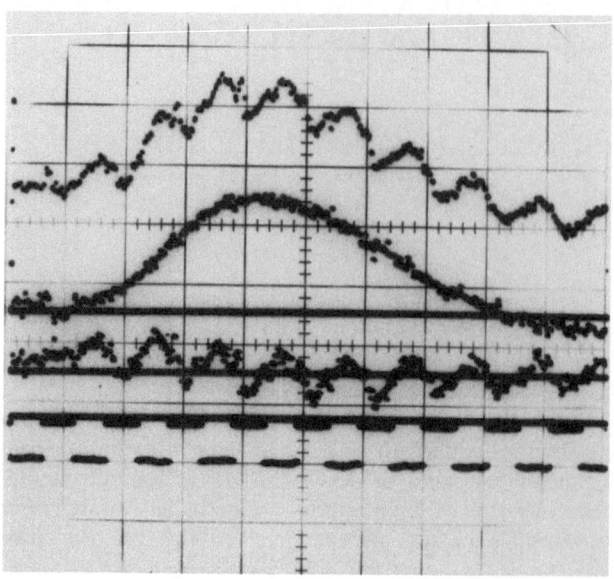

Fig. 1. (A) EOG elicited by repetitive rectangular light- and dark stimuli of 1.1 min duration each and 3000 asb light intensity. (B) EOG elicited by a rectangular light stimulus of 15 min duration and 1000 asb light intensity. (C) Differential curve of A and B. (D) Light stimulus recording of A.

Each recording was preceded by a phase of dark-adaptation of 35 min. Repetitive rectangular light stimuli of 1.1 min duration and 3000 abs intensity were interrupted by dark stimuli of 1.1 min duration. This mode of stimulation elicited a series of FO superimposed on a SO. Before or following the recording of the combined curve a SO was elicited using a continuous light stimulus of 1000 asb (preadaptation to darkness 35 min). The SO was subtracted mathematically from the combined FO-SO-curve off line using a computer program. This procedure resulted in a series of FO exposed to the influence of the SO but not superimposed on it (Figure 1).

RESULTS

The mean values of the amplitudes of the FO during the time course of the SO are shown in Figure 2. Maximal amplitudes were recorded in the first FO. A linear decrease of the amplitudes was observed up to the 20th min. These changes in amplitudes were not correlated to the time course of the standing potential.

The peak latencies of the FO did not change during an observation period of 20 min (Figure 3).

132

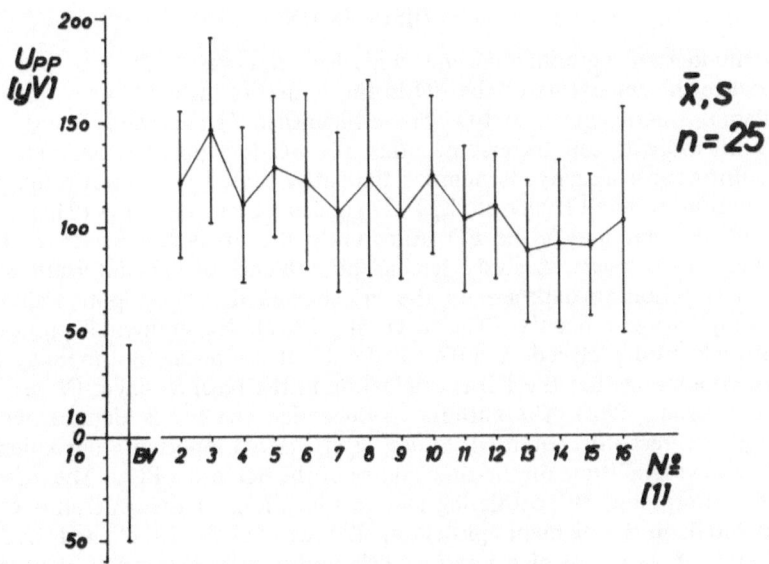

Fig. 2. Mean values ($\bar{x}$) and standard deviations (s) of FO-amplitudes of 25 differential curves (light trough (LT) to dark peak (DP) in μV_{pp} (peak to peak)).
No = number of LT-DP peak to peak values from the beginning of the light stimulus.
BV = base value of steady state.

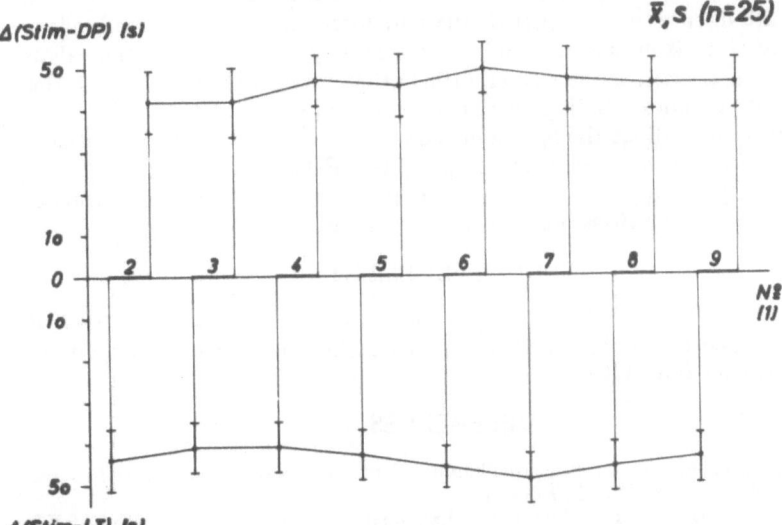

Fig. 3. Mean values ($\bar{x}$) and standard deviations (s) of FO-latencies of 25 differential curves in sec.
Upper curve: Latencies from off-stimulus to DP.
Lower curve: Latencies from on-stimulus to LT.

133

DISCUSSION

A number of experimental and clinical studies was performed in order to localize the generators of the FO in the retina. In night blindness caused by vitamin-A-deficiency the FO was extinguished (Thaler and Heilig, 1979). Conclusively it can be assumed that the FO is dependent on undisturbed photoreceptor activity. Ischemic retinopathy caused by central retina artery occlusion in men (Thaler et al., 1977) and in rhesus monkeys (Thaler et al., 1978) did not impair the FO. Apparently the FO is not influenced by the inner retinal layers. A study testing the influence of light intensity and the pre-adaptation to darkness on the FO showed that these potentials are of photopic origin mainly (Thaler et al., 1982). Experimental studies with microelectrodes placed at different depths of the retina in a monkey led to the conclusion that the FO is originating in the receptor layer (Valeton and van Norren, 1982). The authors assumed that the FO is identical with the cone late receptor potential. Skoog et al. (1974) reported a dependency of the c-wave amplitude on the time course of the SO in the EOG. These findings were interpreted by postulating identical locations of the generators of both potentials in the pigment epithelium. Täumer et al. (1976) elicited the FO by a series of flashes of high intensity. They observed no dependence of the FO on the time course of the SO.

The present study showed no influence of the SO on amplitudes and peak latencies of the FO. These findings are in accordance with the localization of the generators of the FO in the receptor layer.

In indirect recordings of the EOG (using the method of eye movements over a defined angle) the relative amplitudes of the FO are influenced by the level of the light-insensitive part of the corneoretinal potential. The level of the steady state is used as a reference and consequently modifies the calculated FO amplitudes. Rohde et al. (1981) therefore proposed to define the FO in absolute values avoiding relative measurements.

In clinical recordings the light induced increase of the standing potential is of no significance for the calculation of the FO-amplitudes. The FO are predominantly photopic potentials not requiring preadaptation to darkness. Under photopic conditions practically no SO are elicited.

ACKNOWLEDGEMENT

This study was supported by "Fonds zur Förderung der wissenschaftlichen Forschung" and by "Medizinisch wissenschaftlicher Fonds des Bürgermeisters der Bundeshauptstadt Wien".

REFERENCES

Kolder, H., Brecher, G. A.: Fast oscillations of the corneo-retinal potential in man. Arch. Ophthalm. 75: 232–237 (1966).

Rhode, N., Täumer, R., Bleckmann, H.: Examination of the fast oscillation of the corneoretinal potential under clinical conditions. A.v. Graefes Arch. Clin. Exp. Ophthalm. 217: 79–90 (1981).

Skoog, K. O., Nilsson, S. E. G.: The c-wave of the human D.C. registered ERG II. Cyclic variations of the c-wave amplitude. Acta Ophthalm. 52: 1–9 (1974).

Täumer, R., Henning, J., Wolff, L.: Further investigations concerning the fast oscillation of the retinal potential. Biblthca Ophthal. 85: 57–67 (1976).

Thaler, A., Heilig, P., Scheiber, V.: Fast oscillation of the corneoretinal potential in ischemic retinopathy. Ophthalm. Res. 9: 324–328 (1977).

Thaler, A., Snyder, J. E., Kolder, H. E., Hayreh, S. S.: Oscillations of the electrooculogram in experimental ischemic retinopathy. Ophthalm. Res. 10; 283–289 (1978).

Thaler, A., Heilig, P.: Fast and slow EOG oscillations in congenital and acquired night blindness. Ophthalm. Res. 11: 206–211 (1979).

Thaler, A., Lessel, M. R., Heilig, P., Scheiber, V.: The fast oscillation of the electrooculogram. Influence of stimulus intensity and adaptation time on amplitude and peak latency. Ophthalm. Res. 14: 210–214 (1982).

Valeton, J. M., van Norren, D.: Intraretinal recordings of slow electrical responses to steady illumination in monkey: isolation of receptor responses and the origin of the light peak. Vision Res. 22: 393–399 (1982).

Mailing address:
2nd Department of Ophthalmology
University of Vienna
Alserstrasse 4
A-1090 Vienna, Austria

135

THE FAST OSCILLATION OF THE ELECTRO-OCULOGRAM IN SECTORIAL RETINITIS PIGMENTOSA

A. R. G. THALER, M. R. LESSEL AND P. HEILIG

(Vienna, Austria)

ABSTRACT

A series of 9 patients with sectorial retinitis pigmentosa was examined electro-physiologically. The rod components in the ERG (scotopic a- and b-wave) were reduced to approximately 50% of the normal values according to the extent of the retinal changes in the lower half of the fundus. The cone components (photopic a- and b-wave, late receptor potential, d-wave) were impaired to a lesser amount. This is in accordance with the preserved macular area. The slow component in the EOG was reduced to 30% of the normal values. These results suggest a deficiency of the complete retinal pigment epithelium. The fast oscillations of the EOG were reduced to 21% and 11% of the normal values. These findings are contradictory to the theory of Valeton and van Norren (1982) who suggested a common origin of the fast EOG oscillation and the late receptor potential.

INTRODUCTION

Clinical recordings of the fast oscillation (FO) in the electro-oculogram (EOG) in patients with localized retinitis pigmentosa can reveal results which are not consistent with the up to date concept of the origin of this potential.

METHODS

A series of 9 patients with typical sectorial retinitis pigmentosa was examined electrophysiologically. In all patients the ophthalmological visible retinal changes were limited to the lower half of the fundus sparing the macular region. Visual field examination revealed an upper hemianopia. Visual acuity and colour vision were normal. The patients were followed clinically from 1 to 25 years. During this period no involvement of the upper half of the fundi was observed.

The *scotopic ERG* was elicited by rectangular light stimuli of 200 asb and 10 msec duration. Following 5 min of darkness 10 ERG's were evoked and averaged. The *photopic ERG* and the off response were recorded following

Table 1. Mean values ($\bar{x}$) and standard deviation (s) of ERG-amplitudes (in μV) and EOG-amplitudes (in % of the base value) of 9 patients with sectorial retinitis pigmentosa. (d-wave measured from the peak of the following f-wave).

		scotop. a	b	photop. a	b	LRP	off d	SO	FO dark	light
normal values	$\bar{x}$	228	453	76	105	89	39	201	116	82
(n = 50)	s	66	106	14	28	23	15	30	10	7
sect.R.p.	$\bar{x}$	110	216	49	58	54	20	130	103	98
(n = 18)	s	36	92	23	25	19	14	30	20	17
reduction to	%	48	48	65	55	61	52	30	21	11

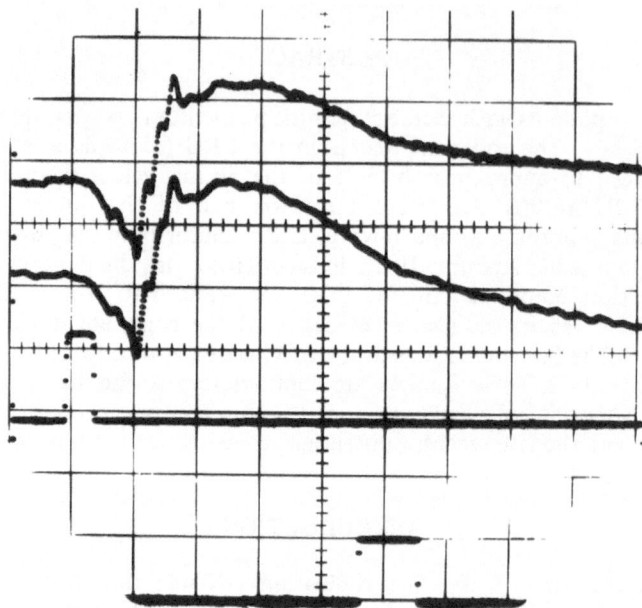

Fig. 1. Scotopic ERG insectorial P.p., Light stimulus 10 msec. Calibration 0.1 mV, 30 msec.

3 min of light adaptation (200 asb intensity). 100 responses were elicited by a rectangular dark-light sequence of 0.3 sec duration each and averaged.

The *slow oscillation* (SO) of the EOG was elicited following 30 min of dark adaptation by a rectangular light stimulus of 3000 asb intensity. The *fast oscillation* (FO) was triggered by rectangular dark-light stimuli of 1.1 min duration each (light intensity 3000 asb). 5 responses were averaged following the recording of the SO.

RESULTS

The mean values of the scotopic a- and b-waves of the patients with sectorial retinitis pigmentosa were reduced to 48% of the normal values (Figure 1).

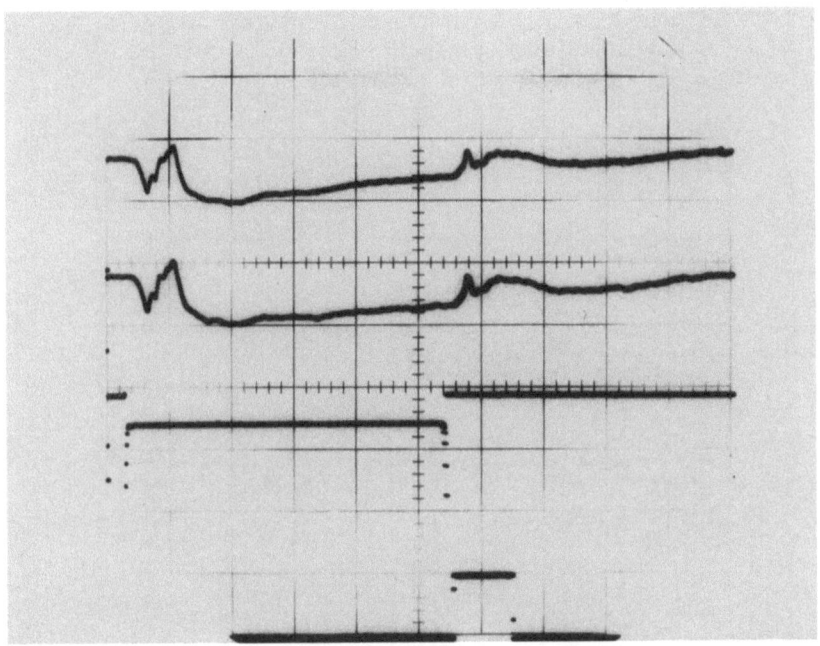

Fig. 2. Photopic ERG in sectorial R.p., Light stimulus 300 msec., Calibration 0.1 mV, 60 msec.

The mean values of the photopic components were impaired to a lesser degree (photopic a-wave 65%, photopic b-wave 55%, d-wave 52% of the normal values) (Figure 2). The level of the negative potential induced by light stimuli of 0.3 sec (cone late receptor potential and D.C. component, Brown K. T., (1968)) was reduced to 61% (Figure 2).

The mean value of the SO in the EOG was reduced to 30% of the normal values (Figure 3), the amplitudes of the FO in darkness (triggered by off stimulation) were reduced to 21%, the amplitudes of the FO in light to 11% compared to the normal values (Figure 4).

DISCUSSION

In sectorial retinitis pigmentosa the amplitudes of the scotopic ERG components are reduced to approximately 50% of the normal values. This reduction is corresponding to the affected fundus area in the equatorial and post-equatorial zone of the fundi. The photopic ERG components are impaired to a lesser amount. These findings can be interpreted by the intact macular regions. The light induced SO of the corneoretinal potential is reduced to a greater amount than expected. These findings suggest that the retinal pigment epithelium of the upper half of the fundus may also be involved in sectorial retinitis pigmentosa (Thaler et al., 1973).

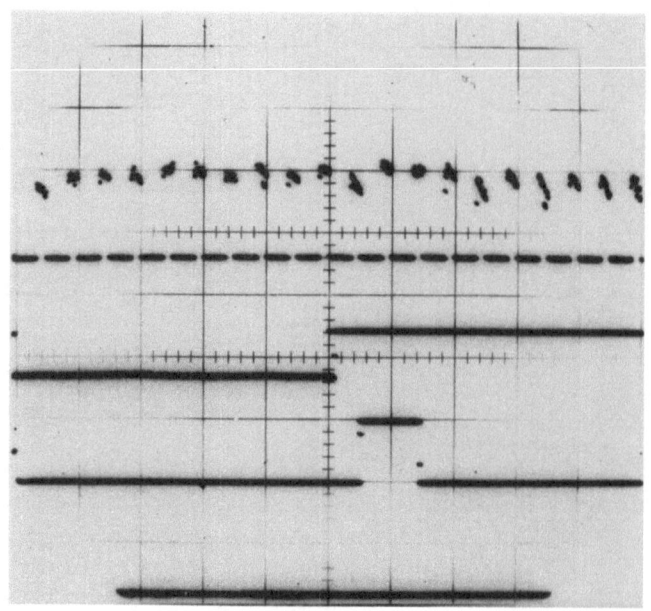

Fig. 3.

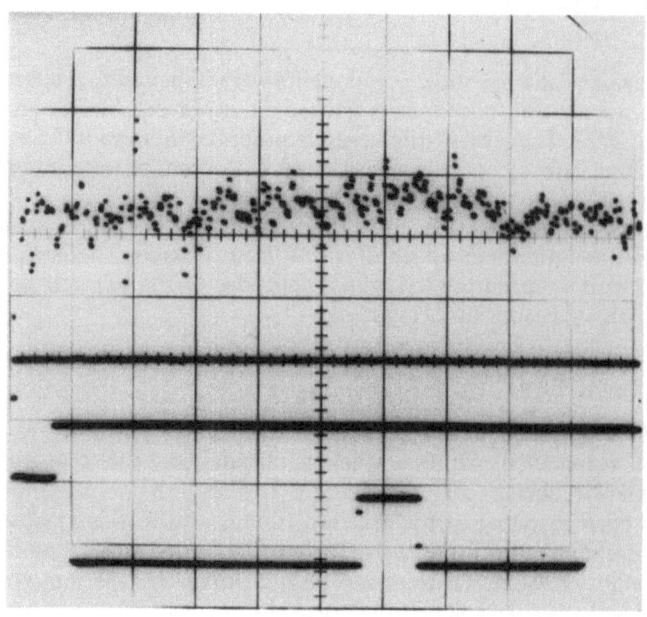

Fig. 4.

The fast oscillation of the EOG was localized at the level of the receptor layer by Valeton and van Norren (1982). The authors assumed that the FO is identical with the cone late receptor potential shaped by the decay of the c-wave and the rise of the light peak of the SO of the corneo-retinal potential. Previous findings are in accordance with this theory. In ischemic retinopathy caused by central retinal artery occlusion the FO is undisturbed (Thaler et al., 1978, a, b). The FO appears not to be dependent on normal functioning inner retinal layers. In night blindness caused by vitamin-A deficiency the FO is extinguished (Thaler and Heilig, 1979). Apparently the FO required normal photopigment activity. The amplitude of the FO is influenced by stimulus intensity but not dependent on dark adaptation time (Thaler et al., 1982). It appears to be primarely a photopic potential. In sectorial retinitis pigmentosa the late receptor potential is preserved to about $\frac{2}{3}$ of the normal values. The FO is virtually extinguished. These results are not in accordance with the assumption that the FO and the cone late receptor potential are representing the same retinal potential.

ACKNOWLEDGEMENT

This study was supported by Fonds zur Förderung der wissenschaftlichen Forschung and by Medizinisch wissenschaftlicher Fonds des Bürgermeisters der Bundeshauptstadt Wien.

REFERENCES

1. Brown, K. T. (1968). The electroretinogram: Its components and their origins. Vision Res. 8: 633–677.
2. Kolder, H., Brecher, G. A. (1966). Fast oscillations of the corneoretinal potential in man. Arch. ophthal. 75: 232–237.
3. Thaler, A., Heilig, P. (1979). Fast and slow EOG-oscillations in congenital and acquired night blindness. Ophthal. Res. 11: 206–211.
4. Thaler, A., Heilig, P., Scheiber, V. (1978). The initial phase of the EOG-oscillation in ischemic retinopathy. Docum. Ophthal. Proceedings Series 15: 151–153.
5. Thaler, A., Heilig, P., Slezak, H. (1973). Sectoral retinopathia pigmentosa. Involvement of the retina and the pigment epithelium as reflected in bioelectric response. Docum. Ophthal. Proceedings Series 2: 237–243.
6. Thaler, A., Snyder, J. E., Kolder, H. E., Hayreh, S. S. (1978). Oscillations of the electroretinogram and electrooculogram in experimental ischemic retinopathy. Ophthal. Res. 10: 283–289.
7. Valeton, J. M., van Norren, D. (1982). Intraretinal recordings of slow electrical responses to steady illumination in monkey: Isolation of receptor responses and the origin of the light peak. Vision Res. 22: 393–399.

Mailing address:
2nd Department of Ophthalmology
University of Vienna
Alserstrasse 4
A-1090 Vienna, Austria

CHANGES OF THE FAST OSCILLATIONS IN DIABETIC RETINOPATHY AND USE OF A NEW COMPUTERIZED EOG DEVICE

H. KURIHARA AND T. NIKARA

(Toyama and Hirosaki, Japan)

ABSTRACT

We made a new computerized automatic device for producing EOG time courses. This device involves recording the potential change produced by an eye movement every ten seconds timed sequentially in a computer memory unit using a conventional AC amplifier. At the end of the recording period the recorded data were compiled by computer print-out as EOG time courses. This device allowed a more detailed investigation of EOG, clearly showing the delayed potential of the c-wave, the second c-wave, the light peak, the dark trough, and the fast oscillation. We recorded the fast oscillation from various grades of diabetic retinopathy.

INTRODUCTION

The ERG and EOG are very important as objective indicators in retinal function. However, electrooculography is not as widely used in routine clinical examinations as electroretinography. The main reason for its unpopularity is the complexity of the procedure and the duration of the EOG test. Recently simplifications of the recording process were made but the results are not fully satisfactory. In this paper, we report on a new semi-automatic recording system for the EOG. We present the characteristics of our instrument and some of the EOG registrations obtained from healthy subjects and patients with diabetic retinopathy.

METHOD

Our recording system is quite movable and composed of a microcomputer housing the data discriminator. The data storage, the time controller, a light control unit which changes the intensity of the illumination of the background, an aiming light spot which evokes an eye movement and the X-Y plotter are indicated.

Figure 1 shows the block diagram of our instrument. The potential changes produced from eye movements are stored in memory after analogue-digital

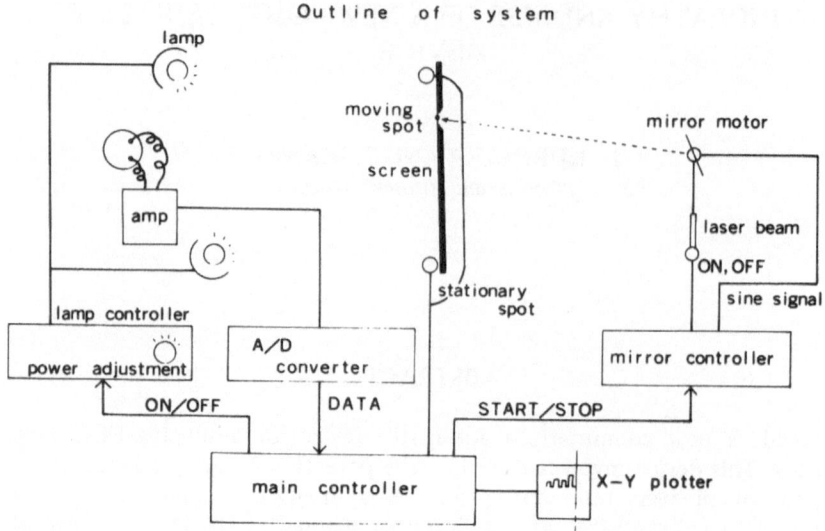

Fig. 1. Block diagram of EOG recording system.

conversion. A laser spot is reflected from a mirror and moves horizontally and sinusoidally. In order to prevent an overshoot of the eye movement, subjects were conditioned by a click to pay attention to the starting point of the laser spot which appeared 200 milliseconds later. The trigger signal for start or stop of the mirror was supplied by the main controller.

Figure 2 shows details of the main controller. It includes the EOG storage unit, the timing unit for starting and stopping the light spot for eye movements, a light adapting controller unit and the drive unit for the X-Y plotter.

Figure 3 shows the time sequence of the instrument. A push button starts the program. A few seconds later, a tone is given to alert the subject for the laser spot. Two hundred milliseconds later both the moving spot unit and the data collecting unit work together.

Figure 4 shows details of the program illustrated in Figure 4. T_1 is set up to 200 milliseconds. T_2 is set to 1, 1.5 or 2.5 seconds. T_3 is between two buzzer signals.

Figure 5 shows the data stored in the memory unit when displayed on the X-Y plotter. Its pen writes 500 uV calibration voltages and indicates when the memory unit is saturated. For the next step, the time course of the EOG potential is written as histogram. We see the EOG potential changes as an imaginary curve connecting the top of the individual EOG signals.

RESULTS

Figure 6 indicates an EOG, obtained from a healthy subject, during dark adaptation and light stimulation with 1000 Lux. We can see clearly not only a dark trough and a light peak but also a tail of the c-wave and the rising

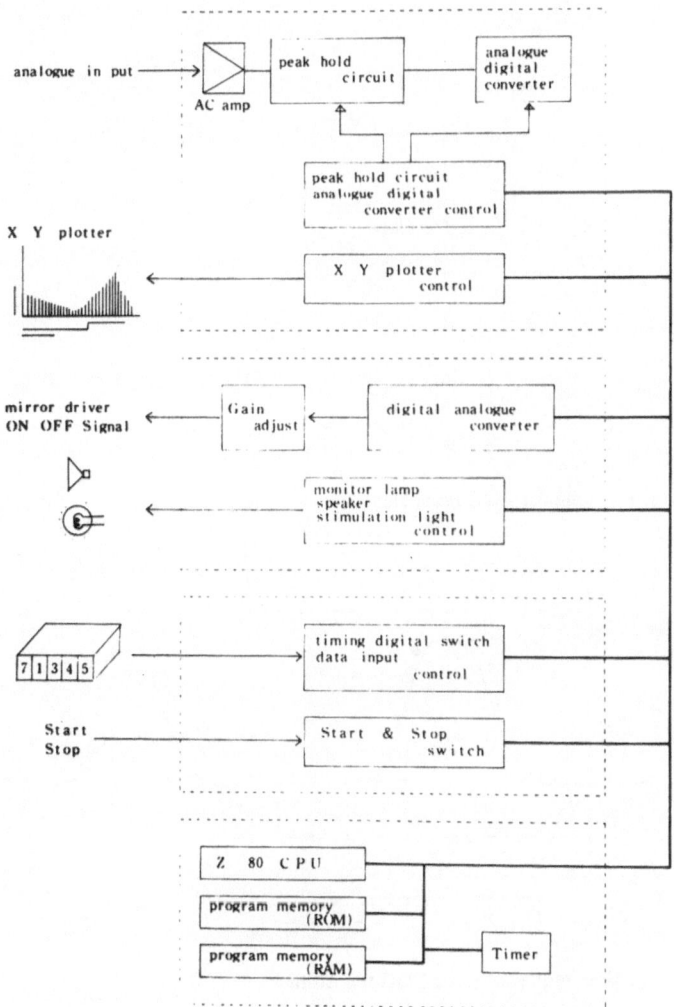

Fig. 2. Internal control unit for EOG recording.

phase of the 2nd c-wave which are hardly recorded using the ordinary recording system.

Table 1 lists average values of the EOG in ten healthy subjects. The value of the dark trough and the light peak fell into the standard range of the EOG in the normal subject.

Figure 7 shows two registrations of the fast oscillation, described by Kolder and Brecher. The fast oscillation on the left was obtained with 45 second light and dark periods, that on the right with 66 second periods.

We reported changes of EOG components in various retino-choroidal

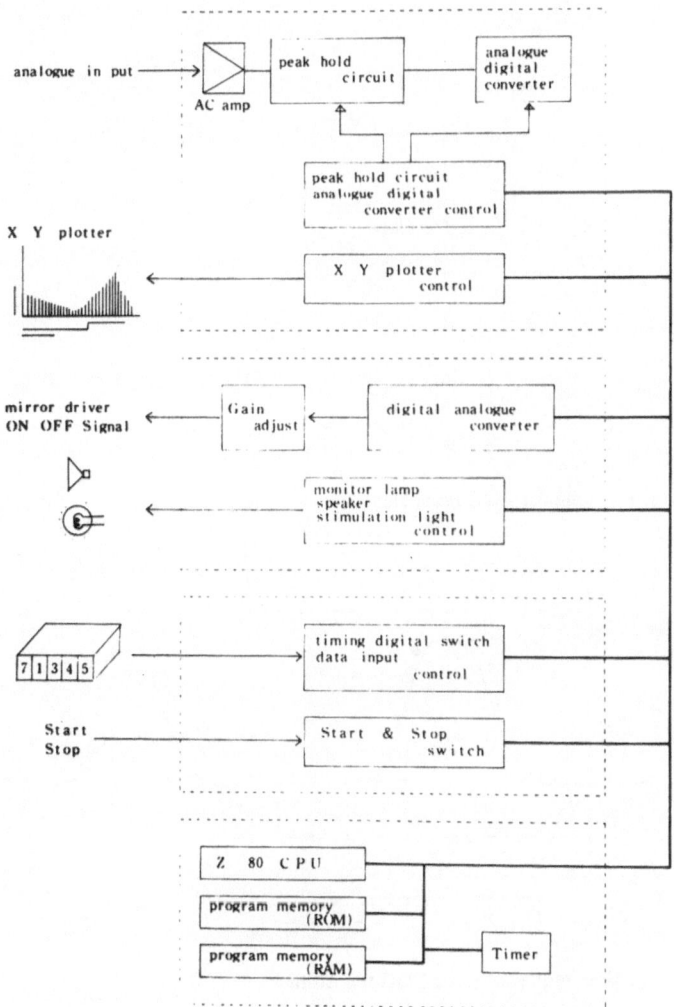

145

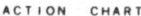

ACTION CHART

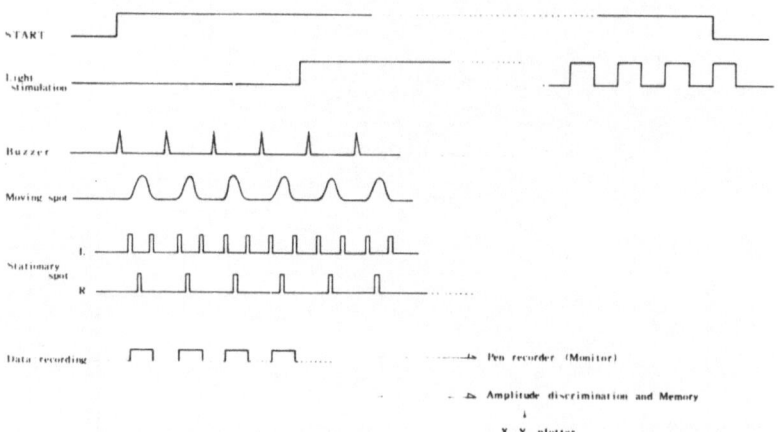

Fig. 3. Time sequencing for EOG recording.

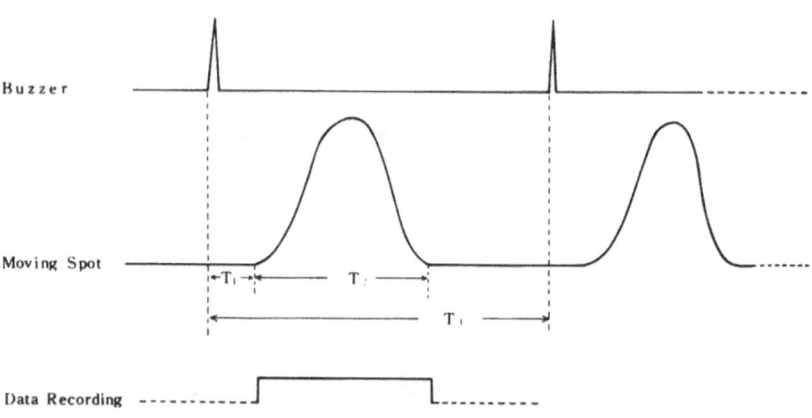

Fig. 4. Details of time sequencing for EOG recording.

diseases. The fast oscillation remained distinct despite the lack of a light rise in patients with diabetic retinopathy of Scott's third grade. We rearranged the severity of diabetic retinopathy into three groups based on Scott's classification of 1953. As shown in Table 2, Group A includes Scott's first and second grades. Group B is a combination of the third and fourth grade of Scott and Group C sums his fifth and sixth grade.

Table 3 lists the appearance and disappearance of the fast oscillation and the light peak in patients with diabetic retinopathy. The more severe the disease, the smaller the amplitude of the fast oscillation and the light peak. For cases in Group B and C, the threshold of the fast oscillation increases with the retinal involvement.

146

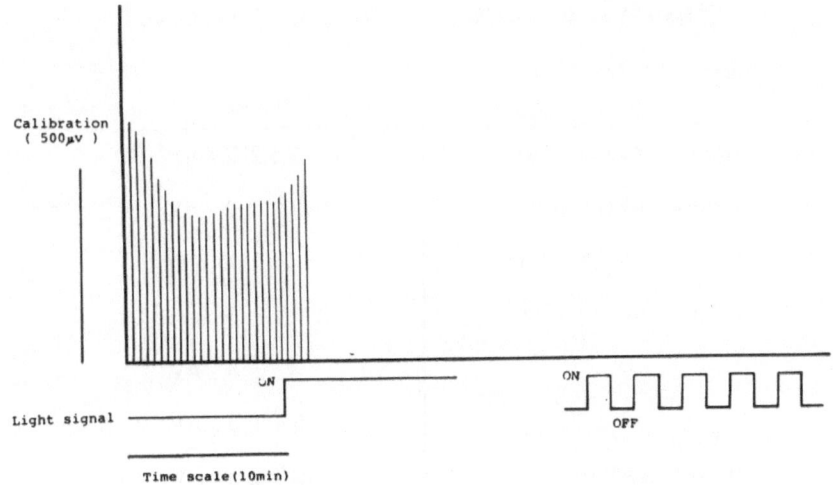

Fig. 5. Schematic record of EOG tracing.

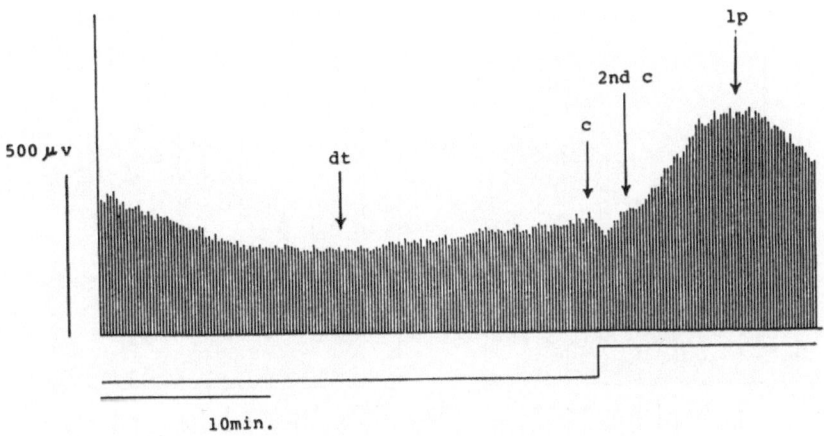

Fig. 6. Actual computer generated EOG tracing.

DISCUSSION

Several publications report improvements of the EOG recording (Henkes, Tazawa, Rhode, et al.). Some methods permit recording the fast oscillation and the slow potential changes simultaneously. Our system was developed for practicality, low noise and moderate cost.

The results in diabetic retinopathy show a positive correlation between the reduction of the first oscillation and the severity of the disease. The diabetic retinopathy progresses from a disturbance of choroidal function to the inner layers of the retina. It is assumed that the activity of the neuroepithelial layer produces the fast oscillation. Therefore, decreases of the

147

Results of EOG in Normal Subjects

	average
Dark trough pot.	352.2 μV
Light peak pot.	900.0 μV
Dark trough time.	12.7 min
Light peak time.	7.0 min
Q	2.6 μV
d	548.6 μV
base value	500.3 μV

Table 1. EOG normative data.

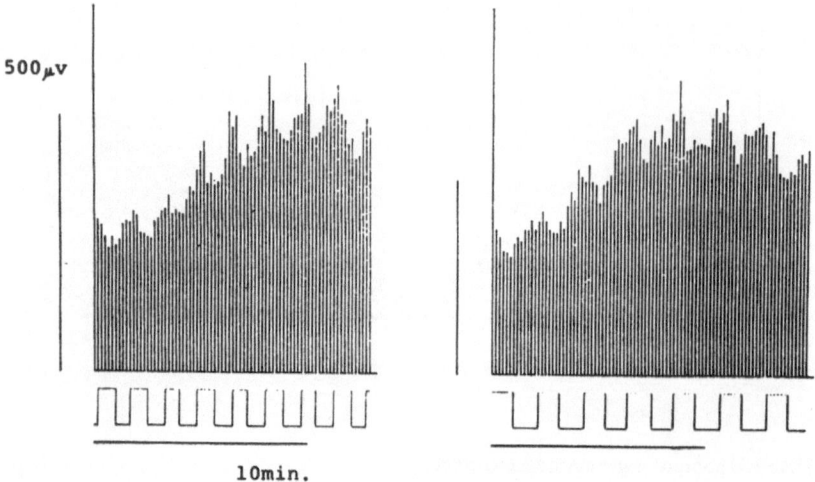

500μv

10min.

Fig. 7. Computer generated record of fast oscillations on EOG.

amplitude of the fast oscillation are significant for the assessment of the progression of diabetic retinopathy.

REFERENCES

Kolder, H. and Brecher, G. A.: Fast oscillations of the corneo-retinal potential in man. Arch. Ophthal, 75, 232–237, 1965.
Kolder, H. and North, A. W.: Oscillations of the corneo-retinal potential in animals. Ophthalmologica 152, 149–160, 1966.

Classification of diabetic retinopathy

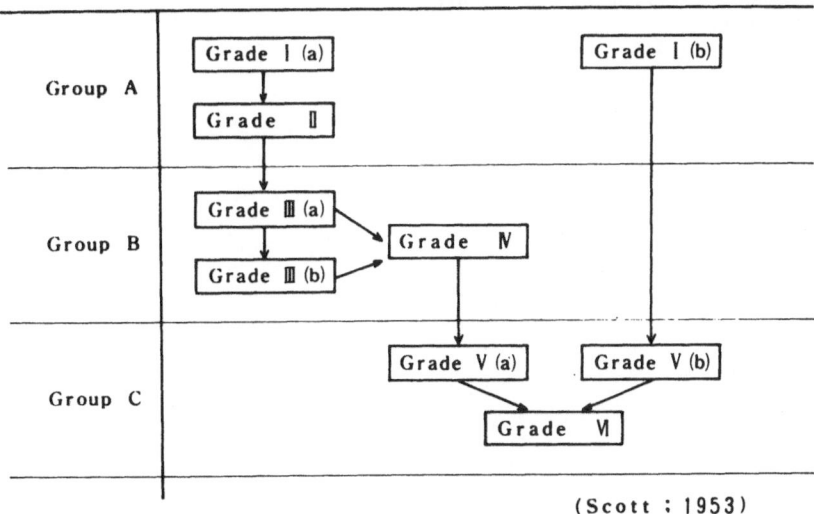

(Scott : 1953)

Table 2. Classification scheme of diabetic retinopathy.

Group	Apperance of fast oscillation			Amplitude of EOG light rise peak
	500 lux	1000 lux	1500 lux	
Normal subject	+	+	+	high
A	+	+	+	high
B	−	+	+	lower
C	−	−	+	invisible

Table 3. Summary data for slow and fast oscillations of the EOG on diabetic retinopathy.

Nikara, T. et al.: Clinical observation of the 2nd c-wave in various retinal diseases., Invest. Ophthalmol. Vis. Sci. in Press, 1982.

Nikara, T. et al.: A new wave (2nd c-wave) of the corneoretinal potential. Experimentia, 32: 594–595, 1976.

Henkes, H. E., et al.: Electro-oculography. A semi-automatic recording procedure. Br. J. Opthalmol., 52: 122–126, 1968.

Rohde, N., Täumer, R. & Bass, F.: An EOG computer and stimulator for the investigation of the slow retinal potential. Bibl. Ophthalmol., 85: 75–83, 1976.

Mailing address:
Department of Ophthalmology
Toyama Medical and Pharmaceutical University
2630 Sugitani
Toyama, 930–01, Japan

VARIABILITY OF THE HUMAN C-WAVE

P. A. HOCK AND M. F. MARMOR

(Stanford and Palo Alto, California, U.S.A.)

ABSTRACT

C-waves recorded from normal subjects showed large variability not only between individuals, but for the same individual on different days and within a single recording session. C-wave time-to-peak, in contrast, was relatively stable. Recordings from patients with Stargardt's disease and congenital stationary night blindness exemplify the problem of judging c-wave normality.

Possible sources of the amplitude variability are discussed. Appropriate stimuli may maximize the possibility of eliciting a recordable c-wave or of defining a relative c-wave index, and thus facilitate use of the c-wave in the analysis of retinal disease.

The c-wave of the ERG may have application as a clinical test of the integrity of the RPE. For such a test to be useful we must first be aware of the normal variability of the c-wave. Considerable variability between subjects has been documented by several groups: some normal subjects appear to lack c-waves, and c-wave amplitude varies with changes in the standing potential (Skoog and Nilsson, 1974; Täumer et al., 1976; Marmor, Pockrand and Lurie, 1979). Previous studies have not, however, addressed the question of variation within a recording session or between recording sessions for the same subject. We find that c-wave amplitudes vary widely within individual subjects, and this lack of constancy confounds the problem of making comparisons between individuals. To exemplify the difficulties of making clinical judgements with the c-wave, we present data from one patient with Stargardt's disease and one with congenital stationary night blindness.

METHODS

The recording lens consisted of either a flexible self-adherent plano-concave contact lens (Skia Corp., Saratoga, CA) with a non-polarizable Ag-AgCl pellet embedded within it (Marmor and Hock, 1982), or a Burian-Allen lens with an Ag-AgCl pellet added. Ag-AgCl skin electrodes (Beckman) on the forehead and hand served respectively as reference and ground. Signals were dc-amplified (Gould Universal Amplifier with patient isolation), fed through a

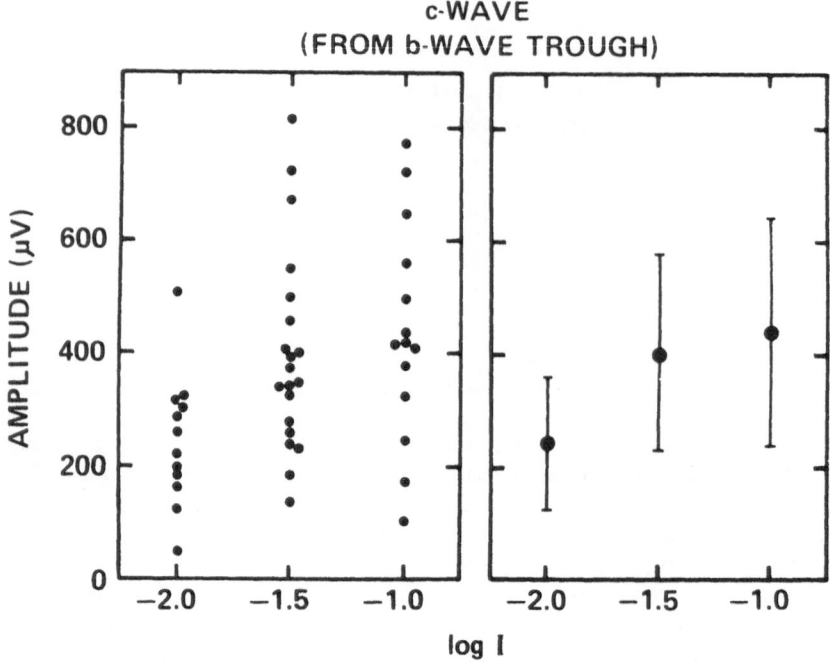

Fig. 1. C-wave amplitudes from 22 normal subjects, at different stimulus intensities. Stimulus duration was 1 sec. Left: Each point represents the average of the responses from one subject during their first recording session. Right: Means of the data on the left ± 1 standard deviation.

60 cycle notch filter (Mentor F-60), and displayed on a paper recorder. Two LED's served as a fixation target. Light from a 100 watt quartz iodide lamp passed through neutral density filters and an electronic shutter (Vincent Associates) and was conveyed by fiberoptics in a ping-pong diffuser close to the eye. The full intensity white light averaged 1.9×10^3 uW/cm^2 at the cornea. All data shown here were obtained with 1 sec flashes presented at 1 min intervals.

All recordings were made with the eye fully dilated (1% tropicamide plus $2\frac{1}{2}$% phenylephrine, or equivalent), after a minimum of 30 min dark adaptation. The self-adherent lens was used over a soft contact lens, with a wire speculum inserted to minimize lid movement.

RESULTS

The *mean* c-wave amplitudes and times-to-peak obtained during the *first* recording session from 22 normal subjects are shown in Figure 1. C-wave amplitude increased monotonically with intensity, but varied widely at each of three intensities studied. The times-to-peak also increased with stimulus intensity (Figure 2), but showed much less variability across subjects.

152

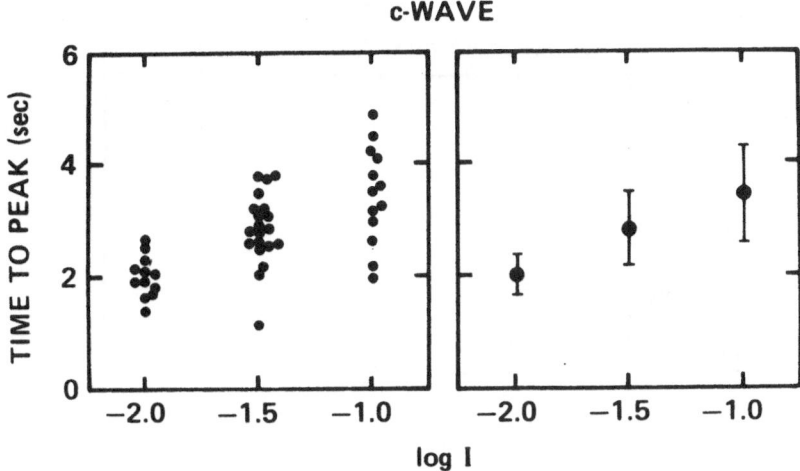

Fig. 2. C-wave times-to-peak from 22 normal subjects, to the same stimuli as in Figure 1. Left: Each point represents the average of the responses from one subject. Right: Means of the data on the left ± 1 standard deviation.

To determine how much of this variability was intra-rather than inter-subject, we analyzed the stability of c-wave amplitudes elicited by a -1.5 log intensity stimulus in the same subject from day to day, and on the same day. Figure 3 shows the session *means* on different days for three individuals chosen as examples because they have moderate (A), small (B), and large (C) c-waves. Note that the c-wave amplitude can vary considerably from session to session. Figure 4 shows that there can also be considerable variation within a single recording session. The subject illustrated, who had the greatest variability in our series, appeared to lack a recognizable c-wave at some times during the session and to have moderate amplitude c-waves at other times. Most subjects did not show this degree of instability and in general, subjects with larger c-waves showed less obvious fluctuations in amplitude. Among 22 subjects shown in Figure 1, variability about the mean value for a session ranged from 11 uV to 146 uV with a median of 50 uV (-1.0 log I), 63 uV (-1.5 log I) and 27 uV (-2.0 log I).

C-wave recordings were also made from two patients with retinal disease. The first was a 28 year old woman with macular Stargardt's disease and a normal conventional ERG. Her c-waves (Figure 5A) appear to be normal. The second was a 40 year old man with myopia and congenital night blindness; his photopic ERG was relatively normal, but his scotopic ERG showed a large a-wave without any rod b-wave. His c-waves (Figure 5B) had low amplitude and a rather prolonged time course.

DISCUSSION

When c-waves are recorded from a large group of normal subjects over a moderate range of stimulus intensities (Figure 1) the amplitude variability is

153

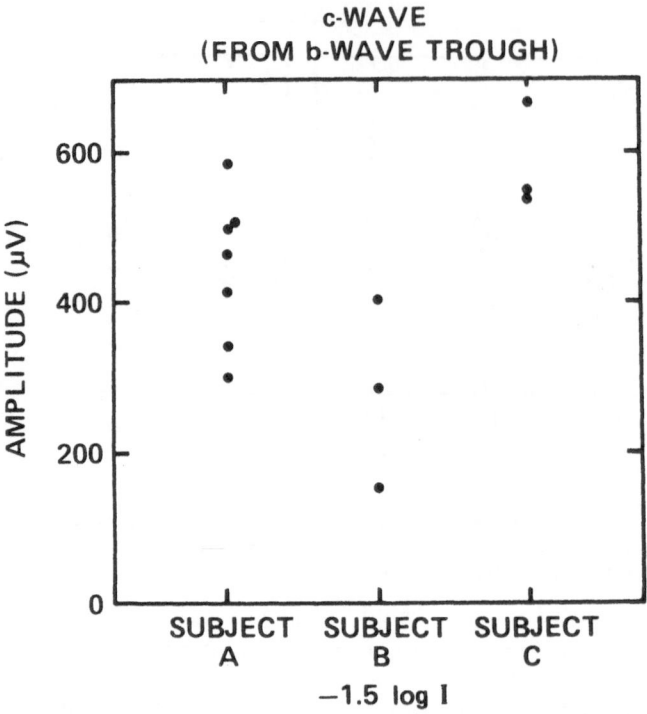

Fig. 3. Day-to-day variability in c-wave amplitude, for three subjects (A, B, C). Each point represents the mean of the responses on a different day. All stimuli were −1.5 log intensity and 1 sec duration.

quite large, as noted previously by several groups. One factor contributing to this interpersonal variability must be the variability in each individual's response amplitude within a session and from one day to the next (Figures 3 and 4).

To consider possible causes for the variability within individuals, it is important to recognize the complex nature of the corneally recorded c-wave. The major positive component is generated by the apical RPE cell membrane in response to K^+ changes originating at the photoreceptors (Steinberg et al., 1970; Oakley et al., 1977), and is influenced by changes at the basal RPE cell membrane responsible for the light rise of the standing potential (Linsenmeier and Steinberg, 1982). The c-wave results from the sum of a large RPE component, a large corneal negative component which is probably generated by the Mueller cells in response to the same K^+ changes (slow PIII) and possibly smaller retinal components of unknown origin (Faber, 1969; Lurie and Marmor, 1982). Even a small percentage change in the RPE or slow PIII components could result in a very large change of the summated c-wave amplitude.

Day-to-day variations in c-wave amplitude may well result from a changing balance between these factors. For example within a recording session, the

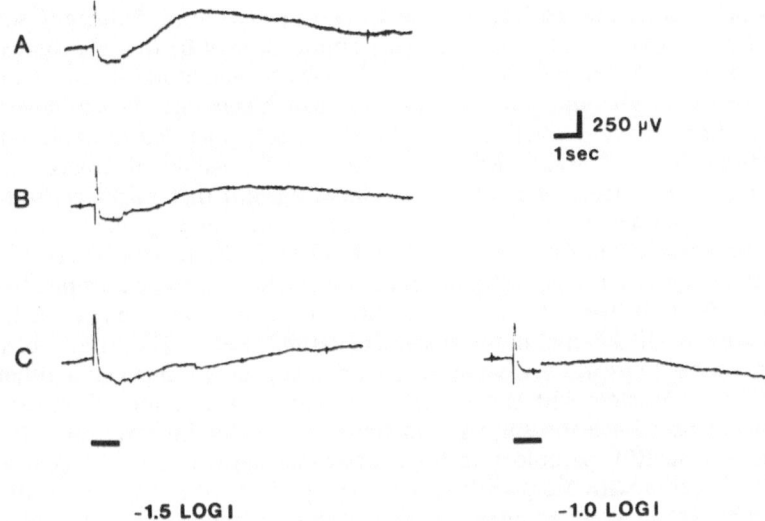

Fig. 4. Within-session variability in the c-wave. These records are all from one subject, and were obtained during the same recording session. The c-waves on the left were elicited by stimuli of the same intensity (−1.5 log unit) and duration (1 sec) Increasing the intensity to −1.0 log unit (right) did not necessarily restore a large c-wave.

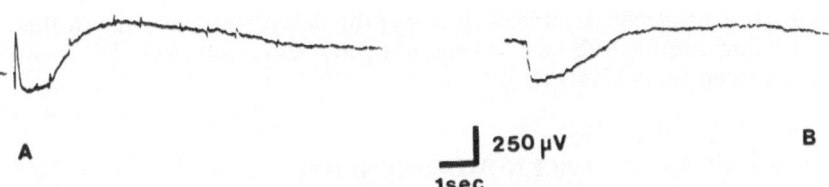

Fig. 5. C-waves in retinal disease. Stimuli were −1.5 log intensity and 1 sec duration. (A) macular Stargardt's disease. (B) congenital stationary night blindness with myopia.

presence of slow oscillations of the standing potential would cause a fluctuation of the c-wave. However, changes in the standing potential cannot account for the variability we report here, since the EOG measured under the same stimulating conditions used to elicit c-waves does not show this variation (Hock and Marmor, in preparation). A more likely explanation for our results is that we have chosen a stimulus intensity (−1.5 log I) which lies at a steep portion of the response-intensity function (i.e. mid-way between the threshold and maximal responses). Minor changes in illumination or adaptation (e.g., from movement, shifts in attentiveness, etc.) would have greater effect using our protocol than using others with higher intensity stimuli.

This variability in amplitude, such that even normal subjects may appear to lack a c-wave on some occasions, confounds the definition of normal and the evaluation of ocular pathology. Several solutions to this problem are possible. A carefully selected stimulus protocol may maximize the probability of eliciting a measureable c-wave. Higher intensity stimuli may help, but at

155

some price of greater patient discomfort and movement, and possibly some loss of sensitivity to pathology. Another approach may be to use a comparative index. For example, the *increase* of c-wave amplitude during a light response of the standing potential may be quantifiable regardless of whether the baseline c-wave is small or large. Further work is needed to explore the conditions of adaptation, light stimulation, and possibly pharmacological alteration (e.g. effects of alcohol or osmotic agents) that might generate a comparative c-wave index. When a c-wave is present, time-to-peak may also be a useful measure since it is more constant within and among subjects. However, the clinical relevence of c-wave time-to-peak has yet to be documented.

Records from two patients are presented in Figure 5 as examples of how the c-wave might be used in the analysis of retinal disease. The c-waves of the patient with Stargardt's disease show no evidence of pigment epithelial pathology, consistent with the normal appearance of her peripheral retina; we would not have been too surprised to find abnormality, however, since there is wide spread RPE pathology in fundus flavimaculatus which falls clinically on a continuum with Stargardt's disease. The patient with congenital stationary night blindness might appear at first glance to lack a recordable c-wave. However, if only the RPE component were absent, the DC-ERG should resemble the slow PIII (a long deep negative potential) and if both RPE and PIII components were absent the ERG should return promptly to baseline after the a-wave. The response obtained was somewhere in between these extremes. We do not know if the low c-wave amplitude is compatible with a healthy RPE or always signifies pathology; the delayed time-to-peak in this patient might suggest RPE involvement, but could also result from changes in the photoreceptors or slow PIII.

ACKNOWLEDGEMENT

Supported in part by National Eye Institute Grant EY01678 and by the Medical Research Section of the Veterans Administration.

REFERENCES

Faber, D. S. Analysis of the slow transretinal potentials in response to light. Ph.D. Thesis, State University of New York, Buffalo (1969).

Linsenmeier, R. A. and Steinberg, R. H. Origin and sensitivity of the light peak of the intact cat eye. *J. Physiol.:* in press (1982).

Lurie, M. and Marmor, M. F. Similarities between the c-wave and slow PIII in the rabbit eye. Invest. Ophthalmol. Vis. Sci. 19:1113–1117 (1980).

Marmor, M. F. and Hock, P. A. A practical method for c-wave recording in man. XVIII. ISCEV Symposium Doc. Ophthalmol. Proceedings Series, 13:67–72 (1982).

Marmor, M. F., Pockrand, P. and Lurie, M. Experiments toward the development of a clinical c-wave test. Proc. 16th ISCEV Symp., Morioka 24–28 May 1978, pp. 107–111. Japanese J. Opthal., Japan (1979).

Oakley, II, B., R. H. Steinberg, S. S. Miller and S. E. G. Nilsson: The in vitro frog pigment epithelial cell hyperpolarization in response to light. Invest. Ophthalmol. Vis. Sci. 16:771–774 (1977).

156

Skoog, K. O. and Nilsson, S. E. G. The c-wave of the human DC registered ERG. II. Cyclic variations of the c-wave amplitude. Acta Ophthal. 52:904–912 (1974).

Täumer, R., Wichmann, W., Rohde, N. and Röver, J. ERG of humans without c-wave. Albrecht von Graefes Arch. Klin. Ophthalmol. 198:275–289 (1976).

Mailing address:
Ophthalmology Section (112B1)
Veterans Administration Medical Center
3801 Miranda Avenue
Palo Alto, California 94304, U.S.A.

157

WHAT DOES THE c-WAVE TELL US IN RETINAL DISEASES?

J. RÖVER, M. MACK AND G. OSCHWALD

(Freiburg, West Germany)

ABSTRACT

The c-wave and the EOG both potentials of pigment epithelial origin show in most diseases a parallel behaviour. However, differences are seen in cases of Best's vitelliform macular degeneration, where the c-wave reflects more subtle affections of the pigment epithelium in carriers than the EOG. Thus, with a reliable recording procedure and a collaborative patient, recording the DC-ERG provides the most important information about the retina including the pigment epithelial layer.

INTRODUCTION

The c-wave is a slow retinal component proven in animals to reflect very closely the function of the retinal pigment epithelium (Marmor et al. 1979, Niemeyer 1976). Since 1978 we have routinely performed DC-ERG recordings in all patients suspected of pigment epithelial diseases in order to eventually establish a quick and reliable electrodiagnostic parameter (Röver et al. 1982).

METHODS

A 315 cd/m² light stimulus is presented for 200 ms in a hemisphere above the patient's eye. Slightly more than 180° of the patient's visual field is covered. The signals are DC-recorded via suction cups on the cornea and on the forehead by means of silver- silverchloride electrode half cells. Before recording, the patient is dark adapted for 20 min, and 3 min of dark adaptation precede each further stimulus.

The normal mean amplitude of the a-wave was $167\,\mu$V, of the b-wave $528\,\mu$V and of the c-wave $464\,\mu$V. The light rise of the EOG, recorded in a conventional manner, was 112% of the average of the dark through (Pernice et al. 1976).

RESULTS

DC-ERG's were recorded from 165 patients with retinal diseases as listed in the following table.

Vitelliform macular degeneration	36
Flecked retina	45
Rod-cone degeneration	17
Cone dysfunction	10
Toxic lesion	8
Other retinal diseases	12
Hereditary choroidal degenerations	12
Other choroidal diseases	25
	165

We selected 7 clinical entities, which are known to affect the pigment epithelium severely. With these data I hope to convince you, that the c-wave reflects the function of the pigment epithelium as closely as the conventional EOG.

The first disease is vitelliform macular degeneration or Best's disease. The electrodiagnostic recordings show normal a- and b-waves, but a severe reduction of the c-wave in comparison to the normal values as given by the open columns of Figure 1. This reduction was significantly correlated to the well known reduction of the light peak of the EOG (Nilsson et al. 1980, Röver et al. 1980, Weingeist et al. 1980).

Five out of 12 female members of a family, in which a dominantly inherited vitelliform macular degeneration was found showed a very faint mottling of the macular pigment epithelium. In spite of minimal clinical findings, they produced clearly reduced c-waves although the EOG light peak was within the normal range. However, in these five female patients, the differences of the c-wave and the EOG, when compared to the normal values, were not significant (Figure 2). In spite of that we may draw the conclusion, that the c-wave has a higher sensitivity in detecting slight disorders of the pigment epithelium, found in carriers (Deutman 1969).

The second retinal disease I wish to discuss is juvenile macular degeneration, a disease closely related to fundus flavimaculatus and Stargardt's disease. We define juvenile macular degeneration according to the criteria given by Krill. Only the macula is involved, pigment epithelial irregularities are visible and the visual acuity is reduced (Krill 1977). In our patients the a- and b-wave was normal. The c-wave significantly correlated with the reduction of the EOG (Figure 3). We further found that the impairment of the visual function was accompanied by a reduction of the slow potentials, indicating that the involved area might be larger than ophthalmoscopically visible. (Pearce 1975). These findings are similar to those in vitelliform macular degeneration, where we found a very pronounced reduction of the slow potentials reflecting vast pigment epithelial dysfunction without receptor involvement.

160

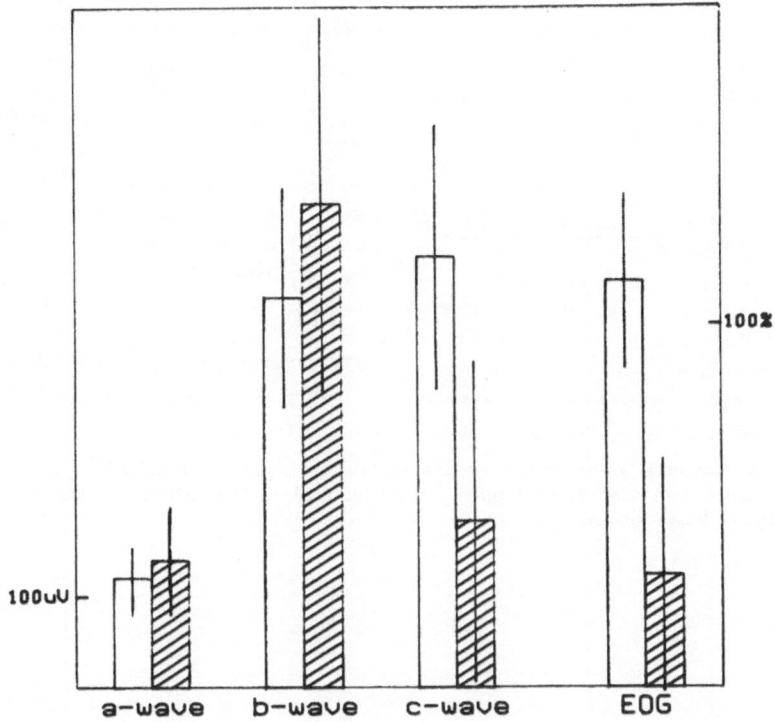

Vitelliform macular degeneration (n=26)

Fig. 1. Mean amplitudes and standard deviations a-, b- and c-wave given in uV and of the light rise of the EOG given in percentage of the base value. Open columns indicate the values of normals, shaded columns of affected subjects. A clear cut reduction of the c-wave and the EOG is visible in patients with Best's disease.

The third disease which we examined is fundus flavimaculatus, which leaves the macula and the visual acuity intact (Eagle 1980). We could only collect a few patients with this disease. They showed a normal a-, b- and c-wave and a close to normal EOG (Figure 4). Here, too, the amplitudes of the two slow retinal potentials were significantly correlated.

The fourth dysfunction of the retina is Stargardt's disease, where both the macula and the perimacula are affected (Noble et al. 1979). Again, as expected from the findings in fundus flavimaculatus, we found a correlation between the values of the c-wave and the EOG. However the mean values of the c-wave and EOG are lower than those in fundus flavimaculatus even though the affected retinal area is ophthalmoscopically larger (Figure 5).

The fifth disease examined is dominantly inherited macular drusen. From the pathologic findings, the pigment epithelium is the structure predominantly

161

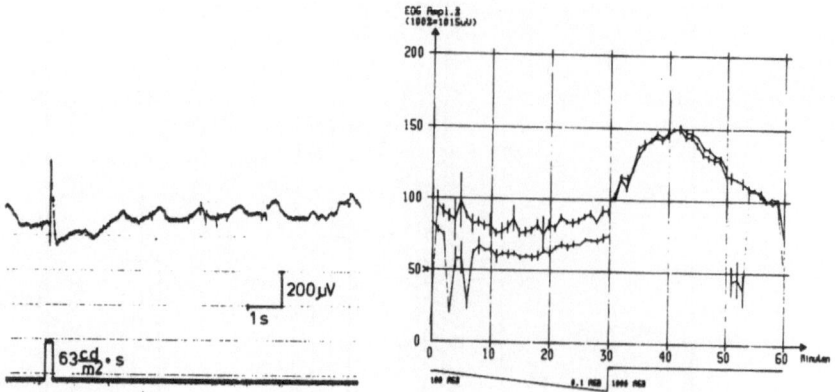

Fig. 2. Normal a- and b-, but a significantly lowered c-wave in the DC ERG (left tracing) associated with a slight reduction of the light peak of the EOG (right tracings) in a carrier of Best's disease.

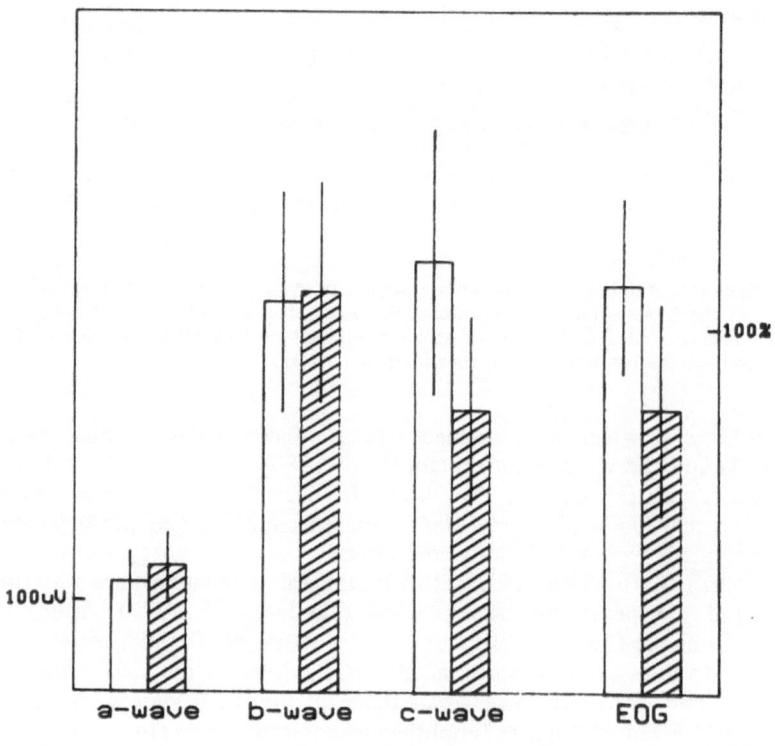

Fig. 3. Reduced c-wave and EOG in juvenile macular degeneration.

162

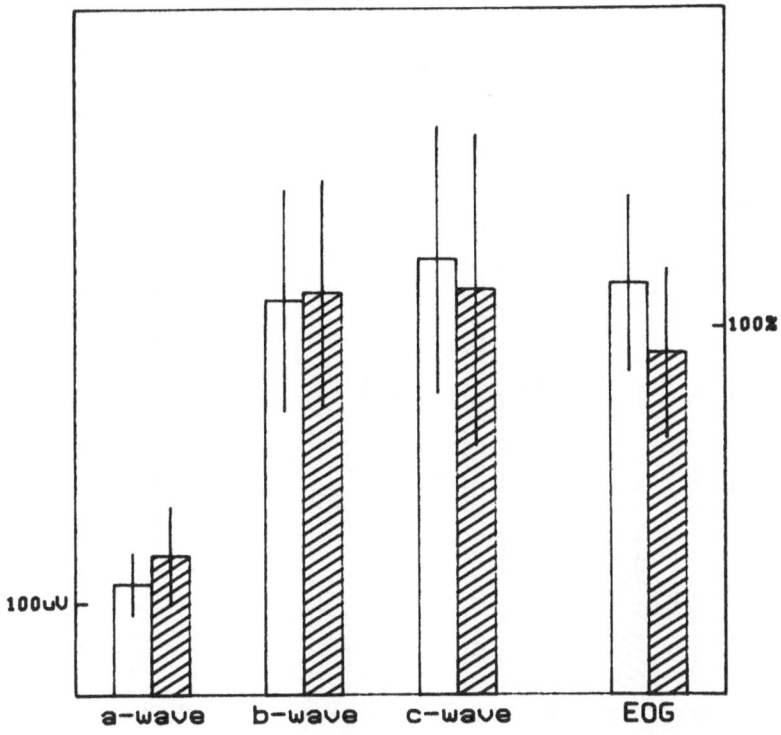

100%

100uV

a-wave   b-wave   c-wave   EOG

Fundus flavimaculatus (n=5)

Fig. 4. Normal a- and b-waves and close to normal c-waves correlated to a normal EOG in patients with fundus flavimaculatus.

involved (Newell et al. 1972). Here again we find a reduction of the c-wave correlated with the lowered EOG. Note that the a- and b-waves are normal (Figure 6).

The next disease group comprises different choroidal atrophies. In these dysfunctions of all retina layers, the reduction of the c-wave is not only correlated to the amplitude of the EOG, but also to the amplitude of the b-wave and to the area of the affected retina (Figure 7).

Let me finally draw your attention to a disease much discussed in recent literature: The bird shot retinopathy, synonymous with vitiliginous chorioretinitis (Gass 1981). We had the opportunity to examine a patient repetitively during the progression of this disease. We found severely diminished a-, b- and c-waves and a reduced EOG even during the early stage of the disease. This would suggest that the pigment epithelium may be the structure most heavily involved, the choriocapillary layer, however, is affected severely and simultaneously, along with changes in the pigment epithelium. Therefore, it appears that the pigment epithelium and the overlying retina is regionally

163

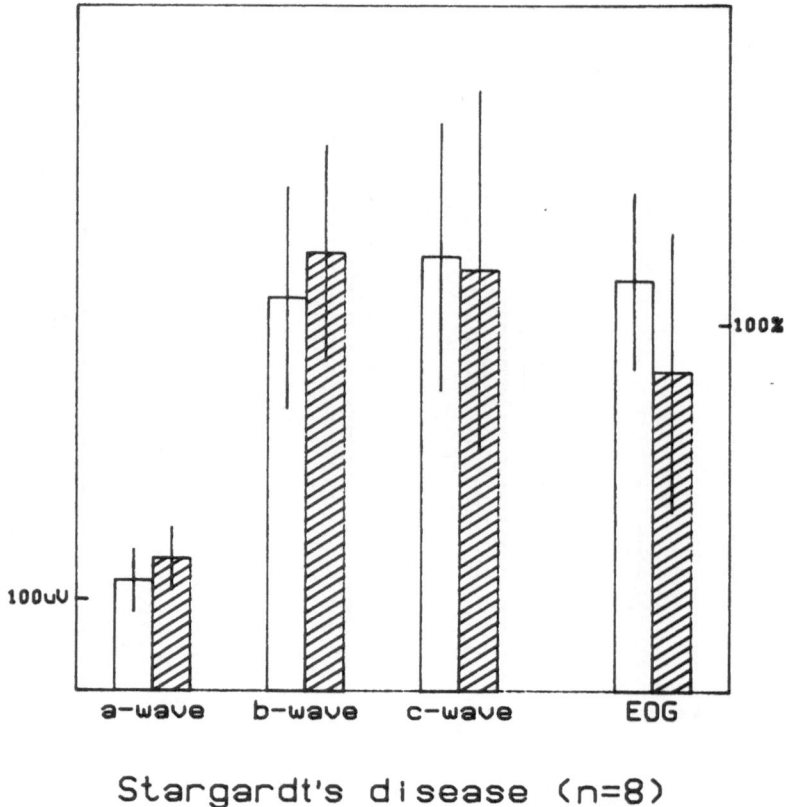

Stargardt's disease (n=8)

Fig. 5. No significant changes of the retinal potentials in Stargardt's disease.

completely destroyed, quite different from vitelliform macular degeneration for example (Figure 8).

Figure 9 gives a summary of our findings, indicating that in most cases the reduction of the c-wave and the EOG is closely correlated.

CONCLUSIONS

We have shown with our recording procedure, that the c-wave reflects the function of the pigment epithelium about equally well — may be sometimes with an higher sensitivity — than the EOG. Therefore we propose to record the c-wave for two reasons. First: In many cases the DC-ERG allows a recording of the most important electrodiagnostic data of the retina and the pigment epithelium within a single session. And secondly: The c-wave seems to detect even subclinical changes of the pigment epithelium when the EOG is still normal.

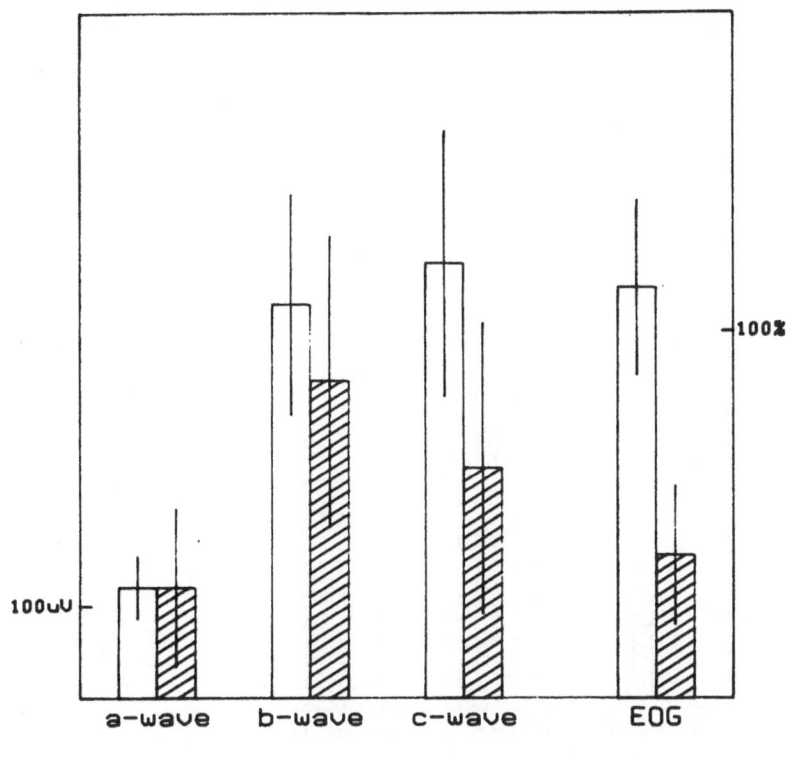

Dominant Drusen (n=7)

Fig. 6. Normal a- and b- waves in hereditary drusen, but severely reduced amplitudes of the c-wave and the EOG.

ACKNOWLEDGEMENT

Supported by Deutsche Forschungsgemeinschaft SFB 70.

REFERENCES

Deutmann, A. F.: Electrooculography in families with vitelliform dystrophy of the fovea: detection of the carrier state. Arch Ophthalmol. 81, 305–316, 1969

Eagle, R. C., Lucier, A. C., Bernhardino, J. R. and Yanoff, M.: Retinal pigment epithelial abnormalities in fundus flavimaculatus. A light and electron microscopic study. Ophthalmology 87, 1189–1200, 1980

Gass, J. D. M.: Vitiligenous chorioretinitis. Arch. Ophthalmol. 99, 1778–1787, 1981

Marmor, M. F. and Lurie, M.: Light induced electrical responses of the retinal pigment epithelium. In: The retinal pigment epithelium. Eds: Zinn, K. M. and Marmor, M. F. 226–246, Harvard Univ. Press Cambridge USA 1979

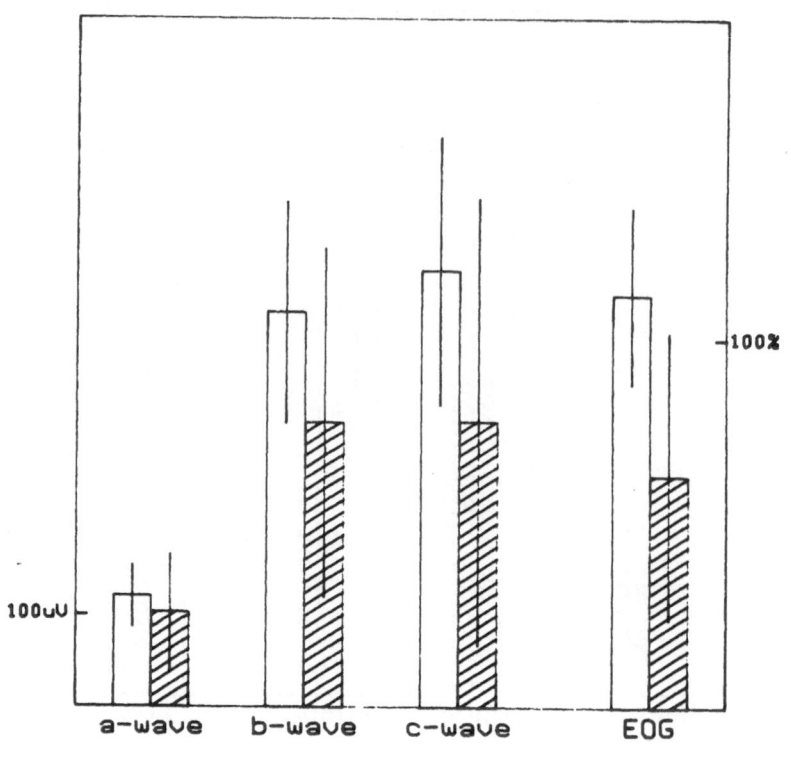

−100%

100uV

a-wave　　b-wave　　c-wave　　　　EOG

Choroidal Atrophies (n=8)

Fig. 7. Lowered amplitudes of the a-, b- and c-waves and the EOG in choroidal atrophies.

Newell, F. W., Krill, A. E. and Farkas, F. G.: Drusen and fundus flavimaculatus: clinical, functional and histological characteristics. Trans. Am. Acad. Ophthalmol. Otolaryngol. 76, 88–96, 1972

Nilsson, S. G. E. and Skoog, K. O.: The c-wave in vitelliruptive macular degeneration (VMD). Acta Ophthalmol. 58, 659–666, 1980

Niemeyer, G.: C-wave and intracellular responses from the pigment epithelium in the cat. in: Electro-oculography- its clinical importance. Biblioth. ophthal. 85, 68–74, 1976

Noble, K. G. and Carr, R. E.: Stargardt's disease and fundus flavimaculatus. Arch. Ophthalmol. 97, 1281–1285, 1979

Röver, J., Schaubele, G., Hüttel, M. und Neppert, S.: Vergleichande Untersuchungen des DC-ERGs und des EOGs bei Best'scher Maculadegeneration. Ber.Dtsch. ophthal. Ges. 77, 425–428, 1980

Röver, J., Hüttel, M. and Schaubele, G.: The DC-ERG: technical problems in recording from patients. Docum. Ophthal. Proc. Ser. 31, 73–80, 1982

Weingeist, T. A., Kotbrin, J. L. and Watzke, R. C.: Histopathology of Best's vitelliform macular dystrophy. ARVO Abstracts p. 259, May 1980

166

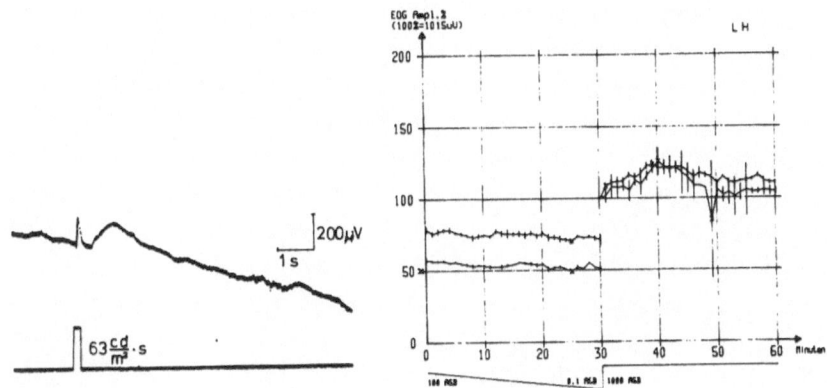

Fig. 8. The reduced c-wave is paralleled by the lowered EOG in vitiliginous chorio-retinitis.

	a	b	c	EOG
Uitelliform macular degeneration	+	+	−	−
„ „ „ family members	+	+	−	+
juvenile macular degeneration	+	+	−	−
fundus flavimaculatus	+	+	(+)	(+)
stargardt's disease	+	+	(+)	(+)
dominant drusen	+	+	−	−
choroidal atrophies	−	−	−	−

+: normal

−: reduced

Fig. 9. Table comparing the c-wave amplitudes and the EOG light rise in the diseases discussed in this paper.

Mailing address:
Universitäts-Augenklinik
Killianstr. 5
D-78 Freiburg, West Germany

ERG c-WAVE AT THE EARLY STAGE OF DIABETIC RETINOPATHY

H. SASAMORI, Y. TAKAHASHI, T. MORI AND Y. TAZAWA

(Iwate, Japan)

ABSTRACT

The ERG, especially the DC-registered c-wave, and EOG were examined in 13 patients with early stages of diabetic retinopathy. The amplitudes of the ERG a-, b-wave and oscillatory potentials and the EOG L/D ratio were almost normal in all cases. The c-wave amplitudes in the majority of the cases were also within the normal range, but in some cases they were supernormal during dark and light adaptation. However, two cases demonstrated considerably low amplitudes. Since no significant change was observed in c-wave and EOG in the early stage of diabetic retinopathy, it is suggested that the effect of the lesion of the inner retina in diabetic retinopathy on the c-wave appears later than that on the oscillatory potentials.

INTRODUCTION

The ERG c-wave is mainly generated in the retinal pigment epithelium, and may indicate retinal and choroidal functions. In our laboratory, basic investigations of the human ERG c-wave (Takahashi 1979, Sasamori 1980) and clinical applications of the c-wave (Tazawa 1980, Mori 1981) have been done for several years. Pigment epithelial damage in diabetic retinopathy has been reported by fluorescein angiography (Okano, 1977) or electrophysiological observations (Yonemura, 1977). Pautler & Ennis (1980) also demonstrated earlier deterioration of the amplitude of the ERG c-wave than the b-wave in diabetic rats' eyes. No study of the human ERG c-wave in diabetic retinopathy has been reported so far. We examined the ERG including c-waves and EOG of human eyes with early diabetic retinopathy.

MATERIALS AND METHODS

The DC-registered ERG c-wave, as well as ERG a- and b-waves, oscillatory potentials and EOG responses were examined in 13 patients, 6 males and 7 females 44 to 65 years old, with early stage of diabetic retinopathy (Scott Ia, IIa).

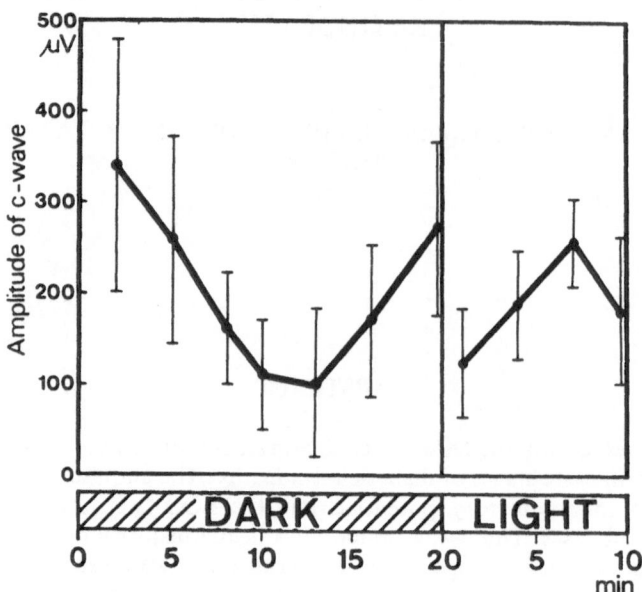

Fig. 1. The ERG c-wave in non-diabetic normal eyes during dark and light adaptation.

The recording procedure of the DC-registered c-wave was essentially the same as described in our previous reports (Sasamoi 1980, Tazawa 1980). Simply, a soft contact lens was placed on the mydriatic eye and a sclerocorneal type hard contact lens was applied over it. The hard contact lens was connected to a non-polarizable $Zn-SnSO_4$ electrode with a silicone tube filled with a chondroitin sulfate solution. The c-waves were recorded every 2 to 5 minutes during a 20 minute dark and 10 minute 5 lux light adaptation course, after 5 minutes of adaptation to 1,000 lux. The light stimuli had an intensity of 50 lux and a duration of 10 sec. The c-wave potentials were DC amplified and recorded on a penwriter.

The time course of the c-wave amplitudes was plotted and compared with that of non-diabetic normal subjects reported previously (Tazawa, 1980). In normal cases, during the dark adaptation course, c-wave amplitudes decrease gradually and reach a low at 10 to 13 minutes after the onset of dark adaptation. Thereafter the c-wave amplitudes increase slowly and recover almost to the initial level. During light adaptation c-waves were low in the initial stage but increased to reach a maximum at about 7 minutes (Figure 1).

The ERG a- and b-waves and oscillatory potentials were recorded by an AC amplifier after 10 minutes of dark adaptation, with single flash stimuli of 20 joule. The EOG measurement was made by a semi-automatic recording system (Tazawa, et al., 1979).

RESULTS

All of the cases with early diabetic retinopathy showed normal ERG a- and b-wave responses. The amplitudes of the oscillatory potentials were normal or

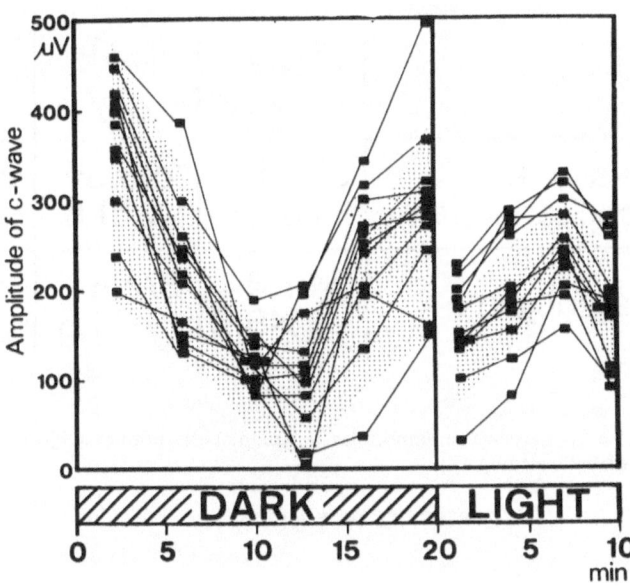

Fig. 2. The c-wave amplitude of eyes with early diabetic retinopathy (solid lines). Dotted areas indicate normal range.

slightly reduced. The EOG L/D ratio were also in the normal range of 2.02 to 4.16 (average 2.81 ± 0.69).

Regarding the ERG c-wave amplitudes, the majority of the cases (11 out of 13 eyes) were within the normal range (Figure 2). The c-wave time course was also almost normal in these cases: they formed minimum amplitudes at 10 to 13 minutes in the dark and a maximum at about 7 minutes in light.

The average c-wave amplitudes of the 11 cases at 2 and 20 minutes of dark adaptation and 7 minutes of light adaptation were 359 ± 83, 293 ± 111 and 247 ± 56 μV respectively, whereas those of the non-diabetic normal subjects were 344 ± 145, 272 ± 113 and 247 ± 40 μV respectively. Although no significant difference was recognized, the c-wave amplitudes in eyes with early diabetic retinopathy were slightly larger than those of normal subjects (Table 1). In a few cases supernormal c-waves were obtained at the early and later part of the dark adaptation and throughout the light adaptation. The cases with supernormal amplitude during dark adaptation had a tendency to show larger amplitude during light adaptation too. Figure 3 indicates a representative case showing the supernormal amplitudes.

Two out of 13 cases, however, demonstrated considerably lower c-wave amplitudes during the dark and light adaptation as indicated in Figure 4.

DISCUSSION

From electrophysiological findings of diabetic retinopathy it is well known that the peak latency of the oscillatory potentials is delayed in early

171

	Dark 2'	Dark 20'	Light 7'
Patients with diabetic retinopathy	359.1 ±83.1	293.3 ±111.6	247.3 ±56.3
Normal subjects	344.4 ±145.5	272.8 ±113.6	247.1 ±40.0 μV

Table 1. The average c-wave amplitudes in non-diabetic normal subjects and patients with early diabetic retinopathy.

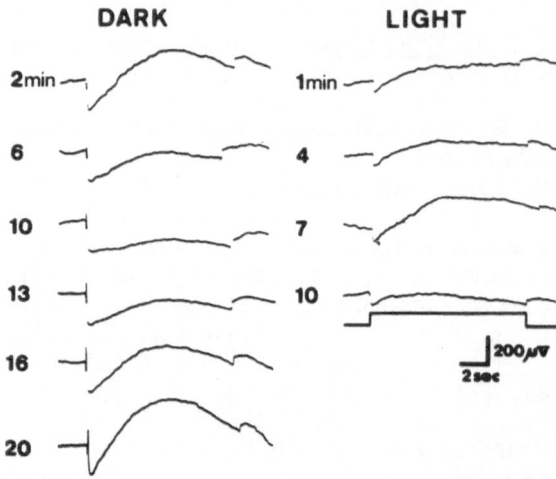

Fig. 3. Actual wave forms of the c-waves which showed a supernormal amplitude.

retinopathy. Recently, Kawasaki and his collaborators (1977) suggested lesion in the pigment epithelium by demonstrating suppression of the hyperosmolarity response induced by intravenous infusion of a hypertonic solution into patients with diabetic retinopathy, graded Scott II. Okano (1977) proved the pigment epithelial lesion in his fluorescein angiographical study on diabetic retinopathy.

We have demonstrated previously that the c-wave amplitude was reduced with the progression of the disease (Tazawa, 1980). In the present study we examined the ERG c-wave and EOG, which indicate function of the pigment

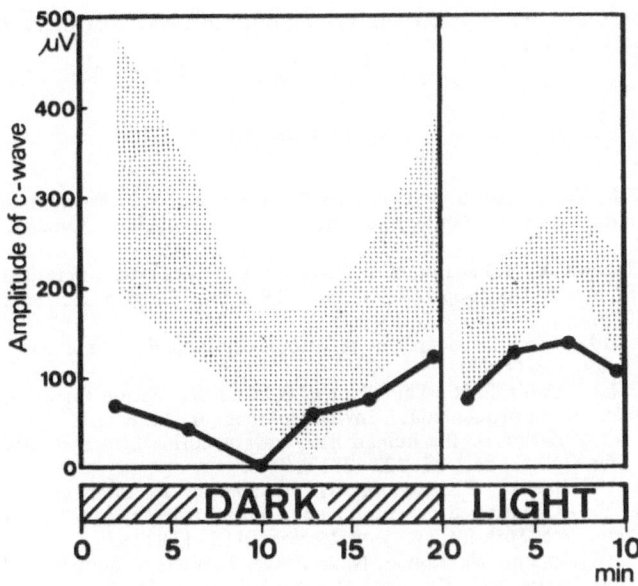

Fig. 4. The time course of the c-wave of two eyes which showed considerably low amplitudes.

epithelium, as well as ERG a- and b-waves and oscillatory potentials in early diabetic retinopathy.

Normal ERG a- and b-waves, normal L/D ratio, normal or slightly decreased oscillatory potentials were obtained from patients. The c-wave amplitudes were also normal in the majority of the cases and supernormal in some cases. Consequently, our results indicate functional abnormalities in the pigment epithelium and its neighboring tissues. Furthermore, it is suggested that, in diabetic retinopathy, the effect of the lesion in the inner layer of the retina on the c-wave seemed to be later than on the oscillatory potentials.

Yonemura and others (1976) observed diminished b-waves but increased c-waves in albino rabbits by intravenous injection of a hypertonic solution. The average serum osmotic pressure of the patients studied in the present experiment was 299 mOSM/1, which was the upper normal limit or slightly higher than the normal level. The supernormal c-wave may be a reflection of the high serum osmotic pressure, though the correlation between the c-wave amplitude and the serum osmotic pressure level was not significant.

Considerably low amplitude c-waves were recorded from 2 out of 13 cases throughout dark and light adaptation. As we reported previously, a small group (20 per cent) of normal subjects showed low amplitude c-waves, although no abnormality was found in their eyes (Sasamori, 1980). Täumer and others (1976) also reported that no c-wave response was obtained from 16.7 per cent of their normal subjects. The 2 cases who showed low amplitude c-waves may belong to the small group of cases which shows the low c-waves despite normal visual function. It was, therefore, difficult to

173

determine presently whether the low amplitude c-waves of these 2 cases were pathological or not.

REFERENCES

Kawasaki, K., Yamamoto, S. & Yonemura, D.: Electrophysiological approach to clinical test for the retinal pigment epithelium. Acta Soc. Ophthalmol. Jpn., 81: 1303—1312 (1977).

Mori, T., Tazawa, Y., Takahashi, Y. & Sasamori, H.: ERG c-wave in retinal detachment recorded pre- and post-operatively. Proc. 19th ISCEV Symp. Horgen-Zurich, 177—184 (1981).

Okano, T.: Fluorescein angiography in diabetic retinopathy. Acta Soc. Ophthalmol. Jpn., 81: 69—134 (1977).

Pautler, E. L. & Ennis, S. R.: The effect of induced diabetes on the electroretinogram components of the pigmented rat. Invest. Ophthalmol. Vis. Sci., 19: 702—705 (1980).

Sasamori, H.: Variation of the human ERG c-wave during light and dark adaptation. Jpn. J. Clin. Ophthalmol., 34: 223—231 (1980).

Takahashi, Y., Ohtsuka, T., Sasamori, H., Takamatsu, T., Inomata, K., Mita, T. & Tazawa, Y.: DC-registered c-wave in human normal eyes and possibility of its clinical application. Proc. 16th ISCEV Symp. Morioka, 113—118 (1979).

Täumer, R., Wichmann, W., Rohde, N. & Röver, J.: ERG of humans without c-wave. Albrecht v. Graefes Arch. Klin. exp. Ophthalmol., 198: 275—289 (1976).

Tazawa, Y., Mera, H., Kondo, T., Sasamori, H., Ogasawara, K. & Yui, H.: Development of a semi-automatic recorder for visual electric responses. Jpn. J. Clin. Ophthalmol., 33: 661—666 (1979).

Tazawa, Y.: Human ERG c-wave; Its characteristics and clinical application. Folia Ophthalmol. Jpn. 31: 1223—1248 (1980).

Yonemura, D., Kawasaki, K. & Ishikawa, C.: Enhancement of the c-wave and abolition of the b-wave by intravenous injection of hypertonic solution. Acta Soc. Ophthalmol. Jpn., 80: 1610—1616 (1976).

Yonemura, D.: An electrophysiological study on activities of neuronal and non-neuronal retinal elements in man with reference to its clinical application. Acta Soc. Ophthalmol. Jpn., 81: 1632—1665 (1977).

Mailing address:
Department of Ophthalmology
Iwate Medical University
19—1 Uchimaru, Morioka, Iwate 020, Japan

THE EOG AND THE ERG IN THE AORTIC ARCH SYNDROME

J. RIBEIRO-da-SILVA AND A. CASTANHEIRA-DINIS

(Lisbon, Portugal)

ABSTRACT

The authors studied the EOG and the ERG in patients with ocular pathology related to the aortic arch syndrome; both records, the EOG and the ERG showed abnormalities. The importance of the EOG is emphasized by the authors as a clinical test to recognize the early choroidal vascular pathology in these cases and to understand better the associated pathology of the pigmentary epithelium of the retina.

INTRODUCTION

The unusual aortic arch syndrome is a condition related to the great vessels in which the insufficient blood supply to the head and upper extremities is the major cause of symptoms and signs.

Ocular manifestations of the disease are common in this syndrome and they include frequently amaurosis fugax, retinal vascular oclusive phenomena and sometimes ischemic optic neuritis due to a slowly and chronic hypoxic effect that appears in the retina, in the optic nerve and in the brain.

According to this we understand that the retinopathy represents the result of a very slow circulation that produces retinal and choroidal hypoxia and probably the choroidal hypoxia causes damage in the outer retinal layers.

Three patients with aortic arch syndrome have been studied at the Lisbon Institute of Ophthalmology. All of them had been previously examined in several Departments of our Faculty and the diagnosis of aortic arch syndrome was only established after arterial angiography. The angiography confirmed the clinical diagnosis and through these tests we understood better the signs and the symptoms of the three patients.

RESULTS

Then we thought it would be interesting to analyze the retinal activity of our patients with electrophysiological tests.

We used an Alvar Electroretinograph and the ERG was recorded under

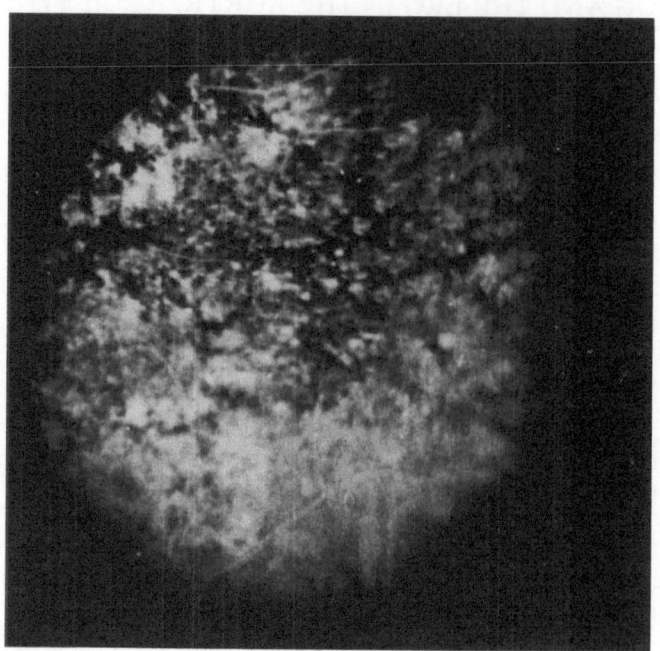

Fig. 1. Aortic arch syndrome. Fluorescein angiography of the fundus eye. Central area.

light and dark adapted states. For the EOG we used the François technique.

In all cases we found fundus pathology and the fluorescein angiography revealed central or peripheral circulatory disturbances in which the pigmented epithelium was always involved (Figure 1 and Figure 2).

In all patients a low central retinal arterial blood pressure was found by ophthalmodynamometry and the average intraocular pressure was under 10 Hg mm.

1st Case

In Table I the photopic and the scotopic ERG are shown to be abnormally low in both eyes.

For the EOG the Arden Index shows also a pathologic result. (115/120).

2nd Case

The photopic and the scotopic ERG are subnormal.
The Arden Index of the EOG is subnormal also (134/134) (Table II).

3rd Case

As in the other patients the photopic and scotopic ERGs were found to be subnormal.

176

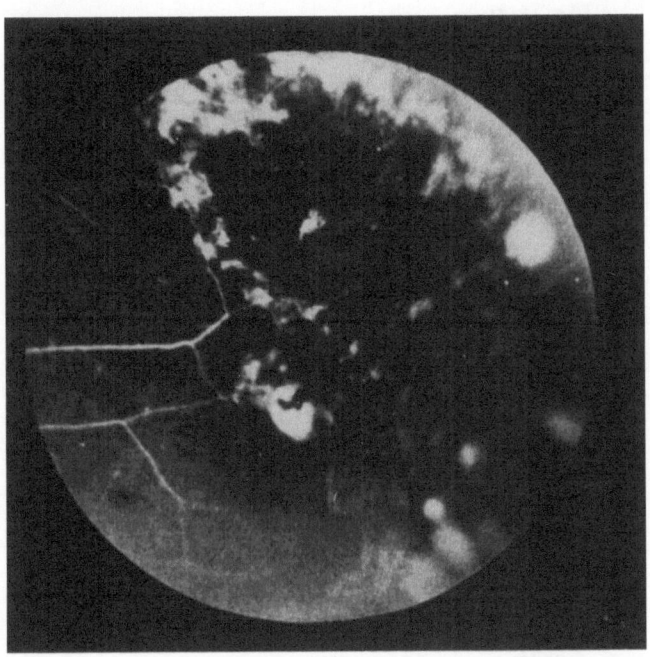

Fig. 2. Aortic arch syndrome. Fluorescein angiography of the fundus eye. Peripheral area.

Table I

CASE I
Amplitudes of the ERG components (μV)

	Right Eye	Left Eye
Photopic ERG		
a wave	20	30
b wave	50	70
Scotopic ERG		
a wave	150	190
b wave	190	220
EOG		
L/D × 100	115	120

The Arden Index of the EOG was low (143/150), but was higher than in the two other cases (Table III).

It is important to point out that in all three cases the oscillatory potential was not present.

In Conclusion: In all patients with aortic arch syndrome we found retinal pathology and retinal dysfunction.

The uveal chronic hypoxia is probably the cause of the low intraocular pressure that we found in our patients and by ophthalmodynamometry we confirmed their low central retinal arterial blood pressure.

177

Table II

CASE 2
Amplitudes of the ERG components (μV)

	Right Eye	Left Eye
Photopic ERG		
a wave	30	40
b wave	70	75
Scotopic ERG		
a wave	200	210
b wave	250	250
EOG		
L/D × 100	134	134

Table III

CASE 3
Amplitudes of the ERG components (μV)

	Right Eye	Left Eye
Photopic ERG		
a wave	38	40
b wave	80	95
Scotopic ERG		
a wave	230	235
b wave	290	290
EOG		
L/D × 100	143	150

From the electrophysiological tests we understand better the retinal dysfunction caused probably by retinal and choroidal chronic hypoxia. Not only the ERG was subnormal with an absence of the oscillatory potentials but also the EOG.

That means, probably, that not only the retina, but also the choroid and its circulation were involved in the aortic arch syndrome.

REFERENCES

Arden, S. B., Barrada, A. and Kelsy, J. H.: New clinical test of retinal function based upon the standing potential of the eye. Br. J. Ophthalm. 46: 449–467, 1962.

Ashworth, B.: The electro-oculogram in disorders of the retinal circulation. Amer. J. Ophthalm. 61, 505–508, 1966.

Bird, A. C.: L'ischemie choroidienne. Bull. et Mem. de la Soc. Fr. Ophthalm. Masson Paris 419–422, 1982.

Castanheira-Dinis, A.: Modificações electro-oftalmológicas na patologia vascular da retina- IV Congresso Luso-Hisp.-Bras. de Oftalm.-Lisbon 1980 (In press).

Dowling, J. L. and Smith, T. R.: Ocular study of pulseless disease Arch. Ophthalm. 64: 236, 1960.

Font, R. L. and Naumann, G.: Ocular histopathology in pulseless disease, Arch. Ophthalm. 84: 784, 1969.

François, J., De Rouck, A., Verriest, G. and Szimigielski, M.: An extended clinical test of the ocular standing potential and its results in cases of retinal degeneration. Proc.

4th ISCERG Symp. Hakone 1965. Japan J. Ophthalm. 10 Suppl. pp. 257–268, 1968.
Hedges, T. R.: The aortic arch syndrome. Arch. Ophthalm 71: 28, 1964.
Knox, D. L.: Ischemic ocular inflammation. Am. J. Ophthalm. 60: 995 1965.
Suyama, T.: A case of pulseless disease. Fol. Ophthalm. Jap. 18, 1110–1105, 1967.
Takayasu, M.: Case report of a peculiar abnormality of the retinal central vessels. Acta. Soc. Ophthalm. Japan 12: 554, 1908.

Mailing address:
Institute of Ophthalmology of Lisbon
Travessa Larga, 2
1100 Lisbon
Portugal

SLOW RETINAL POTENTIALS EVOKED BY PATTERNED STIMULI

M. KORTH

(Erlangen, Germany)

ABSTRACT

Electrical potentials evoked by square-wave stripe patterns of varying spatial frequencies presented as onset-offset stimuli were recorded from the human eye using an amplification with long time constant. Besides the phasic responses at onset and offset a steady potential shift of positive polarity (plateau potential) was noted that persisted as long as the pattern was present. The level of the plateau was highest at spatial frequencies around 5 c/deg. This component seems to indicate mainly a decrease of the receptor process P_{III} initiated by local decreases in retinal illumination. The spatial selectivity of the amplitude of the plateau might indicate that pattern-related processes take place at the receptor level.

INTRODUCTION

Studies of the electroretinogram (ERG) and the visual evoked potential (VEP) obtained with patterned stimuli were concerned only with the transient components of the response. Tonic components lasting as long as the stimulus is presented have been investigated so far only with unpatterned on-off light stimuli. The recording of the animal-ERG in response to a long-lasting light stimulus has led to suggestions that the compound potential waveform could be broken up into 2 to 4 separate phasic and tonic processes of different polarities (Einthoven and Jolly, 1908; Waller, 1909; Piper, 1911; Granit, 1933; Rodieck, 1972). Slow potentials analogous to the ones obtained in animals have been recorded also from the human eye (e.g. Dodt, 1951; Schweitzer and Troelstra, 1963; Hanitzsch et al., 1966; Skoog and Nilsson, 1974).

In the present study, pattern onset-offset stimuli were used in order to study slow potential shifts that might be present for the duration of the presentation of the pattern. Since such stimuli are not associated with global changes in retinal illumination slow responses that might be related to the different local intensity distributions of the pattern can be studied.

METHODS

Square-wave stripe patterns (contrast 0.99) of varying spatial frequencies were presented in the onset-offset mode (Spekreijse et al., 1973) using a Maxwellian-view system. The light source was a 75 Xenon high-pressure arc lamp. The diameter of the stimulus field was 40° and cross hairs in the center of the display served as the fixation point.

Pattern onset-offset stimulation without changing space-average luminance was achieved with a small vibrating mirror mounted on the vertical shaft of a galvanometer. During vibration (800 Hz, triangular waveform) of the mirror the pattern was invisible after proper adjustment of the amplitude of vibration. When the vibration of the mirror was stopped (pattern onset) the pattern appeared, when the vibration started again (pattern offset) the pattern disappeared. The time period during which the pattern was present and absent was 800 ms and 1250 ms respectively. The space-average retinal illumination was 5×10^4 photopic Td.

In certain experiments, by using a separate light path, extra amounts of light of varying intensity were added to or subtracted from the light path entering the eye. In this manner the luminance of the bright, or of the dark, stripes or of both stripes could be increased or decreased at pattern onset or at offset. The addition or subtraction of the extra light was controlled by a shutter which, in turn, was operated by the same function generator that determined the duration of the mirror vibration. Since such stimuli are associated with changes in space-average luminance a ganzfeld (luminance 200 cd/m^2) surrounding the stimulus field was placed in front of the final lens of the viewing system.

The ERG was recorded using an Ag-AgCl electroded mounted in a scleral contact lens. The reference point was the chin and both ear lobes served as ground. In order to detect slow potential shifts a slow time constant of 1.8 seconds of the amplifying system (HP 8857A and Tektronix 502) was used. The high-frequency cutoff was 1 kHz.

For response averaging a digital computer (PDP 11/40) was used. An artifact-rejection algorithm prevented the addition of signals from sources not related to the stimulus. Averaged potentials were read out on an XY-plotter.

The left eyes of two male observers were used. The results obtained from the two eyes which were free of abnormalities were virtually identical.

RESULTS

Figure 1 shows an ERG and an occipital VEP obtained by the presentation of a stripe pattern with a spatial frequency of 5.4 cycles/degree (c/deg). At pattern onset a biphasic response is noted followed by a gradually developing potential shift of positive polarity (plateau potentials). At pattern offset another, small phasic response is seen associated with a rapid decay of the slow potential. In the VEP, besides the phasic components, a slow component of positive polarity is observed that lasts as long as the pattern is presented.

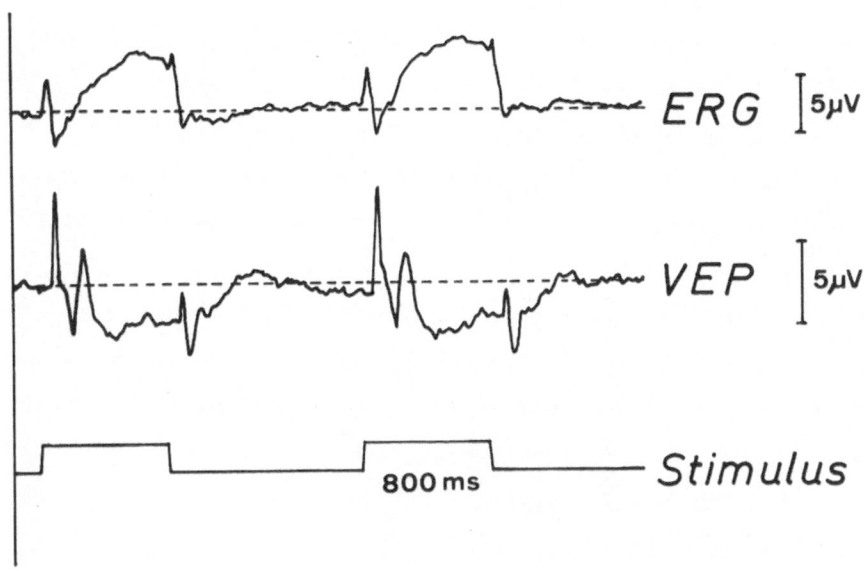

Fig. 1. Onset-offset ERGs and VEPs obtained with the repeated presentation of a stripe pattern of 5.4 c/deg. The records are averages of 128 sweeps. The duration of the pattern presentation is indicated by an upward deflection of the stimulus trace.

In Figure 2 records are shown obtained with a number of patterns differing in spatial frequency. The phasic response at pattern onset has an amplitude around 3 c/deg. the positive plateau potential is most pronounced around 5 c/deg. In contrast, the phasic response at pattern offset (probably in a-wave and a b-wave) shows a monotonic decrease in amplitude with increasing spatial frequency.

The following series of experiments dealt with the question as to how the ERG-waveform in response to a patterned stimulus compares with an ERG-response to changes in homogenious luminance, because such stimuli lead to an ERG of fairly well known origin.

In the experiment illustrated in Figure 3 an unpatterned light was switched on, then the pattern onset-offset stimulus was presented and, finally the light was turned off. The pupil of the subject's eye was immobilized by using parasympatholytic eye drops. As long as the light is kept on, a constant negative P_{III} of high amplitude is recorded. When the pattern is presented the plateau potential presents itself as a shift of the level of P_{III} towards the base line. The increase of the plateau is relatively slow as is the decrease of P_{III} after light-off. The decrease of the plateau is rapid as is the increase of P_{III} after light-on. Thus, the plateau potential seems to originate from those retinal areas receiving local decreases in luminance at pattern onset.

In another experiment (Figure 4) unpatterned light stimuli representing luminance changes from the space-average luminance (L_0) to the level of the dark or of the bright stripes were presented as block-shaped stimuli. The pupil was immobilized. The response to the increase-decrease stimulus shows a small

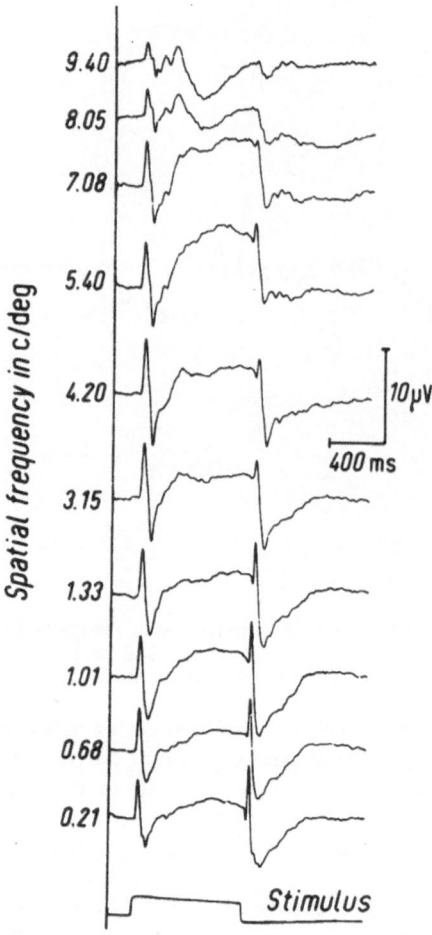

Fig. 2. Onset-offset ERGs obtained with different spatial frequencies of the pattern. All records are averages of 5 experiments with 128 stimuli each.

increase of P_{III} and the decrease-increase response shows a large decrease of P_{III}. The added waveform ('Pattern onset-offset') is dominated by the decrease of P_{III} and resembles in certain respects the waveform obtained with low spatial-frequency stripe patterns (Figure 2). This result suggests that the plateau potential obtained with patterned stimuli is mainly the result of an additive superposition of two receptor processes generated by dark and bright stripes. Since both processes are not balanced in amplitude but the decrease of P_{III} outweighs its increase, the plateau potential is formed.

In a final experiment the pattern onset-offset stimuli were combined with increases or decreases in space-average luminance (see Methods). Figure 5 shows different response waveforms obtained with various luminance profiles shown underneath each record. In a) the typical onset-offset response without

184

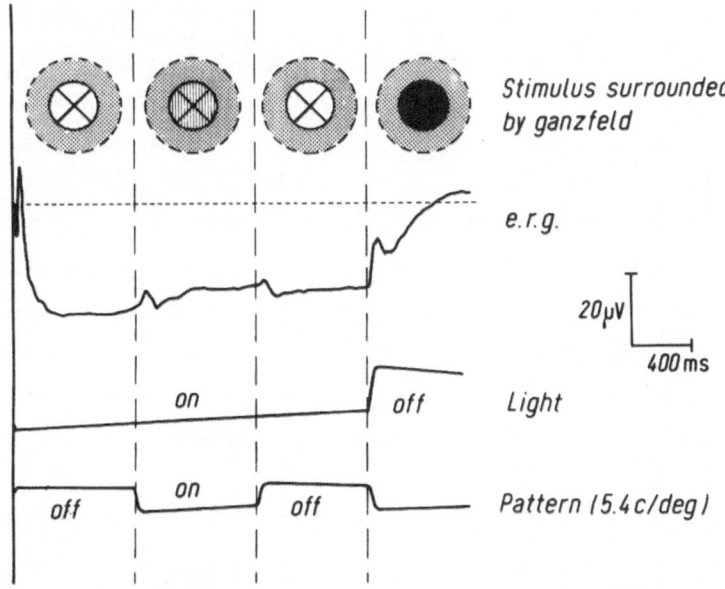

Stimulus surrounded by ganzfeld

e.r.g.

20 μV

400 ms

on   off   Light

off   on   off   Pattern (5.4 c/deg)

Fig. 3. Averaged ERG-response to a light-on, pattern-onset, pattern-offset, and light-off stimulus. The shape of the stimulus traces give an impression of the time constant of the amplifying system. The record shows an average of 5 experiments with 128 stimuli each. The pupil was immobilized.

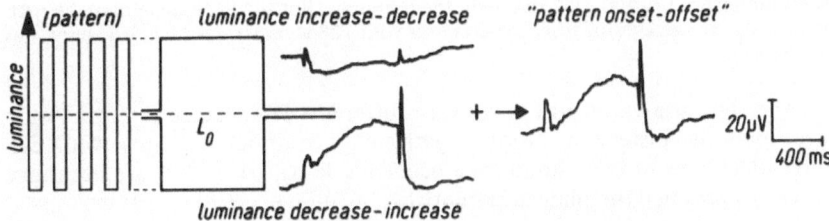

(pattern)   luminance increase-decrease   "pattern onset-offset"

luminance

L_0

+ →

20 μV

400 ms

luminance decrease-increase

Fig. 4. ERGs in response to luminance increase-decrease and decrease-increase stimuli. The intensity of a homogeneous field was increased from the level of the space-average luminance (L_0) to the level of the bright stripes or decreased to the level of the dark stripes. The response shown on the right is the algebraic sum of the two responses shown on the left. The records are averages of three experiments with 128 stimuli each. The pupil was immobilized.

change in space-average luminance (L_0) is shown. In b) L_0 was decreased by a factor of 2, such that only local decreases in luminance, without increases, were presented. The resulting waveform, however, still looked much like the typical onset-offset response shown in a). In c) L_0 was increased by a factor of 2 and local increases and decreases were presented. The resulting waveform still had a pronounced plateau potential and looked similar to the onset-offset response shown in a). In d) L_0 was increased also by a factor of 2, however only increases without decreases in local luminance were presented.

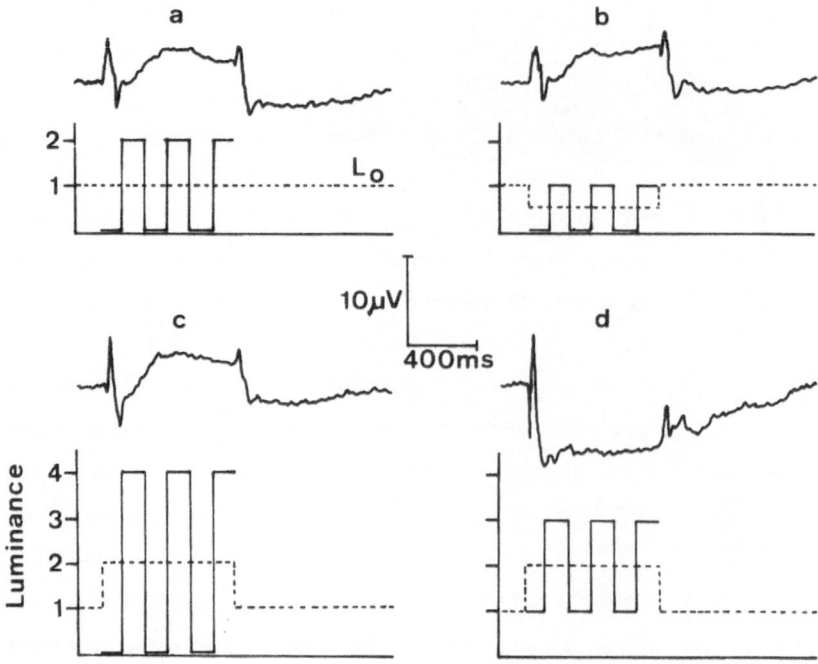

Fig. 5. Averaged ERGs in response to pattern onset-offset stimuli combined with changes of the space-average luminance (L_o). The graphs underneath each record indicate the various luminance profiles used to obtain the responses. For further explanation see text. The records are averages of three experiments with 128 summations each. The pupil was immobilized.

Now the response waveform looks very different. The plateau potential is no longer present, instead a steady negative P_{III} component is observed. Evidently, decreases in local luminance occurring in a), b), and c) are necessary in order to produce the plateau potential.

DISCUSSION

One of the criteria that distinguishes a pattern-evoked occipital response form a luminance-evoked response is the behaviour of the amplitude of a response component as a function of the spatial frequency of a pattern (Padmos et al., 1973). Pattern-evoked responses produced by units having an antagonistic center-surround organization of their receptive fields show an amplitude maximum at a certain spatial frequency of the pattern used (spatial selectivity). Luminance-evoked responses, however, produced by units lacking such an antagonism decrease monotonically in amplitude with increasing spatial frequency. If this concept holds also for the ERG obtained with stripe patterns the plateau potential studied here seems to be pattern-related.

The experiments of the present study suggest that the plateau potential originates from the retinal receptors. This conclusion is based mainly on a qualitative comparison of the different time constants of the increase and decrease of the plateau potential and of the P_{III} component. The plateau potential certainly is not generated by process P_I (c-wave) since the latter has a different time course and can be recorded only from dark-adapted eyes. The DC component of the human ERG described by Schweitzer and Troelstra (1963) and by Schweitzer and Padmos (1966) is unlikely to be involved since it occurs only with low-intensity stimuli under conditions of dark adaptation. A contribution of iris-muscle activity associated with pupillary movements has been excluded also since the plateau potential can be recorded with the pupil immobilized (Figures 3, 4 and 5).

Thus, if the plateau potential can be regarded as an expression of P_{III} activity, pattern-related processes might occur at the receptor level. Figure 5 indicated that decreases in local luminance are the essential stimulus for evoking this component and one might speculate that local decreases in luminance without increases might be sufficient to elicit pattern-evoked responses in the human ERG.

REFERENCES

Dodt, E. (1951). Beiträge zur Elektrophysiologie des Auges. 1. Mitteilung. Über die sekundäre Erhebung im Aktionspotential des menschlichen Auges bei Belichtung. v. Graefes Arch. Ophthalmol. 151, 672–692.

Einthoven, W. and Jolly, W. A. (1908). The form and magnitude of the electrical response of the eye to stimulation by light at various intensities. Quart. J. Exper. Physiol. 1, 373–426.

Granit, R. (1933). The components of the retinal action potential in mammals and their relation to the discharge of the optic nerve. J. Physiol. 77, 207–239.

Hanitzsch, R., Hommer, K. and Bornschein, H. (1966). Der Nachweis langsamer Potentiale im menschlichen ERG. Vision Res. 6, 245–250.

Padmos, P., Haaijman, J. and Spekreijse, H. (1973). Visually evoked cortical potentials to patterned stimuli in monkey and man. Electroenceph. Clin. Neurophysiol. 35, 153–163.

Piper, H. (1911). Über die Netzhautströme. Arch. Anat. Physiol., Physiologische Abt. (Leipzig), 85–132.

Rodieck, R. W. (1972). Components of the electroretinogram – A reappraisal. Vision. Res. 12, 737–780.

Schweitzer, N. M. J. and Troelstra, A. (1963). An end effect in the human ERG. Ophthalmologica 145, 119–122.

Schweitzer, N. M. J. and Padmos, P. (1968). The microstructure of the human scotopic ERG. In: The clinical value of electroretinography. New York: Karger, 198–204.

Skoog, K.-O. and Nilsson, S. E. G. (1974). The c-wave of the human d.c. registered ERG – 1. A quantitative study of the relationship between c-wave amplitude and stimulus intensity. Acta Ophthal. Kopenh. 52, 759–773.

Spekreijse, H., van der Tweel, L. H. and Zuidema, T. (1973). Contrast evoked responses in man. Vision Res. 13, 1577–1601.

Waller, A. D. (1909). On the double nature of the photoelectrical response of the frog's retina. Quart. J. Exper. Physiol. 2, 169–185.

Mailing address:
University Eye Hospital
Erlangen University
D-8520 Erlangen
Schwabachanlage 6
West Germany

DATA TO THE ELECTRO-OCULOGRAPHY OF RETROLENTAL FIBROPLASIA

A. BOHÁR, G. RADÓ AND M. VÉLI

2nd Eye Clinic of the Semmelweis OTE, Budapest, Hungary

The authors studied the EOG of children 6–10 years old with retrolental fibroplasia. Only one eye was involved. It was therefore possible to compare the EOG of a normal eye to that of the afflicted eye.

THE LONG-TERM OBSERVATION OF THE ERG c-WAVE AND EOG IN CASES OF POSTOPERATIVE RETINAL DETACHMENT

T. MORI, Y. TAZAWA, Y. TAKAHASHI AND H. SASAMORI

Department of Ophthalmology, Iwate Medical University 19–1 Uchimaru, Morioka, Iwate 020, Japan

We reported the changes in the ERG c-wave in cases of pre- and postoperative retinal detachment at the 19th ISCEV Symposium in Zurich. The present study is the second in a series of electrophysiological investigations on the function of the pigment epithelium in retinal detachment. The ERG c-wave and EOG were recorded from 5 patients postoperatively who had undergone successful surgery 1–2 years earlier; the ERG a- and b-waves, visual acuity, visual field and fluorescein angiography were also examined. The DC-registered ERG c-waves were recorded through 20 minute dark- and 15 minute light-adaptation courses after 5 minute 1,000 Lux pre-adaptation. The intensity and duration of the light stimulus employed were 50 Lux and 10 seconds respectively. The EOG amplitudes were recorded and analyzed by a computerized semi-automatic EOG recorder.

The c-wave amplitudes and the EOG base values obtained from all patients remained low, and the time curves of the c-wave and the EOG showed subnormal patterns, whereas the ERG a- and b-waves recovered to almost normal levels. These electrophysiological abnormalities demonstrate the delay of the functional recovery of the retinal pigment epithelium, even 1–2 years after successful reattachment of the retina.

INTERACTIVE COMPUTER PROGRAM FOR CLINICAL ELECTROPHYSIOLOGY

D. VAN NORREN and J. VAN DE KRAATS

(Soesterberg and Utrecht, The Netherlands)

ABSTRACT

When developing a new microprocessor based unit for clinical electrophysiology we made the demand that the system be as user-friendly as possible. This resulted in a set-up in which all visible equipment was reduced to two monitors and a keyboard. The operator receives instructions from one monitor and responds by pressing, in most instances, a single key on the keyboard. The second monitor displays the electrophysiological responses. The operator first chooses the type of measurement (ERG, EOG, VER research or standard procedure) from a menu. A standard ERG program starts with an automatic check of electrode resistances. Next a series of 10 flashes at low intensity is presented to the dark adapted subject. When the operator accepts the averaged results, a new series of flashes at a higher intensity is presented, and so on. The program features overload protection, calculation of oscillatory potentials from standard responses, and interactive assessment of a and b-wave latencies and amplitudes. Results of the measurements together with the patient record is stored on a mini-disk. After completion of all measurements the results are printed on a matrix printer.

INTRODUCTION

A microprocessor based system for electrophysiology of vision offers, in principle, many advantages over hardware systems (Miyake, Solish, Hara and Hirose 1978; Stark, Canty and Johnson, 1981). We might mention automatic adjustment of stimulus parameters, rejection of artifacts, data storage, data manipulation, easy change of routines and addition of new routines.

When developing a new microprocessor based system for clinical electro-physiology we made the additional demand that the system should be as user friendly as possible. This resulted in a setup in which all visible equipment was reduced to two visual displays units, a keyboard and two disk drives. The operator receives instructions from one display and responds by pressing in most instances, a single key on the keyboard. The second unit displays the electrophysiological responses.

In this paper a short description will be given of the performance of the system.

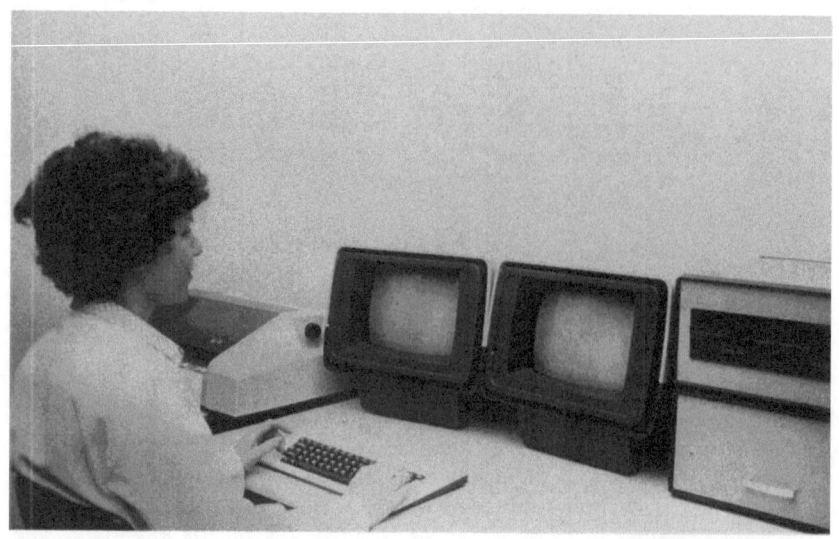

Fig. 1. Microprocessor based system for electrophysiology of vision. The left hand unit displays the instructions for the operator. On the right hand unit the electrophysiological responses (waveforms) are displayed. Two floppy disk drives are visible on the right; on the left hand side of the figure is the printer.

THE PROGRAM

When the power of the apparatus is switched on, the computer automatically starts and asks, on the left hand display, for the date, and the patient's name and number. Next, a menu is presented from which the operator chooses the appropriate program. Available are ERG standard or experimental programs, VEP, EOG programs, and a printout program which incorporates a possibility for the assessment of waveform amplitudes.

In the following, parts of the ERG standard program are present by way of example. Texts between quotation marks are operater responses

```
THIS IS THE ERG STANDARD PROGRAM
ATTACH ERG ELECTRODES; LEFT EYE, RIGHT EYE,
FOREHEAD
C = CONTINUE                                    "C"
ELECTRODE IMPEDANCE IS NOW CHECKED
ELECTRODE IMPEDANCE LEFT EYE:  O.K.
                        RIGHT EYE:  O.K.
WHAT DO YOU WANT?
C = CONTINUE
R = REPEAT                                      "C"
OBSERVE 30 MIN OF DARK ADAPTATION
......MIN    ......SEC
```

The last printed line is in fact a running clock. In our laboratory we follow the practice of placing the electrodes in deep red light after the patient has

194

dark adapted for 20 min. Through the clock the need is stressed for a total period of dark adaptation of 30 min.

The standard ERG program consists of a scotopic series in which three flash intensities (labeled B, D and E) are presented, and a photopic series in which three higher flash intensities (F, G and H) are presented on a light background.

```
C = CONTINUE                                    "C"
FLASH INTENSITY B IS NOW SELECTED
START MEASUREMENT WITH C                         "C"
```

On the right hand display the averaging process (N = 10) can be followed

```
CHECK THE RESULTS. WHAT DO YOU WANT?
C = CONTINUE
R = REPEAT
S = STOP                                         "C"
FLASH INTENSITY D IS SELECTED
```

The results are stored on disk. The program continues until the Scotopic series is completed.

```
SCOTOPIC SERIES COMPLETED
CHECK WHETHER THE AMPLITUDE OF THE B-WAVE IS
AT LEAST 200 μV. IF NOT CONTINUE WITH FLASHES
OF HIGHER INTENSITY.
S = CONTINUE SCOTOPIC SERIES WITH HIGH INTENSITY
FLASHES
P = CONTINUE WITH PHOTOPIC SERIES               "P"
BACKGROUND LIGHT IS SWITCHED ON
PATIENT SHOULD LIGHT ADAPT FOR 2 MINUTES
...... MIN    ...... SEC
C = CONTINUE                                     "C"
FLASH INTENSITY F IS SELECTED
```

The program continues with a series of in total three flash intensities.

```
FLASH INTENSITY H IS SELECTED
START MEASUREMENTS WITH C                        "C"
CHECK THE RESULTS. WHAT DO YOU WANT?
C = CONTINUE
R = REPEAT
S = STOP                                         "C"
THE OSCILLATORY POTENTIALS ARE CALCULATED
FROM THE LAST RESPONSE. CHECK THE RESULTS
```

A digital filtering technique is used to calculate the OP's from the last recorded response. Finally the following lines are displayed

```
ERG STANDARD PROGRAM IS COMPLETED
ADD COMMENTS
```

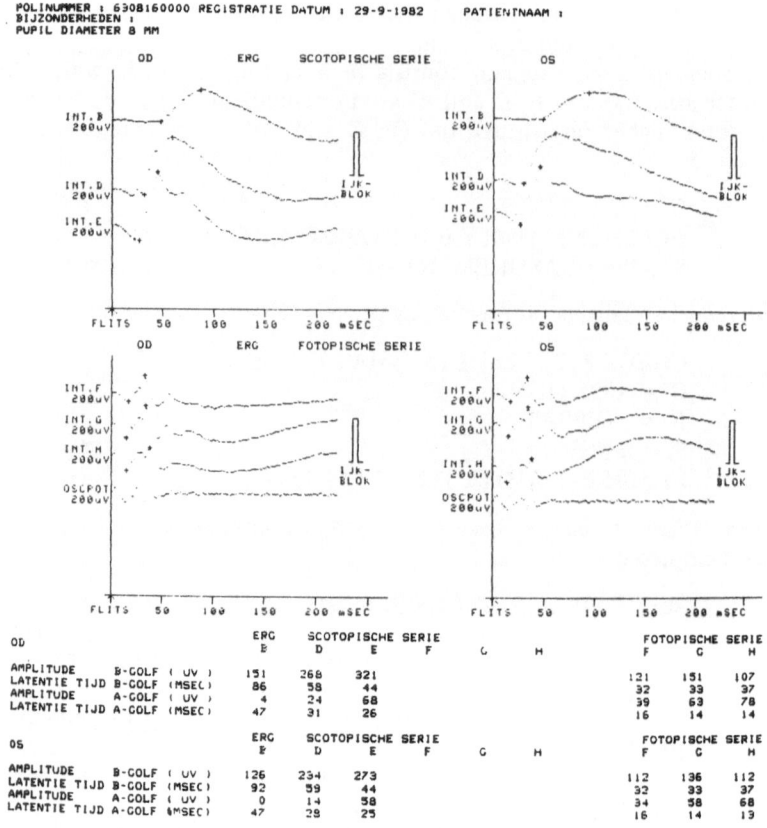

POLINUMMER : 6308160000 REGISTRATIE DATUM : 29-9-1982   PATIENTNAAM :
BIJZONDERHEDEN :
PUPIL DIAMETER 8 MM

Fig. 2. Printout of a standard ERG procedure (in Dutch). The 200 μV printed along the vertical axis refers to the amplitude calibration mark (IJBLOK). The cursor marks (+) were positioned manually at the peaks of the a- and b-waves resp. The calculated amplitudes and latencies are displayed in the table at the bottom of the printout.

If the operator has any remarks about e.g. pupil diameter or a disturbance, these can be added here. The comments are stored on disk with the rest of the results.

Finally, the program returns with the menu. After the patient has left, the printout program is usually selected. Through positioning of a cursor a- and b-wave latencies and amplitudes can be assessed. In Fig. 2 the final printout is displayed. Not incorporated yet is a program which checks for significant deviations from normal results and left vs. right eye differences.

DISCUSSION

The example given above illustrates the possibilities available with a microprocessor system. The apparatus can be handled without any specific knowledge about computers. In fact, operation of the system hardly involves training since the system is self explanatory. We want to emphasize that not only technical features, like computation of a-wave and b-wave amplitudes and of OP's are of importance but equally so the ease with which the system can be operated.

REFERENCES

Stark, D. J., Canty, A. A. and Johnson, I. (1981). The development of a micro-computer system for electrophysiological assessment. Aust. J. Ophthal. 9, 129–133.
Miyake, Y., Solish, A., Hara, A. and Hirose, T. (1978). Clinical application of a digital computer software system to electrodiagnosis. Ophthalmic Res. 10, 268–278.

Mailing address:
Institute for Perception TNO
Kampweg 5, Soesterberg
The Netherlands

USE OF MICROCOMPUTERS TO ACQUIRE ELECTROPHYSIOLOGICAL DATA: DESCRIPTION OF A COMMERCIALLY AVAILABLE SYSTEM IN OPERATION

J. V. ODOM, K. WHITE and G. M. HOPE

(Gainesville, Florida, U.S.A.)

ABSTRACT

VECPs and ERGs have been recorded using oscilloscopes, signal averagers, and/or main frame computers. Each of these pieces of equipment is expensive. Currently available single channel signal averagers are $10k or more.

Modern innovations in electronics have made small general purpose computers both reliable and inexpensive. The wide availability of these computers has led to the emergence of manufacturers of specialized hardware and software which permit control of experiments and/or analysis of electrophysiological data.

There are currently several sources of hardware and software which permit the APPLE II to act as a signal processing system, including averaging, determination of amplitudes and calculation of spectal densities. Details of one such system, Applescope with Scope Driver Library will be given. The advantages and disadvantages of the system in operation will be discussed.

INTRODUCTION

The ability to analyze averaged bioelectric signals is an essential part of the research of most members of ISCEV. Aquiring equipment with these capacities is expensive, typically over $10,000. The recent increase in the availability of low cost, less than $2,000, microprocessors and microcomputers whose memory is as great or greater than the standard averagers introduces the possibility of using these newer devices for electrophysiological recording, averaging, and subsequent analyses. Below we shall outline our strategy for choosing a particular system, the Applescope, describe some of its more salient features, and describe some of its limitations.

Guidelines for Choice

Table 1 lists the systems which we considered purchasing and indications of their cost and some aspects of their hardware and software performance. In making our purchase we were guided by several considerations. First, we wanted an system which would average biological signals. Further processing

199

Table 1. A comparison of various systems for signal processing of clinical electrophysiologic data

	Input Channels	A/D Digitizer Resolution (Bits)	Averaging (Hardware or Software)	Artifact Rejection	Signal Measurement			Stimulus Control (D/A)
					Ampl.	Latency	Other	
Over 10K dollars								
Nicolet	2 (up to 16)	12 (up to 20)	yes	yes (some models)	yes	yes	yes (some models)	no (available)
Grass	2 (up to 4)	8	yes	yes	yes	yes	no	no (available)
Tracor	1	8	yes	yes	yes	yes	no	no
Under 5K dollars								
Applescope (Apple)	2	8	yes	no	yes	no	yes	no
NWIS Model 85 (Apple)	2	8	yes	no	yes	no	no	no
Teyler System (Apple)	2	8	yes	no	yes	yes	no	no
Isaac (Apple)	16	8	no	no	yes	no	no	yes
Datalab (Apple)	16	9	no	no	yes	no	no	yes
Data Logger (AIM-65)	16	12	no	no	yes	no	no	yes

Table 2. Scope Driver options and their limitations.

Option	Description	Limitations
Signal Averager	Acquires average of 1 or 2 channels	Minimum delay of 100 m sec between sweeps; 999 sweeps maximum; no artifact rejection
Digital Volt Meter	Determines voltage of 1 or 2 channels	One cursor; no latency; Original signal level 1 must be calculated; Amplifier gain not considered
Spectrum Analyzer	Analyzes the spectrum of an acquired signal	No dc component; No phase information; No digital printout; Frequency not specified
Autocorrelation	Autocorrelates 1 or 2 channels	No digital printout
Repetitive Sweep	Acquires offset traces	Maximum of 99
Math Pack	Determines a third channel which is some function of 2 channels	
Hardcopy	Prints a) monitor screen b) extrapolated chart record	

was considered desirable but not necessary. Second, we wanted a system which was immediately usable. We did not want to be required to construct our own hardware or software. Thirdly, we wanted to spend less than $5,000. Because it met our guidelines, seemed to have more software for signal analysis, and had been favorably reviewed (MacNicol, 1982), we purchased the Applescope made by RC Electronics with its available software, i.e., Scope Driver Library.

The Applescope consists of two boards, an analogue board and a digital board connected by a 20 conductor cable (hardware and Applescope software costs $595). The two boards fit into any two expansion slots on the Apple II plus. The standard Applescope consists of two independent analogue to digital (A/D) channels which have 8-bit resolution up to 3.5 mHz within one of two selectable input ranges, 0.025 to 0.8 volts and 0.25 to 8 volts, and with horizontal scales of 1 msec to 1000 sec per division (28 samples per division). Recommended options include external triggering and BNC conectors. One may increase either resolution or the upper limit of the frequency sampled (cost $695 per channel). Because one looses a data channel with the improved resolution options we chose not to acquire them.

The Scope Driver Library software (costs $345) contains the following options useful for signal averaging and analysis: Digital voltmeter, signal averager, hard copy, auto correlation, spectrum analysis, repetitive sweep, and math pack in addition to the Applescope. To use the Scope Driver software

201

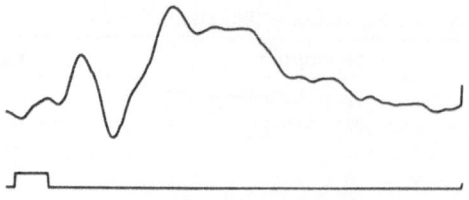

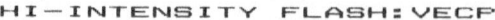

HI—INTENSITY FLASH: VECP

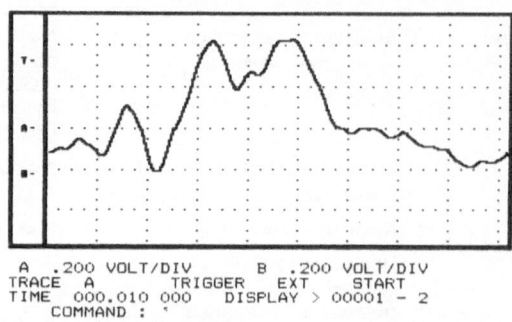

```
A  .200 VOLT/DIV        B  .200 VOLT/DIV
TRACE    A           TRIGGER   EXT      START
TIME   000.010 000     DISPLAY > 00001 - 2
         COMMAND :  '
```

Fig. 1. A comparison of VECPs recorded on a Nicolet MED-80 and the Applescope. The signal marker indicates a positive 1 μv pulse of 25 msec duration. The eliciting stimulus was a 1.5 Hz flash from a Grass P-22 photo stimulator on setting 16 imaged through a fiber optics bundle.

one must have the following hardware: Apple II plus computer with 48K RAM, one disk drive, one video monitor, and an Epson MX-100 printer or equivalent graphics printer.

In operation, one follows the procedure below: one acquires and averages the data, stores the data onto disk, and subsequently analyzes the data using one of the analysis options. Then, if hard copy is desired, one prints the desired data. One needs to keep independent records of the settings under which data were acquired as these are not part of the disk record.

Benchmark Tests

To compare the operation of the Applescope with that of the MED-80 we recorded electroretinograms (ERGs), pattern evoked retinal responses (PERRs) and visually evoked cortical potentials (VECPs) on FM tape. The taped data were then replayed and averages acquired using the Applescope and a Nicolet MED-80. The stimuli elicited by flashes of light were presented at 1.5 Hz, while the pattern reversal stimuli were presented at 4 Hz. The artifact reject option of the MED-80 was not used because the option does not exist as part of Scope Driver. 100 sweeps were averaged on both systems. Obtaining 100 sweeps using Apple Driver required from 3 (1.5 Hz stimulation) to 8 (4 Hz stimulation) times longer than acquiring with the MED-80, presumably because of the shorter intersweep interval required by the Nicolet (10 msec vs. 100 msec).

202

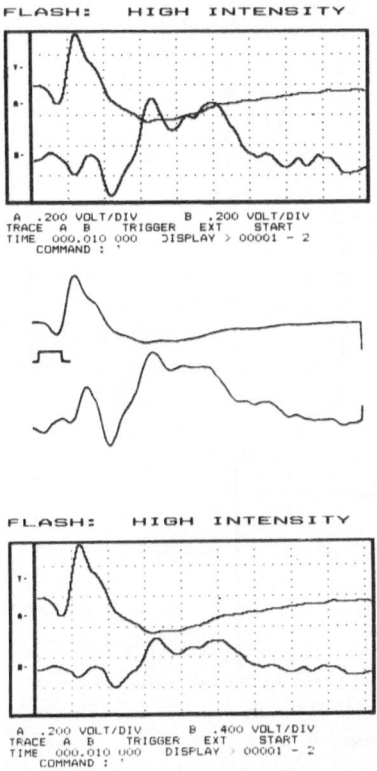

FLASH: HIGH INTENSITY

```
A  .200 VOLT/DIV      B  .200 VOLT/DIV
TRACE  A  B    TRIGGER  EXT    START
TIME  000.010 000   DISPLAY > 00001 - 2
       COMMAND :
```

FLASH: HIGH INTENSITY

```
A  .200 VOLT/DIV      B  .400 VOLT/DIV
TRACE  A  B    TRIGGER  EXT    START
TIME  000.010 000   DISPLAY > 00001 - 2
       COMMAND :
```

Fig. 2. The same stimulus conditions as in Figure 1. The top panel of the figure contains photopic ERGs and VECPs at the same gain for the computer (amplifier gain: ERG = 10K; VECP = 100K). In the bottom panel, the computer gain of the VECP channel has been reduced by half to avoid overlapping the figures. The central panel shows ERGs and VECPs recorded on the MED-80 under identical stimulus conditions. The marker is as in Fig. 1.

Examples of averages and some analysis options are presented in Figures 1 through 6. Figures 1 and 2 present the responses elicited by 1.5 Hz flashed diffuse light while Fig. 4 presents responses elicited by 4 Hz pattern reversal. The responses acquired on the MED-80 and Applescope system (Figs. 1 and 2) are similar but not identical. Presumably the individual responses making up the averages were not the same, because of the difference in intersweep intervals. Use of one (Fig. 1) or two (Fig. 2) input channels yields comparable results for the common response (VECPs). Fig. 2 and Fig. 3 present the same VECP and ERG data printed out in two different formats to illustrate the hardcopy options of the Scope Driver program. The PERRS and VECPs elicited by pattern reversal presented in Fig. 4, are similar to those observed previously and to those acquired using the MED-80.

Two analysis features of the Scope Driver package are presented, the digital volt meter (Fig. 5) and spectral analysis (Fig. 6). The digital volt meter (DVM) option determines the voltage of one or two channels and indicates it

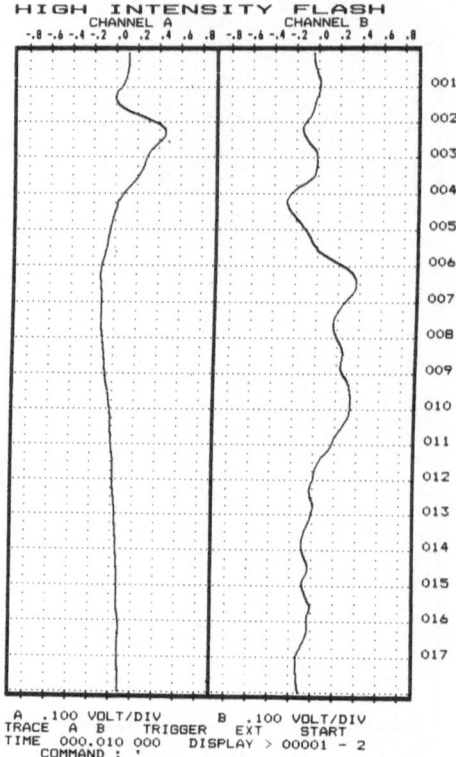

Fig. 3. The tracings are the same as in Fig. 2. Channel A is an ERG; channel B is a VECP. The plotting routine simulates a chart record. The voltage settings on the x-axis are absolute. The time scale on the y-axis is relative.

on the bottom line of the display. The voltage presented is determined from the stored average and is not corrected for gain. Latency information must be estimated from the position of the cursor. Peak to trough measures require the use of two measurements. RC Electronics has indicated in telephone conversations that they plan to modify the DVM package to provide latency measures and possibly to add a second cursor.

Averages and spectra for the pattern reversal waveform and VECP elicited by a square wave grating which subtended 23 arc min. are presented in Fig. 6. The real, imaginary, and magnitude (power) of the spectra may be determined by using the cursor and are displayed on the bottom line of text. The frequency at which these values occur is not presented, nor is a printout of the values. However, such a program may be easily written given knowledge of where the values are stored (provided by RC Electronics in its manual). Phase information is not available. One may average while in the spectrum analysis program. This aspect of the program permits one to acquire data, perform a spectrum analysis, and acquire another data set. Because the spectrum analysis replaces in memory the data it analyzes, one usually chooses to store the averaged data before performing the spectral analysis.

204

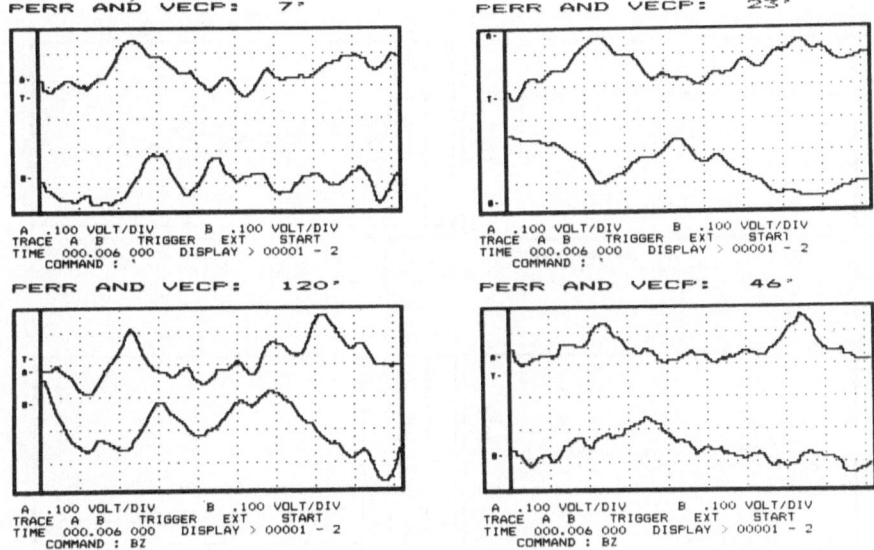

Fig. 4. PERRs and VECPs elicited by 4 Hz pattern reversal of square wave gratings. The gratings varied in angular subtense. Gain for both VECPs and PERRs was 100K. Channel A is the PERR and Channel B is the VECP.

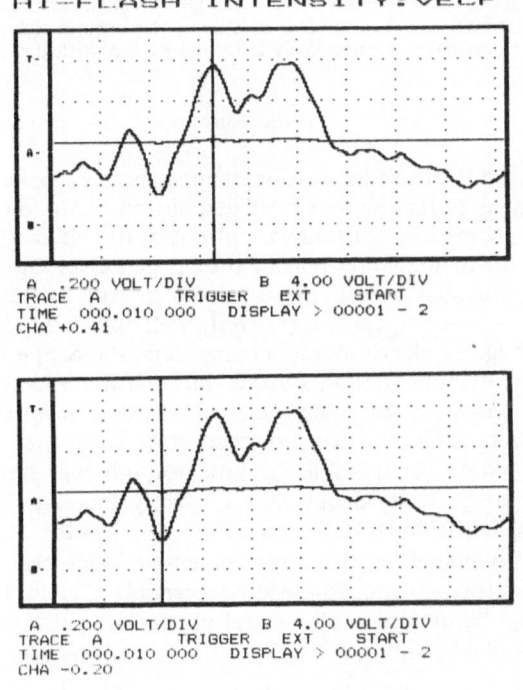

Fig. 5. The Digital Volt Meter is demonstrated. The tracing is the same as in Fig. 1. The peak to peak amplitude is 0.61 volts amplified from 6.1 μV real.

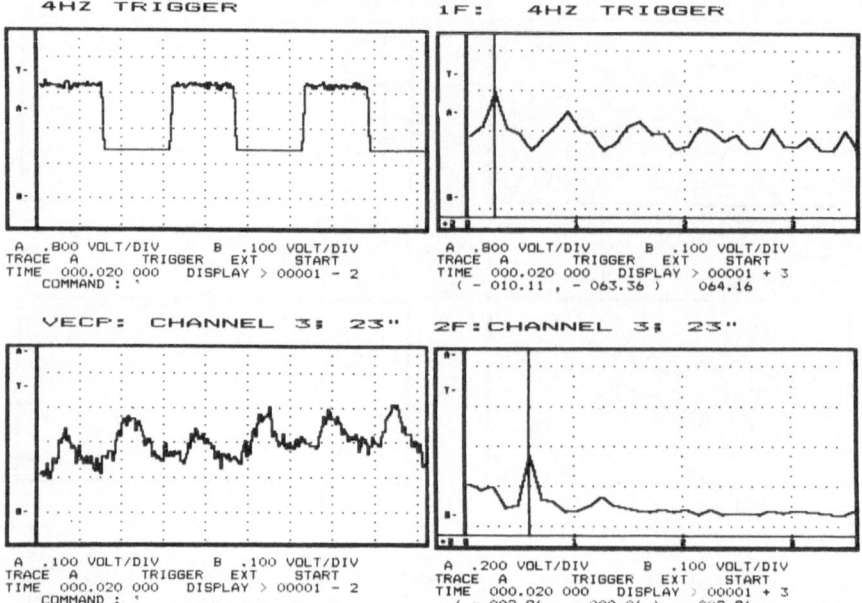

Fig. 6. Spectrum Analyzer is demonstrated. Tracings on the left are data to be analyzed. Tracings on the right are the spectra. The number at the bottom right is the magnitude (square root of the power) of the frequency indicated by the vertical cursor.

Limitations

Scope Driver options of use in averaging and analyzing bioelectrical signals is presented in Table 2 along with a brief description of the options and their limitations when compared with similar options of the MED-80.

There are three major limitations of the Scope Driver Options. First, the documentation provided by RC Electronics is uneven in quality. Although the Applescope reference manual is relatively well documented requiring only minimal knowledge of electronics and computers, the Scope Driver manuals provide minimal documentation. Further information and clarification has been readily provided by RC Electronics on request, however. With an eye to future software maintainence, however, it is clear that more rigorous documentation would be desirable. Second, the inherent limitation of 100 msec between sweeps using Scope Driver, greatly increases averaging time, especially at higher stimulation frequencies, i.e., shorter durations of the average, when compared to the more expensive machines. Third, certain portions of the programs are not readily accessible as data, namely latency information must be determined by visual inspection, phase frequency information is not available, and power information cannot be printed out, except as part of the graphic display which limits one to power at one frequency.

CONCLUSIONS

The preceeding section was devoted to the limitations of the Applescope with Scope Driver options. Clearly there are limitations of the Applescope with Scope Driver Library when compared to a dedicated signal averager; however, comparing the Applescope to the MED-80 which costs 10 times the $4,000 of our system is unfair. The bottom line is that the Applescope and its associated signal averaging software are a bargain at slightly over $1000. Our Apple system ($3000) provides us with computing, programming, and word processing abilities unavailable on most signal averaging systems. Therefore, if one's budget is limited, one needs a small portable system, and one wishes to purchase a commercially available system rather than develope one's own, one may consider the purchase of a microcomputer system such as the Applescope. The rapid improvements in microcomputer hardware and software make the use of microcomputer based averaging systems such as those in our Table 1 a viable option for many clinical and research applications.

REFERENCES

MacNicol, G. Applescope Stores Dual Traces. Byte 1982, 7 (6), 364–372.
Teyler, T. J., Mayhew, W. Chrin, C., and Kane, J. Neurophysiological field potential analysis by microcomputer. J. Neuro. Meth. Methods, 1982, 5, 291–303.

Mailing address:
Department of Ophthalmology
University of Florida
J-284 JHMHC
Gainesville, Florida 32610,
U.S.A.

IMPLEMENTATION OF A PORTABLE PATTERN STIMULATOR AND VEP/ERG RECORDING SYSTEM BASED ON AN APPLE MICROCOMPUTER

B. J. DE WAAL, D. REITS, H. SPEKREIJSE and C. A. GRIMBERGEN

(Amsterdam, The Netherlands)

ABSTRACT

A portable VEP/ERG recording system was developed by utilizing and adapting a commercially available microcomputer. The system was developed to facilitate the testing of patient and subject populations in whom laboratory recordings prove to be difficult and inconvenient. The system was designed to be compact, self-supporting and easily transportable for use at the bedside of clinical wards, in schools, nursing institutions and the like. Two important considerations were also cost-effectiveness and stimulus and recording versatility. The hardware components include a standard television monitor, a stimulus generator, an Apple II microcomputer and I/O peripherals. During the recording procedure the microcomputer simultaneously executes several tasks; sampling and averaging of up to 14 channels, on-line graphic display of averaged responses and pattern stimulation control. The system stimulus generator, though simple in its design, allows luminance flashes or simultaneous presentation of up to four independent, stable and flicker free checkerboard and bar patterns of different sizes and temporal frequencies. The stimulus patterns can be presented in a reversal or appearance/disappearance mode with adjustable timing and modulation depth. The hardware components and software implementation are described.

INTRODUCTION

In an electrophysiological laboratory dedicated to basic vision research and clinical application, experimental and diagnostic protocols often require testing subject and patient groups in which 'in house' laboratory recordings are inconvenient or not possible. For example, in a recent series of studies on maturation of the luminance and contrast evoked potentials (EP) (De Vries-Khoe and Spekreijse, 1982 and Kriss et al., 1983) subject samples spanned the entire age range from neonates to the elderly. Children attending day care centres and local schools (N > 500) were transported to the laboratory, following parental approval, by adult volunteers and laboratory personnel. For either the neonates, many of whom were in temperature controlled infant care units, or the elderly who resided in nursing homes for the aged, laboratory testing was often not possible. For these latter two groups, large and bulky stimulus and recording equipment was moved and maintained at the respective hospital departments and institutions. Although evoked potential recordings were performed under the conditions described, under certain circumstances neither procedure is feasible. In recording evoked potentials to objectively determine e.g. the effects of various anaesthetic drugs administered during open heart surgery, the delicate nature of the operation does not allow auxilliary equipment which by its size or operation interferes with the ongoing surgical procedures.

A viable solution to the difficulties in VEP testing associated with the above subject/patient groups among others is a compact, self-supporting portable stimulus and recording system for 'on site' testing. Such a system should be cost-effective, versatile and flexible. To satisfy our experimental and diagnostic requirements, the system should also:

1. Generate a wide variety of patterns in different parts of the visual field with sufficient resolution, linearity and dynamic range in time, space and contrast.
2. Permit signal recording at a sufficient sampling rate of at least 8 channels simultaneously, with user defined artifact rejection.
3. Include analysis features which
   (a) denote latencies and peak amplitudes of the various components in the averaged signals of transient evoked potentials and
   (b) provide amplitude and phase characteristics of steady state evoked potentials and spontaneous EEG signals by on-line Fourier analysis.
4. Continuously display the averaged signals with optimal automatic scaling for operator visual feedback.
5. Allow continuous operator control.
6. Provide facilities for plotting and printing waveforms and numerical data.
7. Provide long term data storage and retrieval.

To meet these requirements we have developed a low-cost stimulus and recording system which is based on a commercially available video monitor and a general purpose microcomputer, the Apple II. General purpose systems, in general, facilitate hardware design and also provide useful and time-saving software facilities such as operating systems, text-editors, compilers and interpreters. In addition to the useful graphics qualities of the Apple II microcomputer, its serviceability and availability of many I/O interfaces and peripherals have influenced our computer selection. For requirement (1) we have designed a stimulus generator which though simple in its design, allows luminance flash, simultaneous presentation of up to four independent checkerboard and/or bar patterns of the same or different size and/or temporal frequency. One of the advantages of this stimulus generator is that its high quality video signal can generate frame rates of over 100 Hz guaranteeing flicker free and stable pattern images on a monitor of equal frame rate capacity.

To satisfy requirements (3, in part) and (5) our system provides for 14 recording channels response averaging at sample frequencies of 250 Hz; averaging can be interrupted automatically by a present artifact rejector or by the user during subject inattentiveness.

210

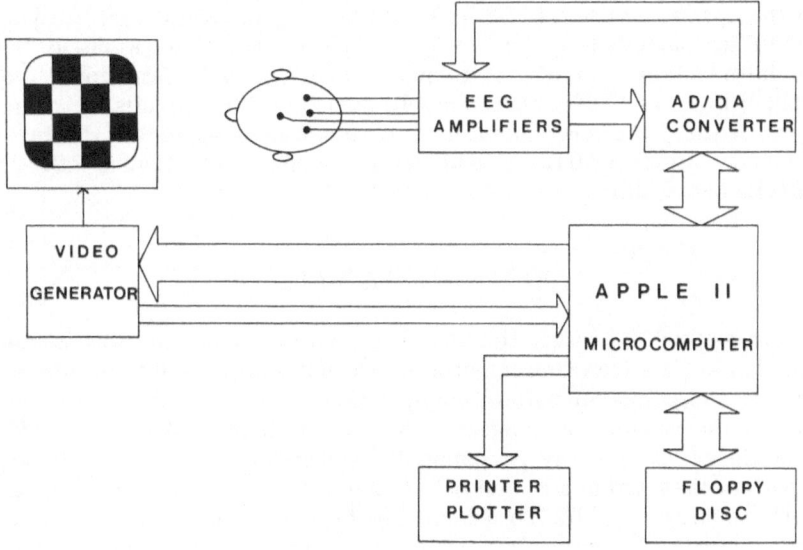

Fig. 1. Schematic overview of the various hardware components of the system.

Requirements (3–7), which are also within the capability of our system are discussed in more detail along with (1–2) in relation to the technical description of the system components and software design.

SYSTEM COMPONENTS DESCRIPTION

The basic computer components consist of a 6502 microprocessor, 48 kbyte RAM and a BASIC interpreter (Fig. 1). A 16 channel AD/DA converter with an 8-bit resolution (Mountain Hardware Corporation) routes the EEG signals into the microcomputer. The 0.4% resolution is more than sufficient for normal EEG signal to noise ratios. The amplification system is calibrated by using a divided ($\times 10^{-5}$) DA signal as input. To provide continuous, on-line response signals for operator visual feedback (requirement 4) one needs fast graphics display facilities. In the Apple II this is realized by integrating the bit representation of 280×192 pixels of the graphics display as the memory pages of the microcomputer. The resultant image is then displayed by a direct memory access (DMA) technique. As the graphics memory, which actually consists of two frames, is a part of the processor memory, it can be altered very fast. In addition to the advantages of this efficient display technique, one of the two image frames is permanently displayed, while the other can be changed allowing averaged response updating. A thermal dot matrix printer (Apple silentype) has been chosen for its low noise and hardcopy output facilities. As the screen dump of the computer graphics display takes only about 30 seconds, the operator is provided with rapid hardcopy printing and plotting of data (requirement 6). A floppy disc drive (5 inch,

211

capacity of 128 kbyte) is connected to the microcomputer to provide storage for the operating system (DOS 3.3), the user programs and the recorded data for off-line analysis (requirement 7). The pattern stimulator as discussed in the introduction with respect to requirement (1) and described in more detail below was built with commonly used integrated circuits to generate video signals for display monitors with frame rates up to 100 Hz. In our system we utilize a 50 Hz Hitachi VM 172 and a 100 Hz Conrac RQB 21C (30 MHz bandwidth).

PATTERN STIMULATOR

As the method for visual stimulation a television technique was selected. Stimulation via a television monitor affords not only versatility in intensity, contrast and choice of pattern configuration (Arden, 1978), but also comfort for the patients and subjects, who are accustomed to watching TV at home. Since visual acuity is commonly estimated by pattern EPs the range of pattern sizes within a $6°$ full-field should subtend, a minimum $1'$ of visual angle (Spekreijse, 1980). To achieve this high resolution at least 360 horizontal lines, each having 360 independent pixels are required, as such a 512×512 pixel array was chosen. To reach a high scanning frequency (to avoid perceptible flicker) and sufficient pixel resolution monitors with a bandwidth of at least 26 MHz are required. Although these requirements can be satisfied with advanced and costly graphics CRT systems, such systems necessitate large and fast random access memory (32 kbyte) for storing display data. Furthermore, manipulating the mode of stimulus presentation, e.g. pattern reversal, a graphic CRT system demands time consuming updating. A complete update including calculations of memory can take more than 0.6 seconds (32k times 20 microseconds for each byte). In contrast, the high speed and efficient memory design of the stimulus technique we have selected takes about 10 milliseconds. The high scanning frequency, pixel resolution and rapid display updating of our stimulus system is more suitable for VEP research. Our alternative memory concept and control of pattern generation is shown in the block diagram of Fig. 2.

The typical patterned stimuli used in VEP testing i.e. checkerboards and bar patterns, require a very small number of different raster lines. A full-field checkerboard pattern can be generated with only two different raster lines; a vertical bar pattern can be generated with only one raster line. Thus memory can be reduced considerably. In the horizontal memory (16×152 bits or 16×64 bytes) 16 different horizontal lines can be stored. Which of the 16 lines will actually be written on the display depends on the value stored in the corresponding location of the vertical memory. The memory contents for a full and two half-field checkerboards are shown in Fig. 3. A more complex pattern, like 4 simultaneous checkerboard patterns of different field sizes in each quadrant, requires 8 horizontal memory lines. A similar memory pattern with the addresses of corresponding lines is stored in the vertical memory. All timing signals are derived from a crystal clock controlled video sync generator which provides optimal sychronization of horizontal

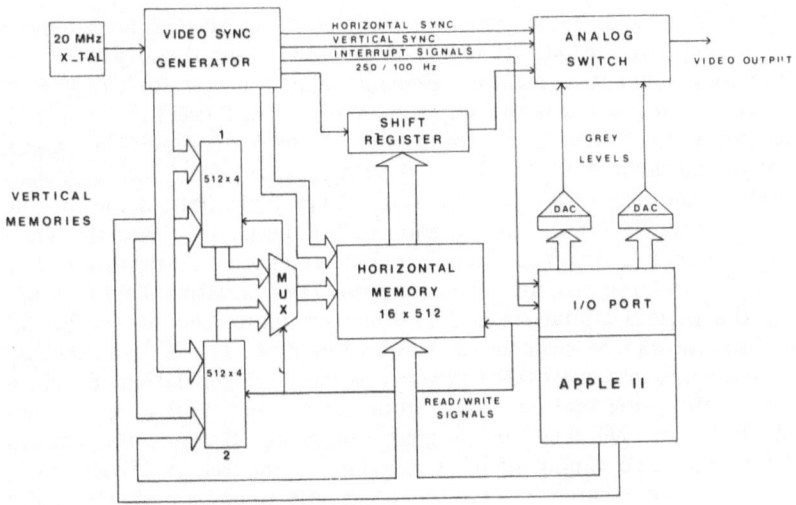

Fig. 2. Block diagram of the video generator.

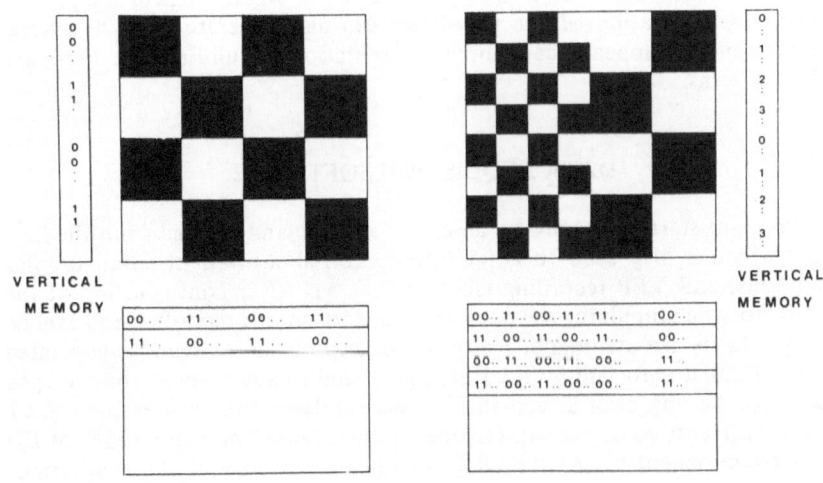

Fig. 3. Memory contents of the video generator for a full- and half-field checkerboard pattern.

and vertical deflection signals with the video signal itself. A shift register is loaded from the horizontal memory according to an address counter (0–63) for its lowest six address bits and according to its 4 highest address bits derived from the vertical memory assigned to a specific line. After loading the shift register, 8 new bits are shifted to an analog switch where the video signal is constructed. The actual length of the shift register must be 9 bits rather than

213

8, to avoid loading artifacts, which result in spurious vertical lines on the display. To improve the bit rate of the video signal without using faster and therefore more expensive memory elements only a longer shift register is needed. As stated previously memory update for a new image takes about 10 milliseconds (512 times 20 microseconds). As in Video-Look-Up Tables, frequently used in state-of-the-art graphics displays, an analog switch assigns grey-levels to the pixels for contrast modulation of the pattern elements. One grey-level is assigned for the logic 0 and one for the logic 1. With this technique the modulation depth can be adjusted in as many as 128 steps controlled by a parallel I/O port of the microcomputer. Two additional interactions between the pattern stimulator and the microcomputer should also be discussed. First, as can be seen in the block diagram of Fig. 2, two identical vertical memories are used. One memory is used for generating the video signal while the other can be loaded from the microcomputer with a new pattern. Both are switched on program command. Second, the pattern stimulator sends two timing signals to the microcomputer. A 250 Hz clock, locked at the frame rates, is used as the sample frequency. An interrupt servicing routine uses the vertical sync to lock the pattern alteration to the vertical retrace of the monitor. This procedure is important for accurate latency estimations (Arden, 1978). Another feature of the grey-level assignment is that in addition to changing the dark and bright levels of the pattern elements, modification of the grey-levels can also generate pattern reversal or appearance/disappearance stimulus presentation of full-field checkerboard or bar patterns.

DATA ACQUISTION SOFTWARE

The program starts in BASIC by an operator command entered from the keyboard which is also used to enter information about patient data, stimulus conditions, and VEP recording (requirement 5). After configuration of the pattern for the stimulator the operator can start on-line recording and averaging by a keyboard command. Every 4 milliseconds an interrupt is generated by the stimulator to sample the EEG signals and to add them to the averaged waveform. During each sweep the last accumulated averaged responses are shown with automatic scaling on one of the graphic memory pages of the Apple (requirement 4). At the same time in the memory of the other frame the new averaged waveform is built up. Besides the 250 Hz sample interrupts the stimulator generator at every vertical sync. The program uses these sync pulses to change the stimulus pattern only during a vertical retrace. A simple form of artifact rejection was added to the real-time programs. When an overflow occurs in one of the AD-channels none of the samples of the actual sweep will be added to the averaged responses (requirement 3). All the interrupt servicing programs and associated routines are written in 6502 assembly language. Efficient assembly programming, AD-conversion time of 9 microseconds and almost processor independent functioning of the stimulator makes it possible to sample and average up to 14 channels. A keyboard command allows the operator to stop the averaging procedure when

214

the responses stabilize. Other commands can restart the program immediately or can plot the final averages (requirement 6). The VEP/ERGs, patient identifying data and stimulus program parameters are stored on floppy disc (requirement 7).

CONCLUSION

A portable and self-supporting VEP/ERG recording system has been developed with commercially available components and a home-made pattern stimulator, which is cost effective (without EEG amplifiers about $4000). The main features of the present system are:

(1) The pattern stimulator can generate a wide variety of rectilinear patterns, e.g. checkerboards and bars, on standard high frame rate monitors. As stimulus modes luminance, pattern reversal and appearance/disappearance can be chosen with adjustable timing and modulation depth.

(b) With a sample frequency of 250 Hz 14 VEP/ERG signals can be averaged and displayed on-line.

(c) The final averaged response profile to a particular stimulus condition is stored immediately on floppy disc. Since data storage takes less than 1 sec the user need not interrupt the experimental sequence; a hardcopy of the result can be printed and plotted at a later time.

All the requirements stated in the introduction with the exception of number 3 have been fulfilled in a system, which is now in an operating state of development. Several new features will be added to the system including auditory stimulation, recording and analysis of high frequency brain-stem potentials and system interfacing to another computer system for more elaborate data analysis and storage. Our continuous design and development efforts are now being directed to meet requirement 3. If more sophisticated on-line analysis techniques are required the Apple microcomputer can be extended by off-the-shelf available plug-in units with fast 16 bits microprocessors (Metamorphic Systems, Inc., 8088 metacard). With the many possible hardware extensions available and user defined programs, the apparatus can be expanded to a general purpose stimulation, data recording and analysis system for a wide range of medical applications.

ACKNOWLEDGEMENTS

The project was supported by the Organization for Health Research (T.N.O.), the Hague. We thank Mr. L. J. de Vries and Mr. P. B. Brassinga for constructing the stimulator and for valuable contributions to its design. We are indebted to Dr. P. A. Apkarian and Dr. O. Estévez for their critical suggestions on this paper.

REFERENCES

Arden, G. B., Faulkner, D. J. and Mair, C. A versatile television pattern generator for visual evoked potentials. In: Visual Evoked Potentials in Man: New Developments, edited by Desmedt, J., pp. 90–109. Clarendon Press, Oxford (1977).

215

Arden, G. B., Bodis-Wollner, I., Halliday, A. M., Jeffreys, A., Kulikowski, J. J., Spek-reijse, H. and Regan, D. Methodology of patterned visual stimulation. In: Visual Evoked Potentials in Man: New Developments, edited by Desmedt, J., pp. 3–15. Clarendon Press, Oxford (1977).

Kriss, A., Spekreijse, H., Verduyn Lunel, H. F. E., Braamhaar, H. G. M., De Waal, B. J. and Barret, G. Pattern onset, offset and reversal responses; effect of age, gender and checksize. In press.

Spekreijse, H. Pattern evoked potentials: principles, methodology and phenomenology. In: Evoked Potentials. Proceedings of an evoked potentials Symposium held in Nottingham, England, edited by Barber, C., pp. 55–74. University Park Press, Baltimore (1980).

Mailing address:
The Netherlands Ophthalmic Research Institute & Laboratory of Medical Physics
University of Amsterdam
P.O. Box 6411
1005 EK Amsterdam,
The Netherlands

216

MICROCOMPUTER PRESENTATION OF PATTERNED STIMULI FOR VISUAL ELECTROPHYSIOLOGY

G. M. HOPE, W. W. DAWSON and J. V. ODOM
(Gainesville, Florida, U.S.A.)

ABSTRACT

This paper describes a series of programs which allow general purpose checkerboard and grating patterns to be drawn, stored on disk, rapidly recalled, displayed and phase reversed as stimuli for electrophysiological recording of visual system activity. The programs are written for a modestly configured system based on the APPLE II PLUS microcomputer. Comparison of Pattern Evoked Cortical Potentials in response to optically projected and computer generated vertical gratings illustrate the efficacy of this approach. Consideration of advantages and disadvantages of this system suggest that this is a viable alternative to currently available approaches to presentation of phase reversing, patterned stimuli.

INTRODUCTION

Inexpensive microcomputers capable of sophisticated graphics offer a convenient mechanism for the generation of patterned stimuli which can be spatially displaced in a periodic fashion. Several papers have described software written for the APPLE II computer for this purpose (e.g., Rowe and Grossman, 1980; Cavanagh and Anstis, 1980; Swihart, 1982). However, these are not entirely satisfactory for routine recording of Pattern Evoked Retinal Responses (PERRs) or Pattern Evoked Cortical Potentials (PECPs) because the patterns are highly specialized (Rowe, 1981; Cavanagh and Anstis, 1980) or require especially constructed external hardware and slowly draw each pattern prior to display (Swihart, 1982). The purpose of this communication is to report a group of programs for the APPLE II Plus microcomputer which allows general purpose grating and checkerboard patterns to be predrawn, stored on disk, rapidly recalled and alternated for visual system stimulation. The software will function on a modest system and requires no specialized, external hardware.

METHODS

Apparatus. The basic components necessary to utilize the software are an APPLE II Plus microcomputer with 48 Kbytes of random access memory

(RAM), one disk drive and a monitor. The features of the APPLE II Plus of interest in this context are its high resolution graphics capabilities, especially that it offers two 'pages' of graphics, each page corresponding to an 8K block of memory. Either page can be displayed on the monitor and it is possible to shift from page to page instantaneously. Each page consists of a matrix of lighted (or dark) spots (pixels), 280 pixels horizontally and 192 pixels vertically. It is necessary to connect one of the integrated circuit (I.C.) pins (pin 8 of I.C. B11) to pin 4 of the input—output (I.O.) socket, as described in detail by Cavanagh and Anstis (1980). This minor modification makes the video retrace sync pulse available to the software so that pattern (page) shifts can be timed to occur during video retrace blanking.

Software description. There are three sets of programs, each set corresponding to a different patterned display (checkerboards, horizontal gratings and vertical gratings). Each set consists of two programs, one which draws and stores the patterns and a second which loads, displays and alternates the pages (patterns). Corresponding programs for the three sets are virtually identical, so only the vertical grating set will be described.

The pattern drawing program first provides information and instructions to the user, then offers the choice of including or excluding a small 'X' as a stable, central fixation point, Element size for each pair of gratings is set by an algorithm which starts with the minimum pattern element ('bar') size, one pixel wide, then raises this minimum to a power (0 to 6).

The program draws two graphics pages, each a complete grating but the inverse, for each 'bar' size. First, graphics page 1 is generated by drawing alternate 'bars'. If the fixation point was elected, the program then darkens a small square in the center of the pattern and draws a small 'X' in the square. The procedure is repeated for graphics page 2, but with precise reversal of light and dark elements. The 16-Kbyte block of memory containing the binary code representing the two gratings is then stored on disk under a file name which includes a number (0—6) indicating 'bar' size. This entire process is repeated for the next larger sized grating patterns, sequentially, until all seven grating pairs are stored on disk. Drawing and storing the seven sets of gratings requires some 20 minutes but they must be drawn only once unless some change is desired (e.g., fixation point removed or added).

The second program in the set is the one routinely used to present the stimuli. The program is menu (options list) controlled and, following instructions, the first (main) menu is presented. This menu offers six options; (1) select specific patterns by size, (2) all sizes in order, (3) calibrate/check timing, (4) calibrate/measure screen luminances, (5) calibrate element size, (6) quit; which are selected by number. Treated in reverse order, the last option, (6) terminates the program. The fifth option produces a line (length equal to the width of the largest 'bar') and requests that the user enter the measured length of the line (in mm) and the distance of the subject's eye from the screen (in meters). These values are stored in two 'text files' on disk and are used later in the program to calculate the visual angles subtended by the various sized grating elements. This option allows recalibration of the pattern sizes for different screen sizes or subject-to-screen distances. The

218

fourth option draws one-half of one screen to allow the luminance of the lighted and unlighted portions to be measured and/or adjusted. The third option activates a subroutine which presents a list from which the user selects an alternation rate, then displays alternating lighted and dark screens to provide sync triggers to allow recording apparatus adjustment and measurement of precise timing of the alternations.

The portions of the program which actually display and alternate the gratings are accessed by options one and two. Option two provides the shift rate selection subroutine, then displays and alternates, at the selected rate, the seven gratings in order of increasing element size. The first option, the one routinely used, presents the user with a second menu or options list offering options (0)–(8), seven grating patterns (sizes, 0–6), each with subtended visual angle; option (7), a set of control screens; and option (8), quit/no more sizes. The visual angle associated with each size is the angle subtended by the width of the 'bar' at the eye-to-screen distance provided to the computer under option (5) above. These are recalled from disk and subjected to an algorithm which calculates the width of each sized 'bar', then calculates the visual angles subtended by the 'bar' width and the horizontal and vertical dimensions of the display. Instructions inform the user that up to 10 of the options (except (0)) can be selected in any order and the corresponding pattern or control will be displayed and alternated in the order chosen. If option (0) is selected first, the program returns to the main (first) menu. If other options have been selected, it proceeds to the display/alternate subroutines.

On entering this group of subroutines, the user is informed that, once each pattern is drawn, the 'return' key will initiate alternation and any keypress will stop alternation. An iterative loop then steps through the selected options. If the current option is the 'Control Set', the program lights the entire field of both graphics pages (with fixation) and, on command, initiates alternation. If the current option is a grating pattern, the appropriate pattern (option number = size number) is loaded into the 16 Kbyte block of graphics memory and, on command, proceeds to the alternation subroutine.

The subroutine which loads the two graphics pages into memory terminates with graphics page 2 on the monitor screen. The alternation subroutine first senses the video retrace sync pulse, then supplies a trigger signal (level change 0.3 to 3.5 volts) to pin 15 of the I.O. socket. It then delays until the next retrace blanking period, then 'switchs' the display to graphics page 1 for the period of time determined by the selected alternation rate. If no key has been pressed (the user termination signal), the entire procedure is repeated to display the next set of patterns or, if the next option was (0), return to the second menu.

Electrophysiological recordings. As a demonstration, visual pattern evoked cortical potentials were recorded from a normal human subject while viewing optically projected vertical gratings and similar gratings on the computer monitor. Signals were recorded from a silver-silver chloride scalp electrode placed 2.5 cm above the inion on the midline, referenced against a similar electrode on the right mastoid, with the forehead grounded. Signals were

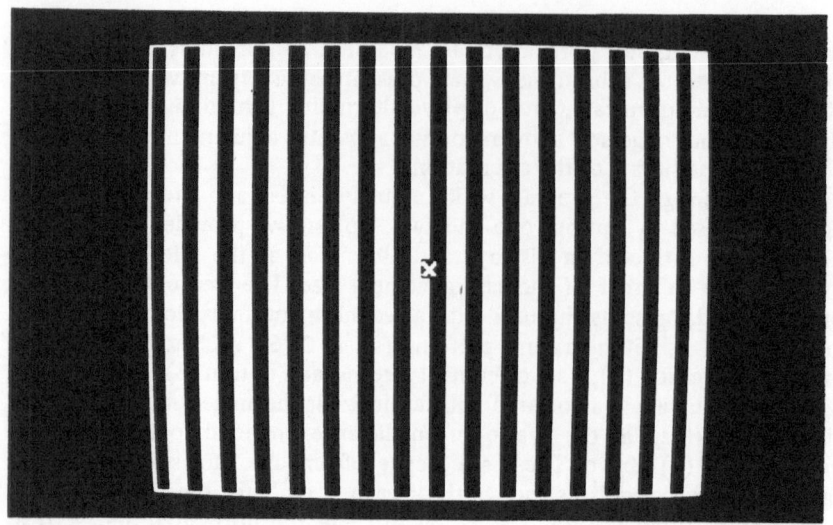

Fig. 1. Example of a computer generated vertical grating pattern. This is an actual photograph of the monitor screen with an intermediate sized vertical grating displayed.

amplified conventionally (10,000 times, Tektronix 122 Preamplifiers), passed through an active 60 Hz notch filter and summed and stored on disk by a general purpose computer (Nicolet MED 80).

The grating patterns were displayed on a 24 inch (diagonal measure) video monitor (Conrac CVB-23), or were transparencies projected (Viewlex) onto a white screen, alternated by opposed speaker coils driven by a square wave generater (Wavetek 110). The optically corrected subject, with natural pupils, was seated in an electrically shielded chamber one meter from the screen or monitor, with the latter placed just outside the open doorway of the chamber. The grating patterns were displayed in ascending order by 'bar' size and were alternated at a nominal rate of three shifts per second. The luminance of the lighted elements on the computer monitor was + 1.2 Log ft. Lamberts and that of the dark elements was − 1.0 Log ft. Lamberts. Corresponding measures for the projected pattern were + 1.75 and + 1.0 Log ft. Lamberts, respectively. Signals in response to 100 cycles (two alternations or phase shifts per cycle) were summed.

Additional analysis of the stored signals was conducted off-line. Analysis consisted of digitally filtering the waveforms to remove a substantial 120 Hz electrical artifact and to determine amplitude and latency values. After filtering, waveforms were plotted on an X–Y plotter (Esterline Angus 575).

RESULTS

Figure 1 presents a photograph of an intermediate sized vertical grating. The most obvious feature is the high contrast between the light and dark bars. Luminance inhomogenieties which are present when viewed on the monitor

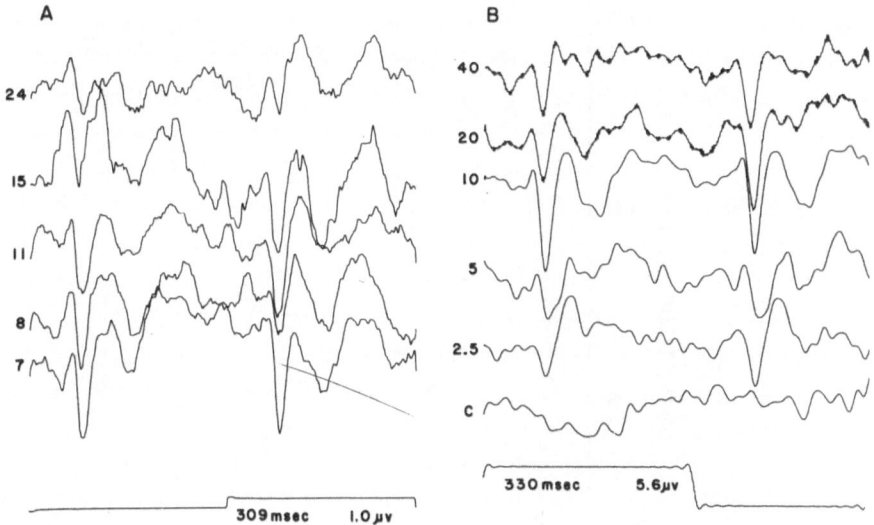

Fig. 2. Pattern Evoked Cortical Potentials in response to an optically produced vertical grating (A) and in response to a computer generated, video displayed vertical grating (B). Visual angles subtended by the light bars of each pattern are indicated to the left of each waveform. 'C' indicates a control recording in response to blank, lighted video displays alternated just as were the patterns.

have been lost in the photographic process. The 'barrel' distortion seen in this figure is also a photographic artifact and is not apparent on the monitor screen.

Figure 2 presents a set of PECPs in response to optically projected and mechanically alternated vertical gratings (Fig. 2A), and computer displayed and alternated vertical gratings (Fig. 2B). Comparison of the waveforms from the two vertical grating displays (2A vs. 2B) reveals that the maximum amplitude of those in response to the computer display are some 50% greater than from the optical display. The amplitudes in response to the computer patterns (2B) vary consistently with pattern element size, as opposed those in response to the optically projected patterns (2A). In both cases, the responses are of reasonable quality.

The amplitudes of these signals were determined digitally by off-line computer analysis and plotted against visual angle (Fig. 3). The amplitudes of the responses to the computer displays increase to a maximum at some visual angle, then decrease with increasing angle. The amplitudes of signals in response to the optically projected patterns are much less orderly. Extrapolation of minimum resolvable angle by least squares regression analysis suggests about 1 minute of arc for data from the computer patterns, but was not possible for this particular set of recordings in response to the optically projected pattern.

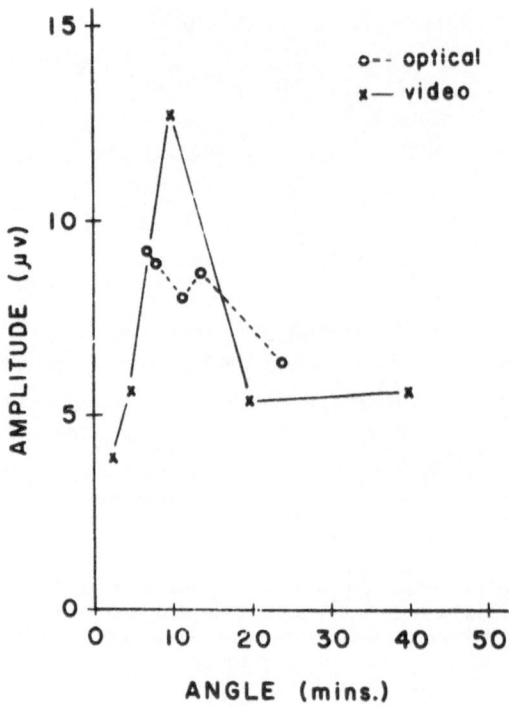

Fig. 3. Amplitudes of the responses in Figure 2 plotted against visual angle. Amplitudes were measured from the first positive peak to the first negative peak.

DISCUSSION

We have found this approach to the generation and alternation of patterned visual stimuli to be convenient and effective. However, as with most visual stimulus generation systems, there are compromises and undesirable features which must be considered. One of the most notable is the injection of electrical noise by the presence of the video monitor in the immediate proximity of the subject. The electrical noise was at two very specific frequencies, 60 and 120 Hz, with the 60 Hz signal being of much higher amplitude. As can be seen in the records presented above, the combination of active and digital filtering effectively removed this noise, yielding very useable records. We have not encountered the 50 Hz visual noise associated with the frame rate (retrace) which has been described by van Lith, Marle and Vijfvinkel-Bruinenga (1979). We have no ready explanation for this, but presume it might be related to the use of alternated patterns, provision of central fixation target or, possibly, differences in phosphor persistance.

Several compromises are inherent in the APPLE II Plus graphics, First, any lighted area on the monitor has a striated appearance. This appears to be due to the discrete nature of the pixels, with the striations reflecting the minute dark spaces between lighted pixels. The striations may appear vertical, horizontal or both, depending on the focus of the monitor. A second, similar, undesirable feature is the tendency for the first pixel of a horizontal string to be brighter than those following it. The reason for this is unclear, but the result is a slightly brighter vertical line along the left edge of each pattern element. Empirically, no effect of these luminance inhomogenieties has been detectable in our data and for routine clinical electrodiagnostic applications, they are probably inconsequential. However, as uncontrolled stimulus complexities, they could present theoretical problems. The relationship between pixel size and the size of the portion of the screen used by the APPLE II Plus for graphics imposes a limitation on the range of visual angles available. The smallest practical element is 2 by 2 pixels for checkerboards and the largest total field is 280 by 192 pixels. However, the total 280 by 192 pixel field can rarely be used because equal numbers of lighted pattern elements must appear on each page — otherwise luminance artifacts will result. Therefore, the maximum total field size is limited to an even-numbered multiple of the largest element. Further, if the total field size is to remain constant for all patterns, smaller element ('checker') sizes must be powers-of-two decrements of the maximum element. Otherwise, smaller elements will not fit completely within the total field and partial — therefore smaller — elements along the margins will compromise element size homogeniety within patterns. Consequently, the total field may be smaller — or the smallest element larger — than might be desired, and element size increments may be somewhat limited. Finally, while the software takes advantage of the video retrace signal to time pattern shifts, in practice we have found that image breakdown can occur at shift rates which are not multiples of the frame rate. Also, Applesoft Basic commands will only allow pattern shifts up to about 20/sec. Above this rate, machine language routines are required (Cavanagh and Anstis, 1981). In general, we have experienced no significant problems as a result of the limitations described, although in some cases, the greater precision afforded by smaller size increments would have been useful.

There are a number of advantages to this method for patterned stimulus alternation, compared to physically displacing a projected transparency — the most commonly employed alternative. First, the video image provides noticeably higher contrast and apparent color temperature than most optical projection systems. These factors probably account for the higher signal amplitudes obtained in the direct comparison of the two approaches. Additionally, pattern shifts are totally electronic and silent, avoiding mechanically generated auditory stimuli — thus auditory signal artifacts — in synchrony with pattern alternation. Finally, the computer controlled pattern alternation is significantly more convenient and rapid than any except the most complex opto-mechanical approaches. The 17 seconds required to change pattern sizes with the computer is much faster than exchanging transparencies by hand, although slower than mechanical exchange, and no adjustment of alternation parameters is required. The video monitor requires neither obligatory projection distances, nor projection beampaths which limit patient placement, nor refocus on movement. The monitor can be physically displaced from the

223

computer by any reasonable distance so that controlling hardware can be both unobtrusive and convenient for use.

In summary, computer controlled video display of alternating patterns as visual stimuli for electrophysiological measurement offers a number of advantages in convenience, simplicity, and some stimulus characteristics, but at the expense of some limitation and compromise. We have found that the advantages significantly outweigh the limitations and this factor, coupled with the modest cost of the system, render this approach a feasible alternative to currently available commercial and optical approaches. The software described, with documentation, is available from the authors, either in printed form or on diskette (furnish APPLE II Plus compatible diskettes) at no cost.

REFERENCES

1. Cavanagh, P. and Anstis, S. M., 1980. Visual psychophysics on the APPLE II: getting started. Behav. Res. Meth. and Instrum. 12, 614–626.
2. Lith, G. H. M. van; Marle, G. W. van and Vijfvinkel-Bruinenga, S., 1979. Two disadvantages of a television system as pattern stimulator for evoked potentials. Doc. Ophthalmol. 48, 261–266.
3. Rowe, M. J. III, 1981. A sequential technique for half-field pattern visual evoked potential testing. Electroencephalogr. and Clin. Neurophysiol., 51, 463–469.
4. Rowe, M. J. III and Grossman, C., 1980. Multiple page graphics for the APPLE II. Kilobaud Microcomput., 39, 66.
5. Swihart, S. L., 1982. Photostimulation with a microcomputer. J. Electrophysiol. Tech., 8, 102–106.

Mailing address:
Department of Ophthalmology
University of Florida
Box J-284, JHMHC
Gainesville, Florida 32610,
U.S.A.

MICROCOMPUTER TECHNIQUE FOR IDENTIFICATION OF ELECTRICAL BIOPOTENTIALS TRANSMITTED ALONG THE OPTICAL PATHWAYS

R. ALFIERI, J.-Y. BOIRE and P. SOLÉ

(Clermont-Ferrand, France)

ABSTRACT

After a light stimulation, the electrical potentials are recorded on the ocular zone (electroretinogram), on the temporal and parietal zones (electroaxogram), and on the occipital zone (electrovisiogram or visual evoked cortical potential). Using mathematical methods (with microcomputer) the morphology and the propagation of electrophysiological signals are studied. Apart from the future possibilities, a clinical application exists now: early detection of demyelinating diseases such as multiple sclerosis.

INTRODUCTION

Electrophysiological research into optic pathways provides us with more detailed information about the anatomical structure. Usually there are two interesting electrical potentials in response to a light stimulation. The first, the ERG (electroretinogram), is due to the photoreceptor, and the bipolar and Müller cells. There are the cones for photopic vision and the rods for scotopic vision. With interference filters it is possible to obtain only the cone response with a red stimulation at 650 nm and only the rod response with a blue stimulation at 450 nm. The second, the VECP or EVG (visual evoked cortical potential or electrovisiogram), depends on the quality of the central part of the retina and more precisely of the cones of the macula because their cortical projection is predominant (Alfieri and Solé, 1979).

Electrophysiological potentials after stimulation may consist of three signals: the ERG; the VECP or EVG and the third the EAG (electroaxogram), which is recorded from the temporal and parietal zones. There are two possible explanations: the EAG could be due to artifacts from a volume conduction of ERG or VECP, or the EAG could in fact come from optic nerve potentials (Siegfried, 1980).

CLINICAL ASPECT

We have two very interesting cases which confirm the second point of view.

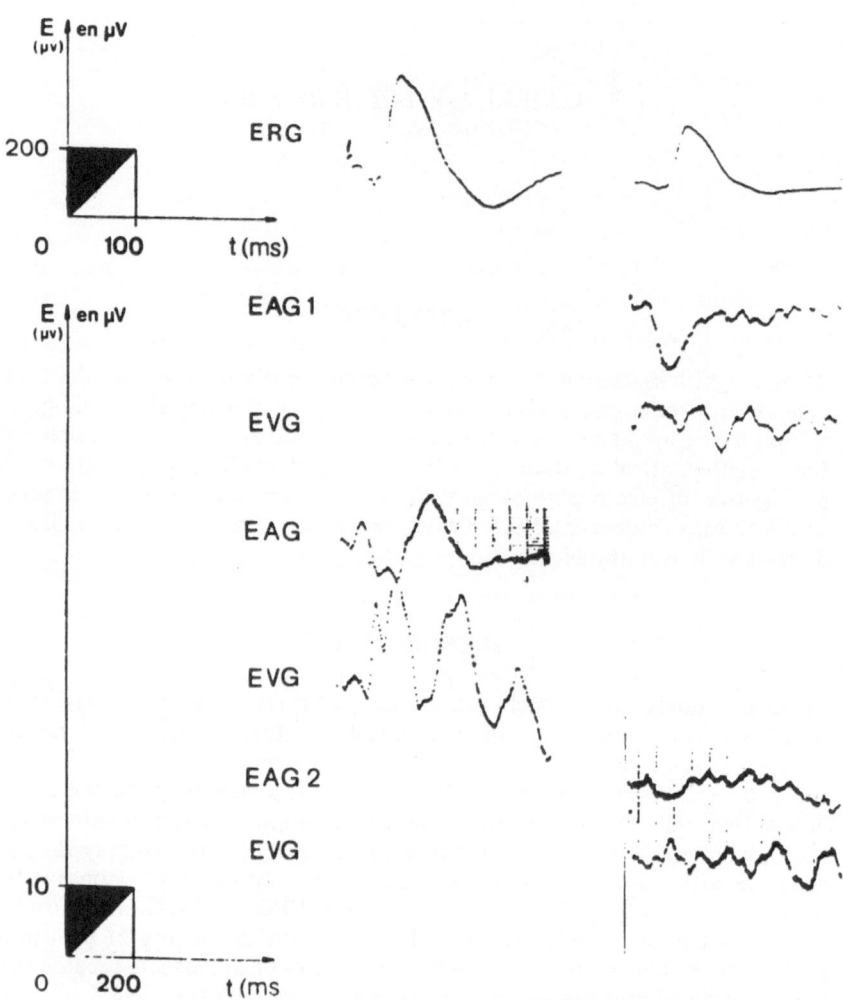

Fig. 1. Optic nerve section. E: potential; t: time; RE: right eye; LE: left eye; ERG: electroretinogram; EAG: electro-axogram (1: before the entry point of the bullet; 2: after); EVG: electrovisiogram.

Case 1

A case of attempted suicide where the bullet cut the optic nerve of the left eye. Figure 1 shows the different signals. For the right eye, ERG, EAG and EVG are normal. For the left eye, the ERG is normal, but the EVG is insignificant; we recorded two EAG on each side of the entry point of the bullet. Only the first EAG from the electrode nearest to the eye (Fig. 1: EAG 1) was significant, which proves that there was no volume conduction from the EVG

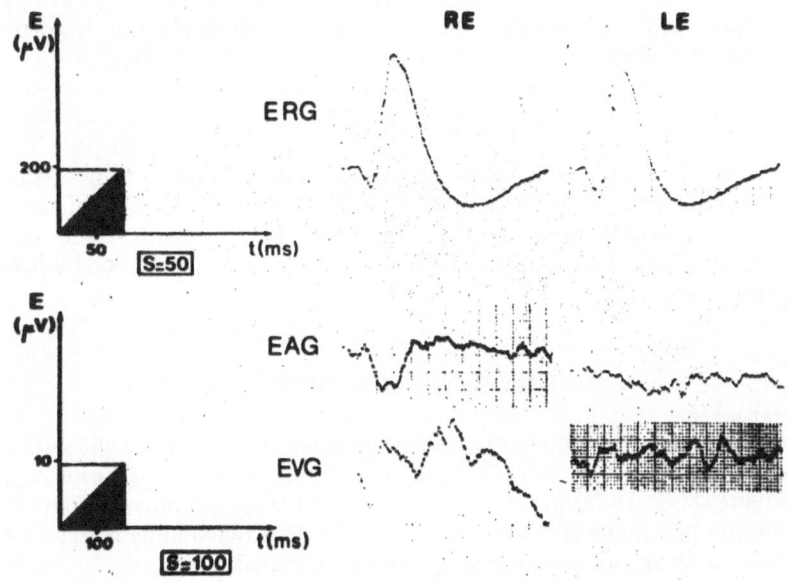

Fig. 2. Optic neuritis at the acute stage. E: potential; t: time; RE: right eye; LE: left eye; ERG: electroretinogram; EAG: electro-axogram; EVG: electrovisiogram.

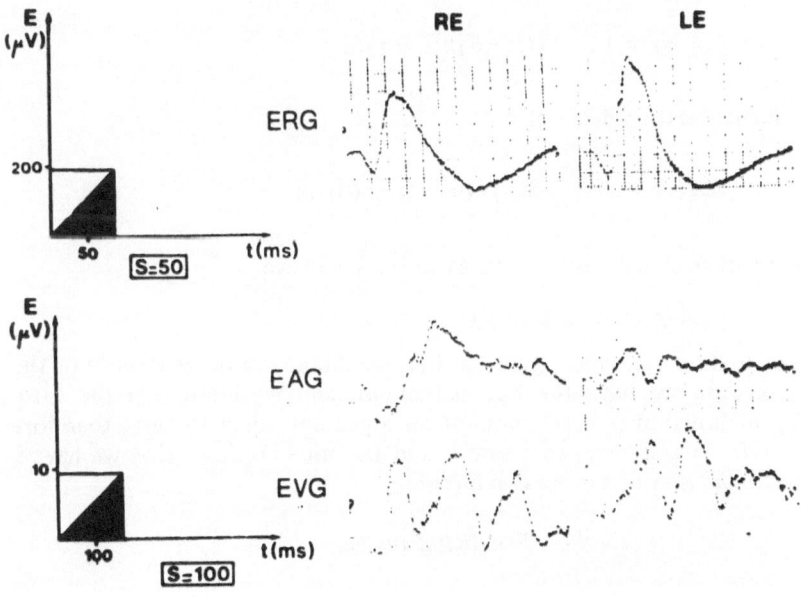

Fig. 3. Optic neuritis at the recovery stage. E: potential; t: time; RE: right eye; LE: left eye; ERG: electroretinogram; EAG: electro-axogram; EVG: electrovisiogram.

227

(because the EVG was not recordable). The second EVG (Fig. 1: EAG 2) is extinguished, which proves that there was no volume conduction from the ERG (while the ERG is normal).

Case 2

A case of optic neuritis with recovery. Figure 2 shows defective transmission along the optic nerve of the left eye since the EAG and EVG are extinguished. Figure 3 shows that after recovery from the optic neuritis there is a *reappearance* of the EAG and the EVG of the left eye, accompanied by light perception.

THEORETICAL ASPECT

We have just seen how the EAG is of great interest, but further theoretical investigation is needed. For example, the calculations of the correlation coefficients (Max, 1981) between these three potentials will prove definitvely this theory: this is the first stage in our work. With the volume conduction hypothesis if we record two signals x(t) and y(t), we will have:

$$y(t) = \alpha x(t - \theta)$$

where α is the attenuation coefficient and θ the conduction delay. The inter-correlation between y and x is:

$$C_{yx}(\tau) = \int_{+\infty}^{-\infty} \alpha x(t - \theta) x(t - \tau) dt$$

with τ the correlation delay. So:

$$C_{yx}(\tau) = \alpha \int_{-\infty}^{+\infty} x(u) x[u - (\tau - \theta)] du$$

with the variate change: $u = t - \theta$. At the end we have:

$$C_{yx}(\tau) = \alpha C_{xx}(\tau - \theta).$$

We have to find τ_m which gives the C_{yx} maximum, to the θ value. For the C_{yx} maximum we have the C_{xx} maximum; and we know that the auto-correlation function is maximum for an argument equal to zero, therefore $\tau_m - \theta = 0$. In this way we know 0 and its value confirms that we have a *volume conduction* or a *nerve conduction*.

The digital system

Recent advances in microcomputers have resulted in better performances and lower prices, which have been of great benefit. It is now possible to design networks with microcomputers each of which performs a special task. Figure

228

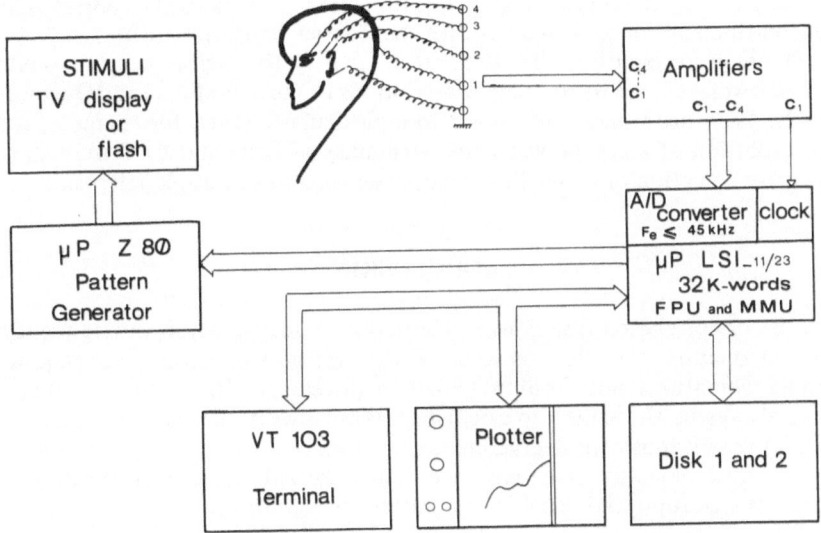

Fig. 4. Schematic block diagram. μP: microprocessor; A/D analog to digital; FPU: floating point unti; MMU: memory management unit.

4 is the block diagram of the system. ERG, EAG and EVG output signals are first sampled and converted into digital form in synchronisation with the stimulus. We have special amplifiers with a very good signal to noise ratio. The converter is used at 35 kHz per channel; the information is stored in memory (with direct access memory technique) for 300 ms. Following this we are able to store the measurements on disk and begin the calculations. The terminal VT 103 with graphic option is used to communicate with the LSI-11/23 (DEC: Digital Equipment Corporation); a plotter is added for the visualisation of the acquired signals. The stimulus system (TV display or flash) is connected to a microprocessor Z 80 which is a pattern generator. It is easy to design any shape (black and white, or color) with this system. The connection between Z 80 and LSI-11/23 presents no difficulty, and RS 232C or IEEE 488 can be used.

Application

We know that the measured data are a set of waveforms from which information must be extracted. In electrophysiology, for example, an electrovisiogram is recorded and interpreted by an ophthalmologist.

In practice, waveforms measured contain far more information than can be fully extracted by the specialist (Chen, 1982). So computer-aid, interactive and fully automatic techniques have been developed for processing and recognition. The results are the outputs of the computer. For the electrovisiogram the processed results may be the spectral display while the recognition results may be an interpretation of the waveforms.

Processing includes: digital filtering of the data to minimize noise like

229

the EEG (electro-encephalogram); interaction for example, correlation, convolution and spectral analysis with the Fourier transform.

The main recognition objectives are to classify the digital waveforms into one of several classes or to obtain descriptions of the data (Faure and Quignon, 1982). Each class may correspond to a particular disease, for example, and the evolution of delay between the beginnings of ERG and EAG may allow the early detection of demyelinating diseases such as a multiple sclerosis.

CONCLUSION

The use of correlation functions and both time-domain analysis and frequency-domain analysis may allow us to avoid the average technique which requires certain conditions not easily satisfied in physiology (the response latency must always be the same); to calculate delays between signals and in this way to have the diagnosis for demyelinating diseases.

Our final objective is to realize a diagnostic aid for an identification of different electrophysiological waves (*pattern recognition*).

ACKNOWLEDGEMENT

We would like to express our thanks to Mrs. S. Roux, Miss C. Warren and Messrs J.-M. Giraud, P. Heydel, G. Rouaisnel and J. Watts for their kind assistance.

REFERENCES

Alfieri, R. and P. Solé. Exploration électrophysiologique fonctionnelle, sectorielle et stratigraphique de la fonction visuelle. J. Fr. Biophys. Méd. Nucl. 3: 63–75 (1979).
Chen, C. H. Digital waveform processing and recognition. CRC, Boca Raton, Florida, (1982).
Faure, C. and J. Quignon. Automatic interpretation of biomedical signal. Communication at 6th International Conference on Pattern Recognition, Munich (1982, in press).
Max, J. Méthodes et techniques de traitement du signal et applications aux mesures physiques. Masson, Paris, 1: 96–98, 161–165, 195–197, 220–222 and 246–248 (1981).
Siegfried, J. B. Early potentials evoked by macular stimulation: optic nerve potentials? In: Schmöger, E. and Kelsey, J. H. (ed.), Visual electrodiagnosis in systemic diseases, 17th I.S.C.E.V. Symposium, Erfurt, 1979. Junk, The Hague, doc. Ophthalmol. Proc. Series 23: 201–207 (1980).

Mailing address:
Faculty of Medicine B.P. 38
Clermont-Ferrand
France

COMPUTER-ASSISTED ANALYSIS OF CLINICAL ELECTRORETINOGRAPHIC INTENSITY-RESPONSE FUNCTIONS

L. WU,* R. W. MASSOF, S. J. STARR

(Baltimore, Maryland, U.S.A.)

ABSTRACT

The amplitude of the human dark-adapted electroretinogram, measured from the trough of the a-wave to the peak of the b-wave as a function of stimulus intensity can be described nominally by the Naka-Rushton equation which has three independent parameters: R_{max}, K, and n. R_{max} is the asymptotic value of the ERG amplitude as a function of intensity, K is the intensity that produces an ERG amplitude that is one-half R_{max}, and n is a dimensionless constant that controls the slope of the function. The advantage of using the Naka-Rushton equation is that the three empirical parameters can be interpreted clinically. For example, changes in R_{max} may correspond to response compression owing to retinal 'gain' changes or to regional losses of retinal function; changes in K correspond to changes in retinal sensitivity or to changes in pre-retinal light absorption; and changes in n may be interpreted in terms of heterogeneous losses of retinal sensitivity. ERG intensity-response functions were obtained from normal subjects and retinal disease patients, and maximum likelihood values were computed for R_{max}, K, and n for each individual's data. The present paper describes these data and the computer system and analysis algorithm for recording and analyzing the ERG intensity-response function.

INTRODUCTION

The typical clinical protocol for recording the electroretinogram (ERG) consists of presenting a fixed set of stimuli to the patient, recording the responses, and comparing features of the ERG waveforms to norms established for each stimulus condition. An obvious short-coming of this practice is that normative data and ERG interpretations are laboratory specific (unless efforts are made to identically replicate conditions). Furthermore, data reductions usually are limited to simple reports of amplitude and implicit-time measures; such one-dimensional measures do not allow for ready interpretation of the data in terms of retinal pathophysiology.

*Research to Prevent Blindness Foreign Scholar Fellowship recipient; from Capital Hospital Chinese Academy of Medical Sciences, Beijing, Peoples Republic of China.

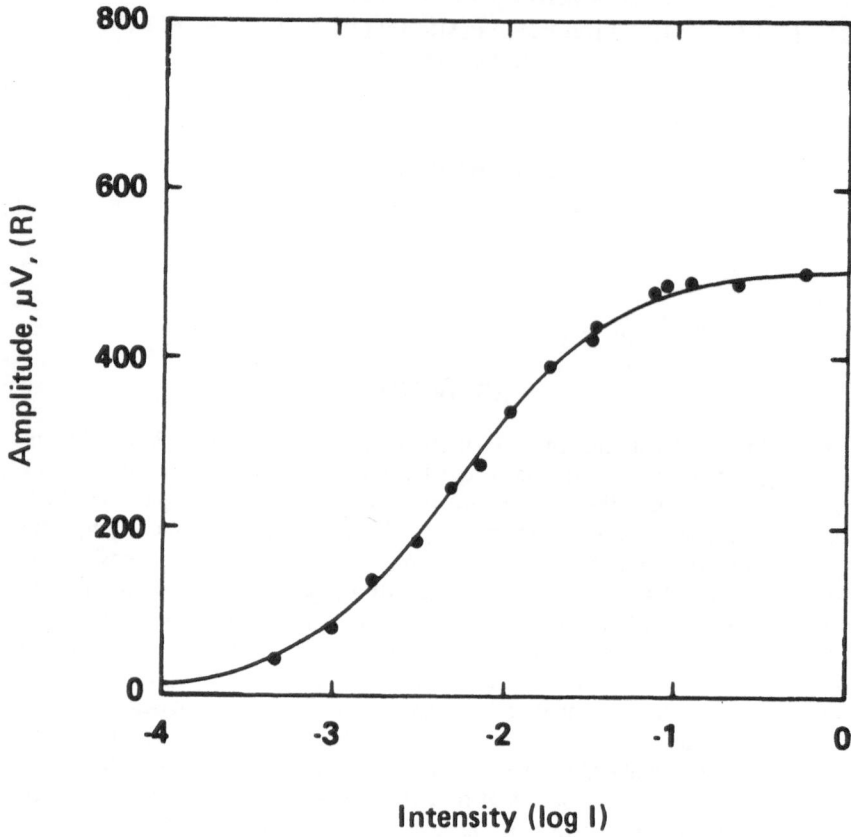

Fig. 1. ERG amplitudes measured from the trough of the a-wave to the peak of the b-wave are plotted as a function of log stimulus intensity (points). The solid curve fit to the data was generated by the Naka-Rushton equation (Eqn. 1).

The purpose of this report is to describe a new technique that we have developed and now routinely employ at the Wilmer Institute for quantitatively assessing retinal function by way of recording and analyzing the dark-adapted ERG as a function of stimulus intensity, viz, the ERG intensity-response function (1–2). It is well-known that ERG amplitude (measured from the trough of the a-wave to the peak of the b-wave) increases in a sigmoid manner as a function of log stimulus luminance (3–5). As shown in Figure 1, ERG amplitude data as a function of log luminance are well-described by the so-called Naka-Rushton equation (6)

$$R(I) = \frac{R_{max} I^n}{I^n + K^n} \tag{1}$$

where R is the ERG amplitude in μV, R_{max} is the maximum attainable or asymptotic ERG amplitude in μV, I is the stimulus luminance of the flash in cd-sec/m², K is the half-saturation constant in cd-sec/m² (if I = K

232

then $R = 0.5 R_{max}$), and n is a dimensionless constant. Reductions in R_{max} serve to compress the ERG intensity-response function, as shown in Figure 2a; elevations of K serve to translate the ERG intensity-response function along the log luminance axis, as shown in Figure 2b; changes in n serve to alter the slope of the ERG intensity-response function, as shown in Figure 2c.

The three ERG intensity-response function parameters, R_{max}, K, and n, appear to be statistically independent (2), and they are easily rendered subject to clinical interpretation. Reductions in the area of functioning retina (for example by photocoagulation) will cause reductions in R_{max}. Reductions in retinal sensitivity or increases in light absorption by pre-retinal media will serve to increase the value of K (any filter weighting coefficient on I in Eqn. 1 can be factored into K). If each small area of the retina can be thought of as generating its own ERG intensity-response function, then the overall ERG intensity-response function recorded in response to Ganzfeld stimulation can be considered the sum (superposition) of ERG intensity-response functions of small retinal areas. The more varied the sensitivities of individual retinal areas are, the shallower will be the slope of the composite ERG intensity-response function (i.e. smaller value of n). It can be seen from an examination of the curves in Figure 2 that a change in any one of the three intensity-response function parameters will cause a change in ERG amplitude as it is usually measured at a single stimulus luminance.

The present paper focuses on the description of our method of recording the ERG intensity-response function and the computer algorithm used to determine R_{max}, K, and n from the ERG amplitude data. We then show some examples of data collected from selected patients to illustrate clinical applications and interpretations of the ERG intensity-response function.

METHODS

Apparatus. The stimulator and recording apparatus is a commercially available microcomputer-based system (LKC Systems UTAS E-1000). The Ganzfeld stimulus is provided by a 40 cm diameter integrating sphere, spray-coated on the interior with multi-layered, high-reflectance, magnesium oxide-based paint, uniformly illuminated by a computer-triggered Grass PS-22 photo-stimulator or a computer-triggered bright-flash unit. The system is self-calibrating and maximum stimulus luminances are 3.9 cd-sec/m² for the photostimulator and 2530 cd-sec/m² for the bright-flash unit. Stimulus luminance is varied in 0.2 log unit steps, over a range of 5.0 log units, by computer controlled, stepper motor-driven filter wheels containing Wratten neutral density filters. A light-emitting diode fixation light that can be set to either 360 or 85 cd/m² is mounted in the Ganzfeld sphere.

The ERG signals are amplified by AC coupled, differential amplifiers for which the gain and filters (range = 0.05 to 8000 Hz) are set by the computer (for the ERG measures we typically employ a 0.3 to 300 Hz band-pass). The amplified signals are input into an analog-to-digital converter (12 bit resolution; 5 μsec conversion time). The converted digital signal is recorded by a Z-80 based, 64K RAM microprocessor, and buffered in memory (1024

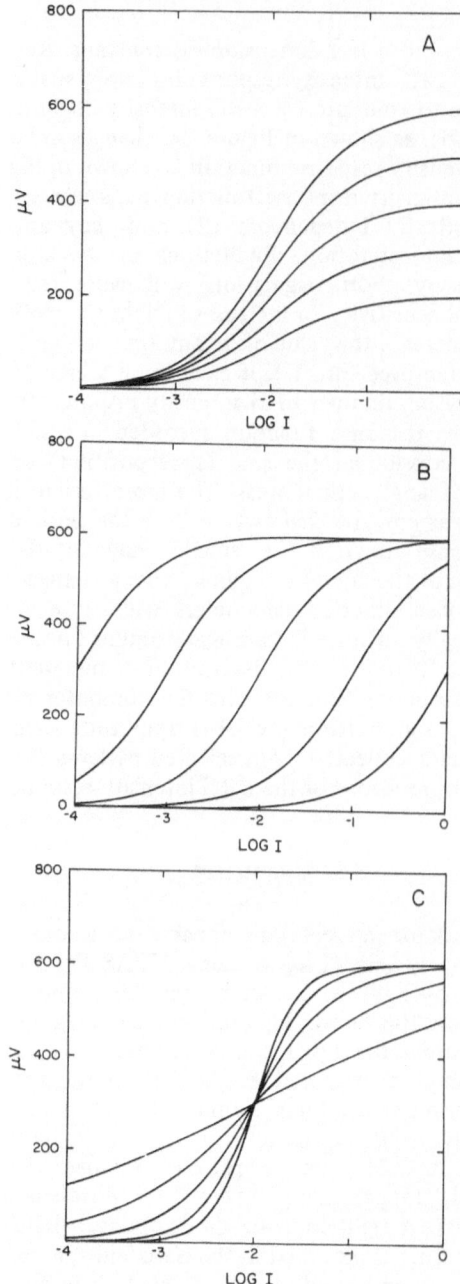

Fig. 2. a) Schematic ERG intensity-response functions generated by Eqn. (1) employing different values of R_{max}. b) Schematic ERG intensity-response functions generated by Eqn. (1) employing different values of K. c) Schematic ERG intensity-response functions generated by Eqn. (1) employing different values of n.

234

double-precision samples per waveform). Every other value in the data buffer is displayed on a high-resolution, Z-80 coprocessor-based, graphic terminal (480 × 510 pixels with 32K RAM screen buffer), and at the discretion of the operator the entire buffered waveform and all attendant parameter and personal patient data can be recorded on diskette. During the recording session signal averaging can be initiated, with or without an automatic artifact reject that uses an operator-defined rejection threshold, amplifier parameters and the timebase can be changed, and stimulus luminance can be controlled, all from the terminal keyboard. Either during the recording session, or later when working on waveforms recalled from diskette, cursors can be positioned on the ERG waveform with amplitudes, implicit-times, and the differences between cursor values displayed. The waveform, plus positioned cursors and cursor information can be printed on a high-resolution graphics printer.

Procedure. Following 45 minutes of dark-adaptation and pupil dilation, the ERG is recorded from both eyes using bipolar Burian-Allen contact-lens electrodes. Single-flash ERGs are recorded at stimulus luminances ranging from $-4.2 \log \text{cd-sec/m}^2$ to $0.6 \log \text{cd-sec/m}^2$ in 0.2 log unit steps, presented in ascending order from dimmest to brightest. If the response is contaminated by a photomyoclonic reflex (7), then the stimulus is repeated at regular intervals (duration ranging from 3 sec at the lowest intensity to 10 sec at the highest intensity) until the reflex habituates. At low intensities the ERG is averaged (with a $30 \mu\text{V}$ artifact reject threshold) from 5 to 25 times, depending on noise level.

RESULTS AND ANALYSIS

A typical set of ERG intensity-response function data are illustrated in Figure 3. If we adopt the assumption that Eqn. (1) is an idealized representation of the ERG intensity-response function, then departures of the data from Eqn. (1) can be attributed to random fluctuations in the parameters and perhaps an added noise source ($^\sigma$a). Thus for any intensity I, the measured ERG response $R'(I)$ theoretically is determined by

$$R'(I) = \frac{(R_{max} \pm {}^\sigma R_{max}) I^{(n \pm \sigma n)}}{I^{(n \pm \sigma n)} + (K \pm \sigma_K)^{(n \pm \sigma n)}} \pm {}^\sigma a. \qquad (2)$$

The regression analysis we employ determines the values of R_{max}, K, and n that minimizes the sum of squares of the differences between predictions of Eqn. (1) and the measured values, represented by Eqn. (2). The sum of squares over all intensities tested (from i to j) is the goodness-of-fit measure

$$\chi^2 = \sum_{I=i}^{j} \left(\frac{R'(I) - R(I)}{j} \right)^2. \qquad (3)$$

The value of χ^2 will vary with the choices of R_{max}, K, and n in Eqn. (1).

235

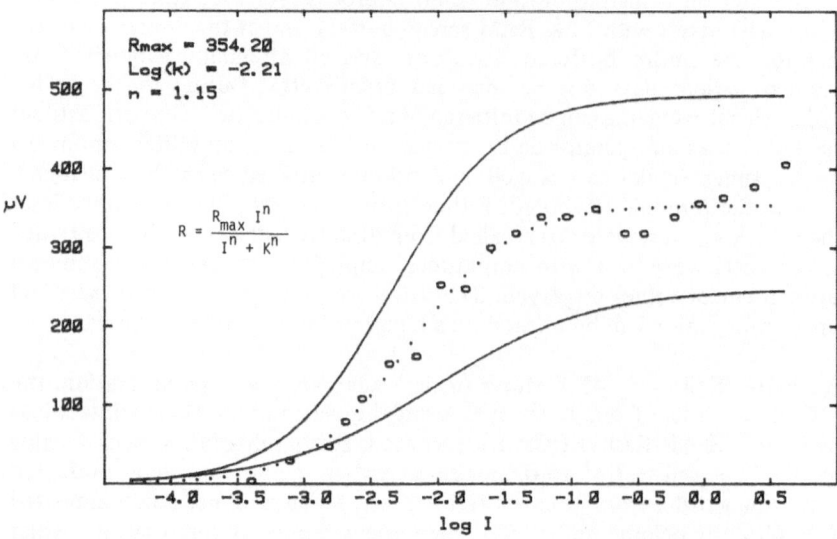

Fig. 3. Typical normal ERG amplitudes measured as a function of stimulus intensity (circles). The dotted curve was generated by Eqn. (1) employing the indicated R_{max}, K, and n values which gave the minimum value for χ^2 in Eqn. (3). The solid curves bound the normal 95th percentile.

Obviously, if $R'(I) = R(I)$ for all values of I, the fit of Eqn. (1) to the data would be perfect and $\chi^2 = 0$.

We have written a computer program that searches for values of R_{max}, K, and n that minimizes χ^2. The analysis consists of a grid search of the hypersurface defined by χ^2 as a function of R_{max}, K, and n to locate the coordinates of the minimum χ^2 value. The dotted curve fit to the data in Figure 3 is the result of this analysis which found that the values of $R_{max} = 354\,\mu V$, $\log K = -2.21 \log cd\text{-}sec/m^2$ and n = 1.15 yield the minimum value of χ^2.

Figure 4 illustrates histograms of intensity-response function parameters for the ERG amplitude data of retinitis pigmentosa patients (Figure 4a), of cone dystrophy patients (Figure 4b), and of macular degeneration patients (Figure 4c). For the retinitis pigmentosa patients, the primary abnormality is in R_{max}; for the cone dystrophy patients, the primary abnormality is in n; and for the macular degeneration patients, the primary abnormality is in K.

DISCUSSION

The advantages of the ERG intensity-response function are: 1) the derived parameter values are independent measures of different aspects of retinal function and therefore are subject to clinical interpretation, 2) the derived parameter values from measurements made in different laboratories will be

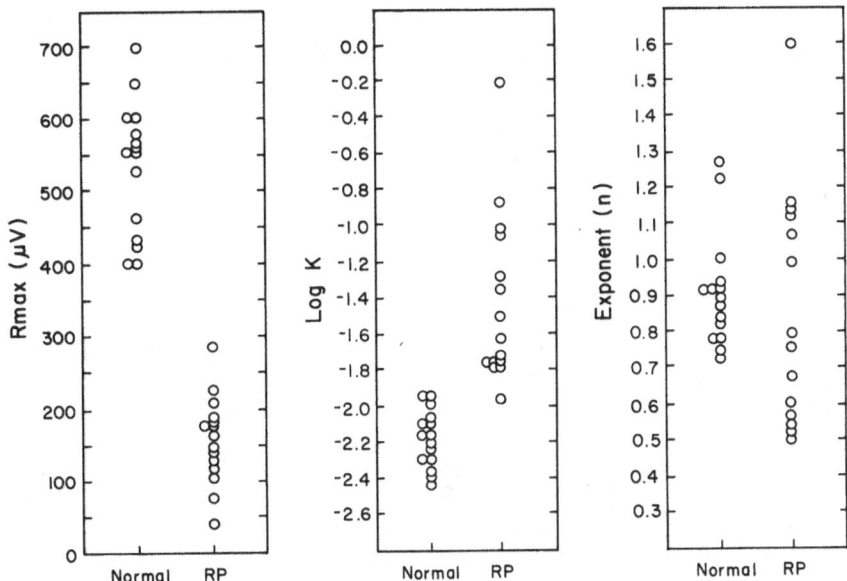

Fig. 4a. Frequency plots of ERG intensity-response function parameters for a) retinitis pigmentosa (RP) patients, as compared to the normal values.

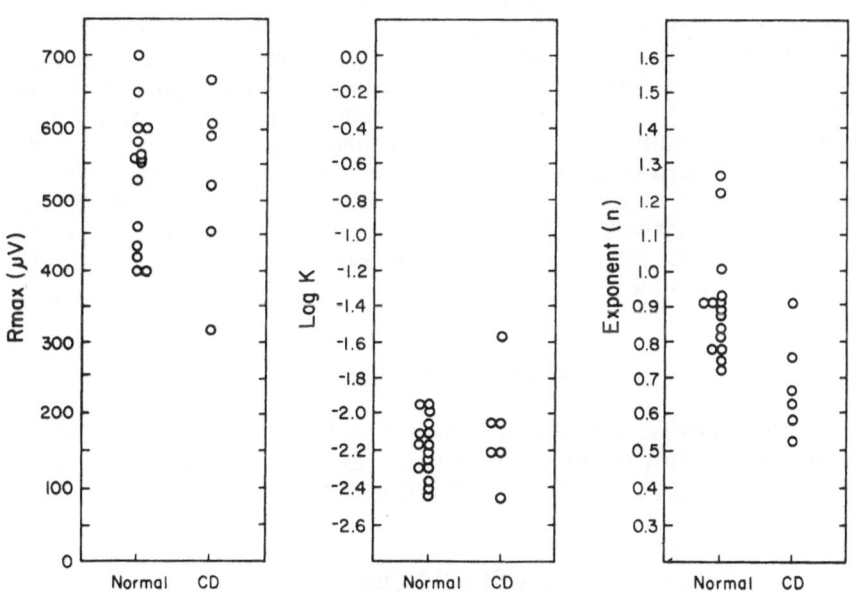

Fig. 4b. Frequency plots of ERG intensity-response function parameters for b) cone dystrophy (CD) patients, as compared to the normal values.

237

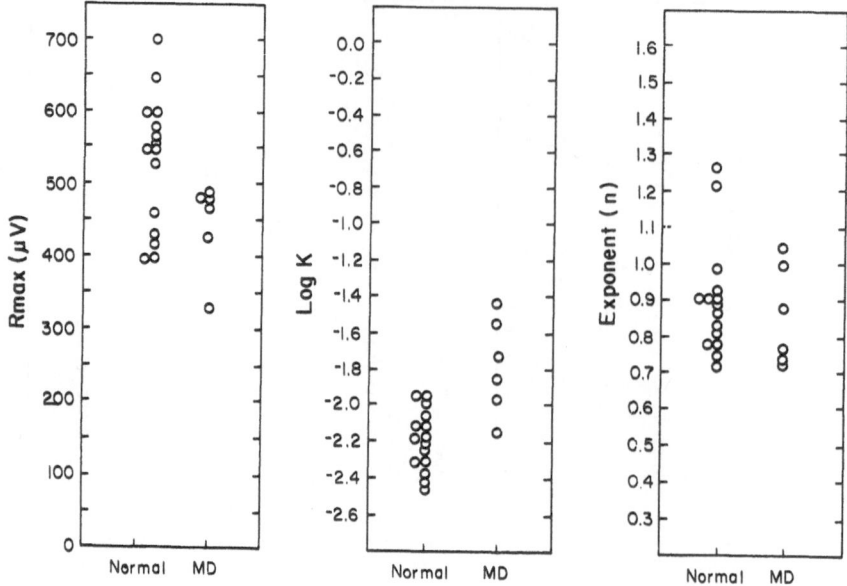

Fig. 4c. Frequency plots of ERG intensity-response function parameters for c) macular degeneration patients (MD), as compared to the normal values.

comparable irrespective of laboratory conditions or apparatus, provided that stimulus luminance and amplifier gain are properly calibrated, and 3) the variability on individual parameters will be less than the variability of single ERG measures. To fully realize the clinical potential of the ERG intensity-response function, however, it is still necessary to obtain normative population statistics on the intensity-response function parameters, to evaluate sources of variability in the data, and to systematically examine the effects of different retinal pathologies on the parameters. Computer-based systems, such as the one described in the present report, will greatly facilitate the collection and analysis of ERG intensity-response function data, and the commercial availability of such systems makes it feasible to use this technique routinely in the clinical setting.

ACKNOWLEDGEMENT

The authors express their appreciation for technical assistance provided by Carolyn Perry. This research supported by research and core facility grants from the National Eye Institute (EY 01791 and EY 01765).

REFERENCES

1. Massof, R. W. and Johnson, M. A.: Prereceptor Light Absorption in Setters with Neuronal Ceroid Lipofuscinosis. Invest. Ophthal. Vis. Sci., 20, 134–136, 1981.

238

2. Massof, R. W., Wu, L., Finkelstein, D., Perry, C., Starr, S. J., and Johnson, M. A.: Properties of the Electroretinogram Intensity-Response Function in Retinitis Pigmentosa. Brit. J. Ophthalmol. (in press).
3. Liu, Y. and Yang, C.: Local and Stray Light Components of the Human Electro-retinogram Due to Stimulation by Light Subtending a 20° Visual Field. Scientia Sinica, 15, 696–705, 1966.
4. Krill, A. E.: Hereditary Retinal and Choroidal Diseases, Vol. I, Harper and Row, New York, 1972.
5. Fulton, A. B. and Rushton, W. A. H.: The Human Rod ERG: Correlation with Psychophysical Responses in Light and Dark Adaptation. Vis. Res., 18, 793–800, 1978.
6. Naka, K. I. and Rushton, W. A. H.: S-Potentials from Colour Units in the Retina of Fish (Cyprinidae) J. Physiol., 185, 536–555, 1966.
7. Johnson, M. A. and Massof, R. W.: The Photomyoclonic Reflex: An Artifact in the Clinical Electroretinogram. Brit. J. Ophthal. 66, 368–378, 1982.

Mailing address:
Dr. R. W. Massof
Wilmer Ophthalmological Institute
Johns Hopkins Hospital
Baltimore, Maryland 21205, U.S.A.

DYNAMIC RANDOM-ELEMENT STEREOGRAMS: A MICROPROCESSOR APPLICATION

K. D. WHITE AND J. V. ODOM
(Gainesville, Florida, U.S.A.)

ABSTRACT

Dynamic random-element stereogram stimuli may be used to elicity psychophysical and/or electrophysiological responses whose presumptive neurogenic basis lies in the cerebral cortex. Such stimuli can be generated at low cost using a 'home' graphics microcomputer, plus a special interface and a TV to provide the binocular display. In effect, any graphics picture made by the microcomputer in black, white, and gray is translated by the interface into crossed disparity ('near'), uncrossed disparity ('far'), or no disparity ('fixation distance') correlates of 3-D depth. An observer actually views a screen full of dynamically changing, randomly occuring elements onto which the selected disparities have been introduced.

The interface for our Ohio Scientific CIP 'home computer' is constructed with 9 common ICs. Its main functions are: a) to generate the dynamic random elements, and b) to control the magnitude of disparity, over a range from about 0 arc sec up to about 30 arc min (at a convenient viewing distance). Graphics information from the microcomputer simply selects the disparity type (crossed, uncrossed, or neither) appearing on particular screen areas. Because the majority of the microcomputer capabilities are not needed to generate the stereograms, the computer is free to time the stimulus presentations, sequence the trials, synchronize a signal averager, collect data, etc. during the course of an experiment.

Dynamic random-element stereograms (DRES) are like other kinds of stereograms in that a pair of highly similar, two-dimensional stimuli is presented respectively to the two eyes. Subtle differences in the retinal images (i.e., retinal disparities) permit perception of apparent three-dimensional depth in the binocularly fused presentation. The interest in using stereograms has been enhanced by findings from neuroanatomical and single unit electrophysiological studies that the cerebral cortex is the site of origin for responses to retinal disparity in primates. Stimuli which utilize retinal disparity exclusively to evoke a response can thus provide a powerful linkage of noninvasive psychophysical or electrophysiological tests to the putative neural substrate. DRES were designed to be such stimuli.

Doc. Ophthal. Proc. Series, Vol 37, ed. by H.E.J.W. Kolder
© 1983 Dr W. Junk Publishers, The Hague/Boston:Lancaster

Each stimulus of a DRES pair resembles the thermal noise ('snow') seen on a poorly tuned television; spots appear unpredictably over the screen and randomly disappear and reappear over time (i.e., dynamic random elements). The DRES pair can depict a stereoscopic target, e.g. a square figure on a background, by causing any element that appears on one stimulus to have a binocular counterpart on the fellow stimulus. On that portion of the display depicting the square target, the binocular counterparts produce a different retinal disparity than do the counterpart elements depicted as background. The 'snow' in the square and the 'snow' in the background seem to be at different depths when the DRES is viewed stereoscopically.

The method for producing DRES stimuli involves an electronic display driven by a digital computer. In this paper we show how inexpensive 'home' microcomputers, or even certain microprocessor based video games, can be used to display DRES stimuli on a color television. The special interface circuit described below required no special software beyond the standard black and white graphics capability of these commercially available micro-processor systems.

For illustration consider a DRES depicting two depths presented on a color TV. The red (R) and green (G) guns of the picture tube respectively supply the two eyes with a stereoscopic stimulus pair when chromatically selective filters are worn over the eyes (anaglyph method). The interface circuit provides separate outputs for the R and G guns, with the signals generated as follows. Part of the circuit randomly produces a sequence of ons and offs at very high speed. In one case the sequence arrives at the two outputs simultaneously so that every time the R gun turns on (creating an element seen by one eye) the G gun also turns on to produce its binocular counterpart. Partner elements generated in this case will have a near-zero retinal disparity (given perfect electronic adjustment of the TV, correct convergence by the observer, and similar provisos) because the raster scan of the TV ideally is at the same position on the screen when the R and G elements appear. The interface also supports another two cases, in which the identical on/off sequences come to both outputs but with a slight delay at one output. This delay permits the TV raster to move a small amount horizontally after turning on the R element before it turns on the G element (or vice versa). The elements remain binocular partners but occur on disparate screen positions, producing a retinal disparity. A DRES stereoscopic target is created when elements from one 'case' fill a delimited area on the TV screen while elements from a different 'case' fill the rest of the screen.

The interface accepts black and white graphics data to control a selector: black selects crossed disparity (R preceeds G), white selects uncrossed disparity (G preceeds R), and gray selects no disparity (simultaneous). If a monitor connected to the microprocessor system showed a bar grating in black and white, the interface generates a DRES depicting near bars and far bars.

How far (or near) the bars seem depends on the amount of retinal disparity; in turn this depends on the amount of delay between R and G outputs of the interface. The longest delay the interface permits is about 500 nanosec. With Advent 710 projection TV and a 2 m viewing distance, the resulting

242

retinal disparity is then about 35 arc min. A near-threshold disparity of 20 arc sec requires a delay of about 5 nsec. The delay between R and G outputs is controlled by an adjustable DC voltage supplied to the interface such that no measurable delay occurs near +5V and long delays, but of opposite sign, occur at +3.5V (graphics white = crossed, 'far', R preceeds G) and at +6.5V (graphics white = uncrossed, 'near', G preceeds R). Small variations in the electronic components, as well as local details like the operating temperature, can introduce over 100 nanosec (several arc min disparity) of unwanted delay, but the adjustable delay designed into this interface will permit one to compensate for the unwanted portion through calibration.

The interface circuit has a second mode of operation allowing one to calibrate the retinal disparities present on a DRES. The part of the circuit which generates elements at random for a DRES can be reconfigured to repeat one sequence of elements over and over. The net effect is to replace the dynamic random elements with a number of stationary vertical stripes, since the very same elements are now repeated during every horizontal line of the raster scan. As these stripes pass through the regions of screen designated for bars (following the above example), there are small horizontal offsets. The offsets

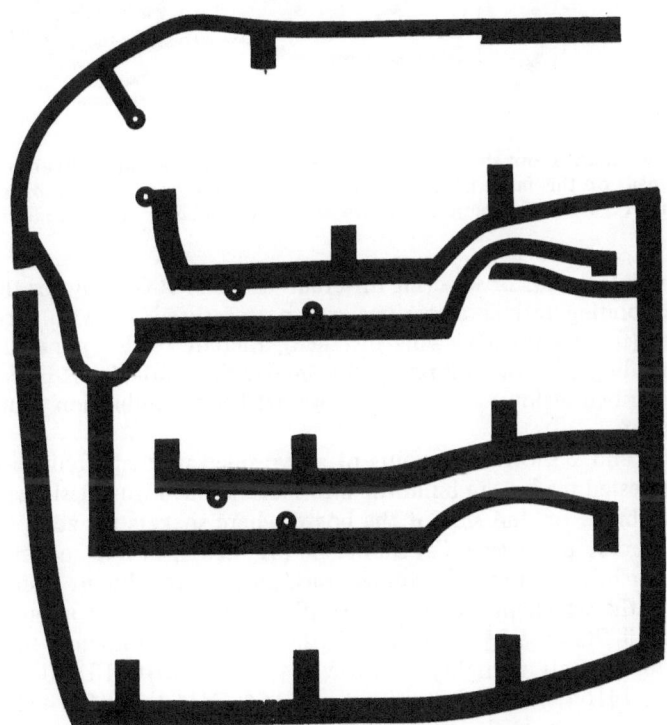

Fig. 1. Printed circuit board layout showing power and ground busses. DIP sockets for 9 integrated circuit packages and one connector mount on this side of the double-sided circuit board.

243

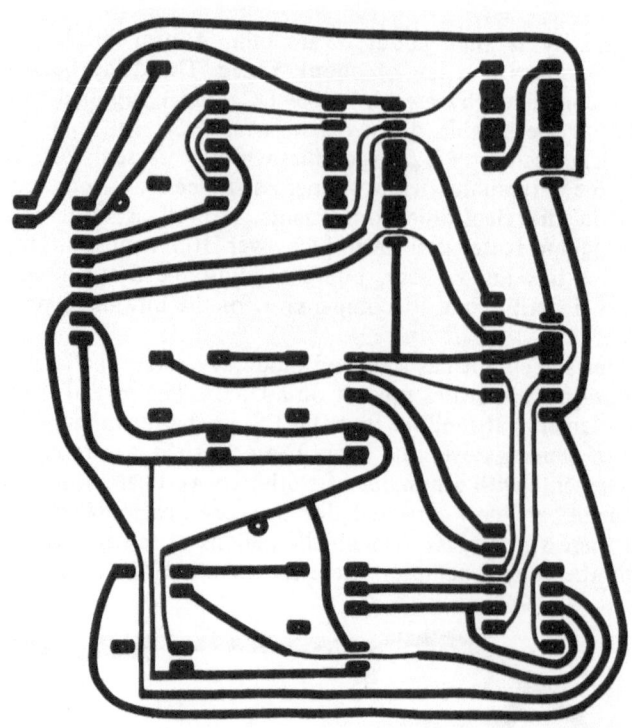

Fig. 2. Printed circuit layout showing interconnections of the integrated circuit packages. Two round pads on this mask permit alignment with corresponding round pads on the mask shown in Figure 1. This permits the two sides of the circuit board to be in register.

are easily visible results of selecting different 'cases' of R-G delay for the bars. The corresponding retinal disparities can be measured off with a ruler or micrometer (for a known viewing distance), thereby rendering needless the more demanding task of calibrating the intervening variable, R-G delay. A switch (described below) lets one choose DRES or calibration modes for the TV display.

Figures 1 and 2 show the layouts of a two-sided printed circuit board so that an interested reader can build the interface circuit. Figure 1 shows power and ground buses on the side of the board where sockets for accepting the integrated circuit packages (ICs) should be installed. Ten DIP sockets, 9 for ICs and 1 for microcomputer's connections, are required. Figure 2 shows the metalized paths which interconnect the IC's with the microcomputer. The printed circuit fits on a $3\frac{1}{2}$" x 4" board; the Figures are shown to scale. The ICs required are (left to right): top row, 74151, CD4010, CD4010; middle row, 74164, 74164, 74153; bottom row, 74164, 74164, 7486. The leftmost DIP socket shown in both Figures is for connecting inputs/outputs of the interface. Pinouts of the connector socket are: + 5 VDC (pins 3 and 4), common ground (pins 6, 7, and 8), adjustable voltage from + 3.5 to + 6.5 VDC (pin 2), black and white graphics input (pin 16), clock input (pin 9), R gun output (pin 13), and G gun output (pin 14). Pin 1 of this connector should be attached to a SPDT switch, permitting the DRES mode if grounded and the calibration mode when at + 5 VDC or open. Note that the DRES mode must be selected, even if only briefly, to insure that the interface will start functioning after powering up the full system.

Virtually all graphics microcomputers and video games make available the + 5 VDC, ground, and black and white graphic signals for the required interface inputs. The adjustable voltage input ideally should come from an external power supply but frequently a 500 ohm potentiometer will suffice if the terminals go to + 5V and ground while the wider goes to connector pin 2. Clock input should be synchronized with the video output, and the best way to do this is by deriving the interface's clock from the same oscillator used to provide video (black and white graphics) synch signals. The synch signals, stripped of graphics information, are sent to the color TV, as are the R and G outputs.

Using the inverface described here, appropriately connected to the microcomputer, ordinary graphics will be translated into DRES stimuli. Any picture made on the graphics will reappear in the DRES as depth changes, and evoke responses due to retinal disparity.

ACKNOWLEDGEMENT

This research was partially supported by NEI grants EY-03640 to K.D.W. and EY-03781 to J.V.O.

Mailing address:
Department of Psychology
University of Florida
Gainesville, Florida 32611, U.S.A.

DIGITAL VS ANALOG FILTERING OF ELECTROPHYSIOLOGICAL DATA UTILIZING MICROPROCESSORS

J. B. SIEGFRIED

(Philadelphia, Pennsylvania, U.S.A.)

ABSTRACT

Digital filtering of averaged evoked potential waveforms by microprocessor is presented and evaluated as a technique for enhancement of signal-to-noise ratio, and compared to analog filtering. It is shown that analog filters inherently produce distortions of amplitude and phase, and that these distortions are virtually eliminated within the bandpass limits of a digital filter. Calibration data are presented, comparing phase and amplitude before and after both analog and digital filtering. Digital filtering is accomplished offline by means of an LSI-11 microprocessor. In addition, filtering effects upon actual data are shown and analyzed.

INTRODUCTION

Analog filtering of electrophysiological visual signals is commonly employed to improve signal-to-noise ratios, as a low pass filter to attenuate high frequency noise, as a band reject or 'notch' filter to attenuate house mains interference, and as a bandpass filter to selectively enhance 'wavelets' ('oscillatory potentials') and other medium frequency phenomena (Siegfried and Lukas, 1981 a, b; Siegfried and Whittaker, 1982; Whittaker and Siegfried, 1983).

The use of analog filters, whether 'passive' as are found in most amplifiers, or 'active' produces predictable distortions of the electrophysiological data both in amplitude and phase. The steeper the slopes of the analog filter, the more extensive and significant the distortion. With passive analog filters set to a 1–1000 Hz passband, with the usual shallow slopes associated with amplifier filters, probably little significant distortion occurs within the frequency range of interest. However, when relatively narrow bandpass filtering is performed, for example 50–200 Hz to selectively enhance 100 Hz wavelets, significant phase distortion occurs. This means that latency or implicit time measurements may be seriously in error. Digital filtering by microprocessor represents another technique to improve signal-to-noise ratios. I calibrated the electrical recording system using sine wave input of various frequencies and analyzed the effects of both active analog filtering and digital filtering. In addition, the effects on actual data are presented.

METHODS

1.73 V rms sine waves were applied as input to a signal averaging computer (Nicolet Instruments Corp., model 1174), both directly and through an active analog filter (Krohn-Hite, model 3323). The filter was set for a bandpass of 50–200 Hz, − 3 dB points, 24 dB/octave slopes. The input to the signal averaging computer was filtered with a passive 2 KHz low pass analog filter. Sampling rate was 40,960 Hz.

Digital filtering was performed upon the averaged data, and was processed after averaging by a microprocessor (Digital Equipment Corp., MINC 11/23). First, the average was subjected to a forward fast Fourier transform (FFT) (Cooley and Tukey, 1965). This procedure yielded a real and imaginary set of 4096 coefficients, corresponding to frequencies, where frequency = (Fourier coefficient)/(epoch). Second, those coefficients corresponding to frequencies outside the bandpass of interest (in this case, 50–200 Hz) are set to zero. And third, an inverse FFT is performed by the computer. This last process returns the data from frequency domain to temporal domain. The data now consist of only those frequencies between 50 and 200 Hz.

RESULTS AND DISCUSSION

Figure 1 shows the original sine wave input ('unfiltered', left column), for frequencies from 20 Hz to 680 Hz, and after filtering, both analog (middle column) and digital (right column). Bandpass is 50–200 Hz for both analog and digital filters. Each record is 100 ms in duration, and amplitude scales are the same for all records. Figure 2 shows plots of amplitude attenuation and phase shift for both analog and digital filtering. Two points should be noted which are illustrated in Figures 1 and 2. The digital filter is much more sharply defined, being essentially rectangular, and the analog filter exhibits very significant phase shifts, both phase advance and phase lag. Even when the analog filter bandpass settings are selected to cause zero phase shift at a particular frequency (in this case, 100 Hz, the approximate repetition frequency of cortical VEP wavelets), very significant phase shifts occur with small increases and decreases in frequency from this value.

Figure 3 illustrates the effect of analog and digital filtering upon VEP wavelet recordings. The original averaged waveform is seen in the top record (A) in which wavelets are seen superimposed on early slow waves, preceding and coincident with 'P$_{100}$'. In B, records have been digitally filtered 50–200 Hz. It can be seen that in the digitally filtered records, wavelet peaks line up precisely with those seen in the original records (A), while slow waves have been attenuated. In C, records have been active analog filtered. Wavelet peak phase shifts, equivalent to as much as 10 ms are evident from a visual inspection of the records.

248

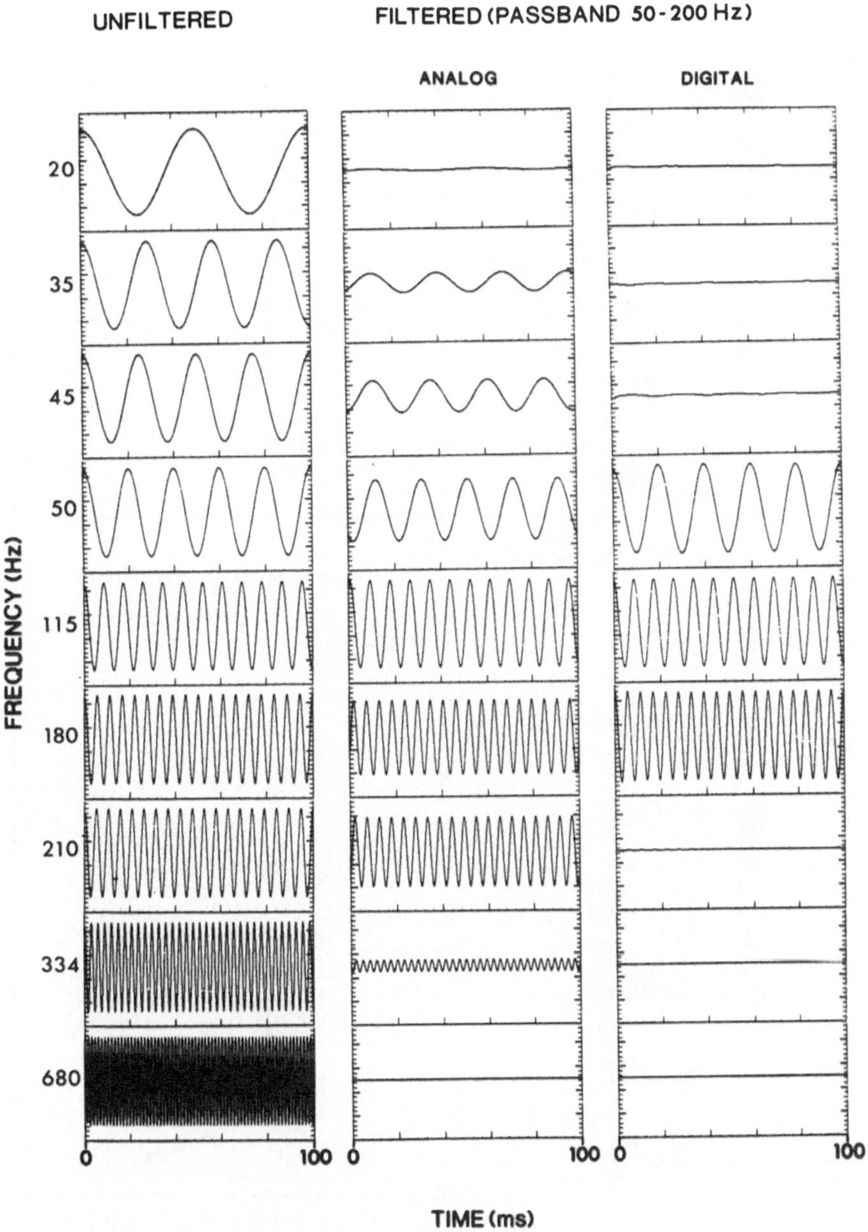

UNFILTERED   FILTERED (PASSBAND 50-200 Hz)

                              ANALOG   DIGITAL

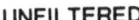

FREQUENCY (Hz)

20

35

45

50

115

180

210

334

680

0   100   0   100   0   100

TIME (ms)

Fig. 1. Sine wave calibration of recording system. Each record is the average of 64 sweeps, of 100 ms duration. Amplitude scale is constant throughout the figure. Left column is sine wave input. Middle column has passed through an active analog filter set at 50–200 Hz, − 3 dB points, 24 dB/octave slopes. Right column has been digitally filtered 50–200 Hz.

249

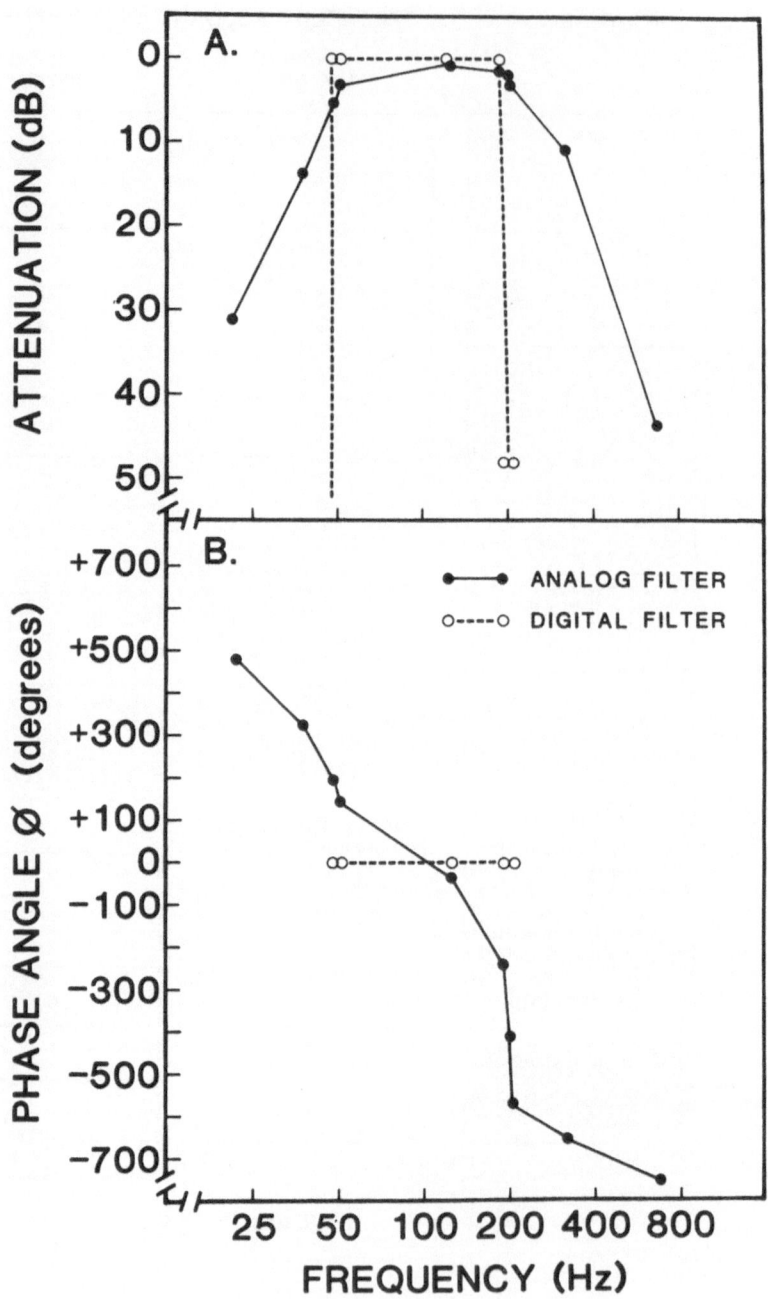

Fig. 2. Amplitude attenuation (A) and phase angle (B) as functions of frequency for the calibration data presented in Figure 1. Positive phase angles represent phase advance; negative phase angles represent phase lag.

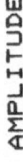

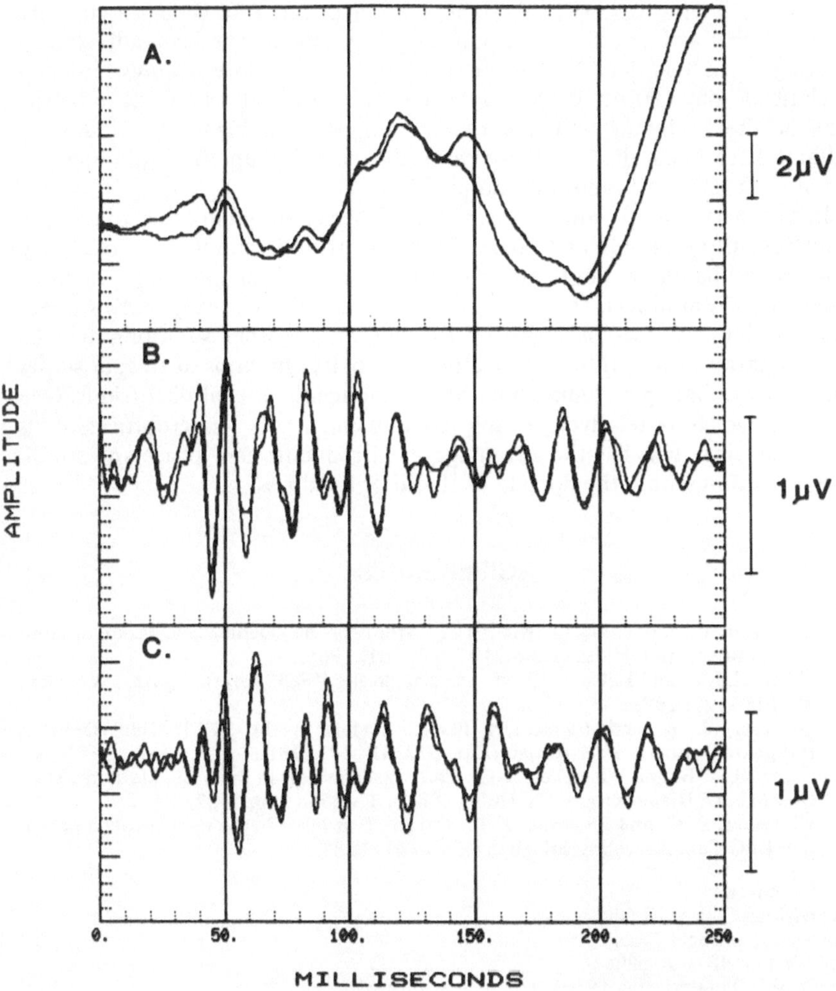

Fig. 3. (A) Two consecutive averages of 256 sweeps superimposed passed through 1–1000 Hz passive analog filter. 20 ms flash duration onset coincident with beginning of record, 2 Hz flash repetition rate. Positively at the occipital electrode (O_z) relative to reference (C_z) is indicated by an upward deflection. (B) Record A after digital filtering 50–200 Hz. (C) Record A after active analog filtering 50–200 Hz, − 3 dB points, 24 dB/octave slopes. Initial sampling rate is 8,192 Hz. Computer input low pass filter setting was 2 kHz.

One serious pitfall of digital filtering should be carefully noted. 'Windowing' artifacts may be easily created due to the implicit iterative assumption of the FFT algorithm. Such effects manifest themselves as damped oscillations at the beginning and end of the digitally filtered record if they are present. They are caused by any differences in DC level or slope of the averaged waveform between the first few data points at the beginning of the record and the last few data points at the end of the record.

251

(Theoretically, the data should begin and end at zero). In order to virtually eliminate this artifact, the averaging sampling 'epoch' has been adjusted to precisely equal the inter-stimulus onset interval, and the inter-stimulus interval is relatively long (500 ms). This forces the averaged VEP waveform to be the same at the beginning and end of the 'window'. In Figure 1, windowing artifacts have been eliminated by carefully matching up the beginning and end of each sine wave input function.

In summary, all recording systems should be calibrated in order to analyze distortions of amplitude and phase. Such distortion is minimal for relatively wide analog bandpass limits and shallow slopes such as are found in most physiological amplifiers. However, when the need for relatively narrow bandpass filtering, or low- or high-pass filtering arises, other solutions may be sought. Active analog filters offer more selectivity, in terms of steeper slopes and narrower bandpass limits, but they introduce significant distortions. One solution, which is relatively simple to implement on a microprocessor, is digital filtering. This has the advantage of introducing zero phase and amplitude distortion within the domain of the filter bandpass.

REFERENCES

1. Cooley, J. W. and Tukey, J. W.: An algorithm for the machine calculation of complex Fourier series. Math. Comp., 19, 297–301, 1965.
2. Siegfried, J. B. and Lukas, J.: Early wavelets in the VECP. Invest. Ophthal. Vis. Sci., 20, 125–129, 1981a.
3. Siegfried, J. B. and Lukas, J.: Early wavelets in the VECP. Doc. Ophthl., H. Spekreijse and P. A. Apkarian (Eds.), 27, 41–47, 1981b.
4. Siegfried, J. B. and Whittaker, S. G.: Early fast wavelets in the VEP: Methods. Doc. Ophthal., G. Niemeyer and Ch. Huber (Eds.), 31, 245–250, 1982.
5. Whittaker, S. G. and Siegfried, J. B.: Origin of wavelets in the visual evoked potential. EEG Clin. Neurophysiology, 55, 91–101, 1983.

Mailing address:
Pennsylvania College of Optometry
Neurovisual Sciences Tract
1200 West Godfrey Avenue
Philadelphia, Pennsylvania 19141, U.S.A.

This research was partially supported by National Eye Institute, N.I.H. research grant RO1-EY03467 and U.S. Army Contract No. DAAG29-79-C-0103.

A MICROPROCESSOR-AIDED TRICHROMATIC ILLUMINOMETER BASED ON GENERAL PRINCIPLES OF RETINAL CIRCUITRY

E. ZRENNER AND J. ABELLAN

Max-Planck-Institute for Physiological and Clinical Research, Parkstr. 1, D-6350 Bad Nauheim, F.R.G.

In order to estimate the effect of visible radiation on the response magnitude of the various neurons in the visual system, a light measurement device was constructed, based on the trichromatic as well as on color-opponent principles of retinal circuitry. By combining several sets of optical filters, the spectral sensitivity of three silicium photodiodes was matched to the pigment absorption spectra of the human blue-, green- and red-sensitive cones, respectively. The photodiodes' responses were combined in several differential amplifiers whose output was matched to the spectral sensitivity of red/green opponent, blue/yellow opponent and non-opponent (V_λ) retinal neurons as determined in rhesus monkeys (E. Zrenner, Neurophysiological Aspects of Color Vision, Monograph, Springer Verlag 1982). Thus the effect of any visible radiation on the several types of receptors as well as on postreceptoral color-opponent neurons and non-opponent neurons can be estimated individually. Recombining the rectified outputs of the color-opponent channels in a summing amplifier yields a three-peaked sensitivity function, which matches very well the three-peaked human increment spectral sensitivity function as it is obtained in normal trichromatic observers in response to bright flashes of long duration (E. Zrenner, Docum. Ophthal. Proc. Series, 1982). This results in a new, physiological measure of retinal illumination. By using identical sets of optical filters in two of the three photodiodes, the effectiveness of visible radiation in eliciting neuronal responses in the visual system of color deficient observers can be estimated as well.

THE DISTINCTION BETWEEN LUMINANCE AND SPATIAL CONTRAST COMPONENTS IN THE PATTERN ERG

F. C. C. RIEMSLAG, J. L. RINGO, H. SPEKREIJSE AND
H. VERDUYN LUNEL

(Amsterdam, The Netherlands)

ABSTRACT

Recent reports about the pattern ERG seem to conflict with our previous investigation (Spekreijse et al., Doc. Ophth. 1973) in which we argued that the ERG to pattern can be attributed to nonlinear distortion of the responses to the individual pattern elements. Contrast as such, i.e. luminance differences between neighbouring elements, did not seem to play a role. In those experiments the quality of visual acuity was degraded by the use of glass contact lens electrodes, so only relatively large (50') checks could be used. In light of the recent reports, we have extended our earlier experiments, now employing the Dawson Electrode which does not interfere with acuity. In our experiments, the stimulus conditions were designed to distinguish between components produced by luminance distortion and those produced by spatial contrast. This distinction was achieved by independent manipulation of local luminance and contrast in the stimulus. For instance, contrast was produced by either local luminance increase or decrease, or, by using chromatic contrast without local luminance changes. Our present results confirm our previous conclusion, that is: contrast per se does not make a substantial contribution to the voltages recorded in the ERG. This differs from the simultaneously recorded pattern EPs, which are dominated by contrast. We have also found that great care must be taken because of the ease with which the cortical potential can be recorded with the ERG electrodes.

INTRODUCTION

Pattern reversal stimulation was introduced in electroretinography in order to be able to record responses from localized parts of the retina (Johnson, Riggs and Schick, 1966). The reversal stimulus consists of the counterphase modulation of two sets of equal area elements, e.g. checks. This way the total flux that reaches the eye is kept constant. The stray light which reaches the periphery of the retina is not modulated since it is the sum of the contributions of the two sets of checks. In the area directly stimulated each set of checks produces fundamental (linear) responses and higher harmonic (nonlinear) responses. By stimulating two equal areas in counterphase, the fundamental and higher odd harmonic components will be in counterphase and hence cancel. The second and even higher harmonic components, however, will be *in* phase and add to form a response. The contrast reverses twice every period in a pattern reversal, so from the contrast stimulation only even harmonic components might be expected. The even harmonics in the ERG recorded to pattern reversal stimulation could contain both pattern specific components and non-linear luminance components. Contrast processing, involving the detection of luminance differences across space, might be expected to require higher order neurons.

Contrast components might, if present, reveal more of the activity of the deeper layers of the retina complementing the flash evoked ERG, which is reported to originate from the outermost layers of the retina (e.g. Arden, 1976).

The existence of non-linear distortion products in the human ERG to luminance stimulation was demonstrated in 1961 by van der Tweel, and was studied more extensively with Wiener kernel representation (Koblasz, 1978; Larkin, Klein, Ogden, and Fender, 1979). Ogden et al., (1980) measured the first and the second order kernel of the rhesus monkey ERG after experimental ocular injury. They recorded a specific effect appearing exclusively in the non-linear part of the luminance response, and suggested that the experimental injury caused a defect post-synaptic to the receptors.

Recent studies suggested that pattern specific components exist (Vaegan, et al., 1982, Arden et al., 1982). From the differences between the pattern and luminance ERGs, under pathological (Sokol and Nadler, 1979; Arden, Vaegan, Hogg, Powell and Carter, 1980; Fiorentini, Maffei, Pirchio, Spinelli and Porciatti, 1981; Arden, Vaegan and Hogg, 1982; Vaegan, Arden and Hogg, 1982) and experimental pathological conditions (Maffei and Fiorentini, 1981, (cat)), it was concluded that inner layer activity is reflected in the pattern reversal ERG. This, however, was disputed by Sherman (1982). The reports on pattern specific components conflict with a previous report which showed that the even harmonic components of the luminance ERG, (these components are non-linear when the stimulus is a square wave), are indistinguishable from the responses to pattern contrast reversal (Spekreijse, Estevez and van der Tweel, 1973).

However, by using a Henkes-glass contact lens ERG electrode, the visual acuity in the experiments of Spekreijse et al. 1973, was reduced, and large checks had to be used to record equal amplitude EPs with and without the contact glass. The recent studies were made possible by the development of new electrodes (Dawson, Trick and Litzkow, 1979; Arden, Carter, Hogg, Siegel and Margolis, 1979) that do not interfere with contrast-vision. In the light of these new developments we reexamined the question whether contrast specific components can be recorded in the human ERG. We manipulated the stimulus parameters in order to change contrast and luminance modulation independently. For instance in one set of experiments we kept the local luminance modulation constant, while the contrast modulation was varied. In the second set of experiments we shifted the phase of the modulation of one set of checks with respect to the other set in order to gradually decrease the second harmonic local luminance responses to zero, through a region where the second harmonic contrast components would increase gradually. The third set of experiments made use of heterochromatic matched lights to produce chromatic pattern reversal without local photopic luminance modulation (Riggs, Johnson and Schick, 1964; Regan and Spekreijse, 1974).

The results confirm the conclusion of Spekreijse et al. 1973, that the ERG to pattern reversal can be explained readily on the basis of non-linear, local luminance components. There is no reason for assuming contrast specific components in the ERG.

METHODS

Recording

The ERGs were recorded with a DTL electrode (Dawson et al., 1979) floating on the lower corneal border (limbus), referred to a CuCuSn electrode placed at the temporal bone near the eye. A ground electrode was placed on the midline of the forehead close to the hairline. The VEP was recorded simultaneously from a CuCuSn electrode, placed on the midline 1 cm above the inion and referred to a midline electrode placed 9 cm up. The signals were amplified with a Van Gogh EEG amplifier, bandwidth .5–75 Hz. An extra fourth-order low pass Butterworth filter with a cut-off frequency of 70 Hz was used in order to avoid backfolding of the higher frequencies. Online signal analysis was performed with a combined HP21MX-HP2100 computer system. With this system both spectral analysis and time-average analysis were performed.

Stimulus

A standard checkerboard mirror arrangement (Spekreijse, 1966) produced the pattern stimulus. The field size was 30°, and checks of 15', 30' and 60' were used. A large bright surround field (> 90°) was used to suppress stray light responses from the periphery. The mean luminance of the checks was 430 cd/m². The luminance of the periphery was equal to the mean stimulus luminance.

Subjects

The experiments were performed with two subjects, having good vision, and no ophthalmological abnormalities.

Results

Figure 1 shows the results of a series of recordings in which only one of the two sets of checks was modulated (square wave). The other set was kept at a constant luminance level either lower, equal or higher than the mean luminance of the modulated checks. Since the modulation of the checks

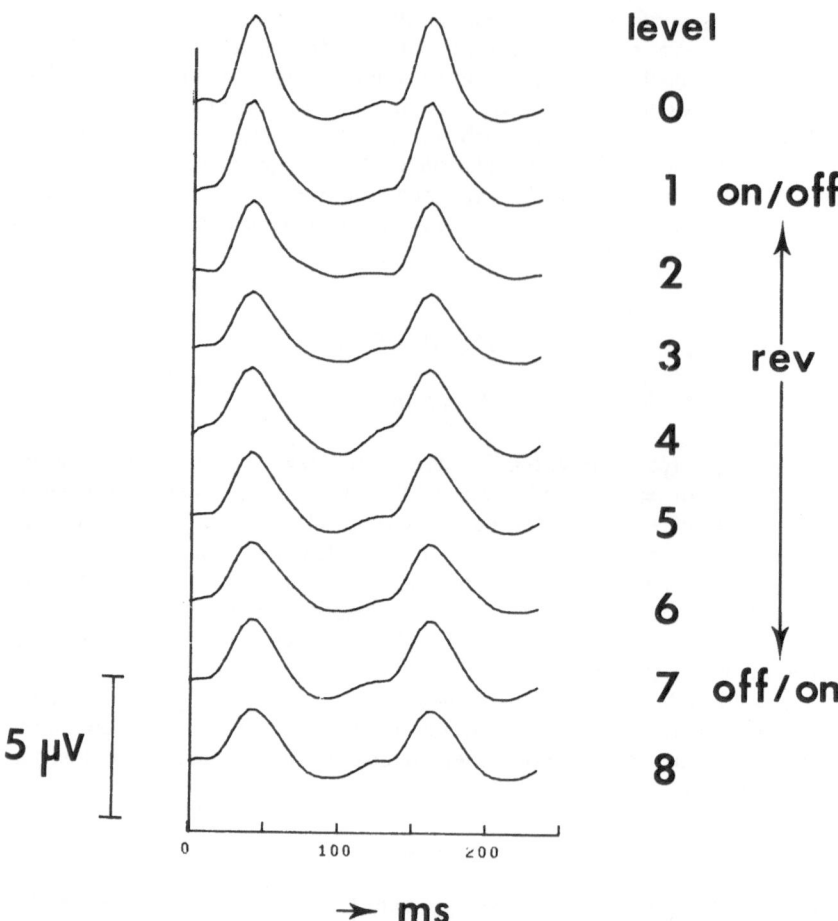

level

0

1 on/off

2

3 rev

4

5

6

7 off/on

8

5 µV

0   100   200

→ ms

Fig. 1. Even harmonic components of the ERG responses. Only one set of checks (size 60', field size 30°) was square wave modulated with a period of 240 ms. The other set was kept constant at various levels, as indicated (1 unit corresponds to 107 cd/m²). The modulation was between the levels 1 and 7. No apparent difference was found between the minimal contrast situations (top and lower trace), where contrast did not reverse at all, and the maximal contrast situation (fourth trace) where the contrast reversed symmetrically twice every period.

remained unchanged the local luminance modulation was constant throughout the series. Since the unmodulated set of checks took a new value every trial the contrast modulation was taking several values throughout the series. Therefore non-linear luminance components would have been constant, while the contrast even harmonic components would have been maximal when a symmetric contrast modulation was given. In this experiment, where the modulation depth was 75%, the contrast modulation was symmetrical, when the luminance of the unmodulated checks was slightly less than 75% of the mean luminance of the modulated checks. This is because contrast is weighted against the instantaneous total luminance level. When the contrast modulation is symmetric, the strongest contrast reversal stimulation is produced. In the situations where even harmonic contrast stimulation was minimal (upper and lower trace) or maximal (fourth trace) the actual responses were quite similar. The simultaneously recorded EP showed a fourfold increase in the 2nd harmonic amplitude for the maximal contrast situation. The ERG can be explained on the basis of local luminance only, while the EP is governed by the contrast stimulation.

In the second set of experiments the two sets of checks were sinusoidally modulated around the same mean luminance. An adjustable phase difference was introduced between the two sets of checks and the second harmonic amplitudes of the responses were recorded as a function of this phase difference. When in such an experiment the checks are modulated counterphase (180° phase difference) a reversal stimulation is produced. Both local luminance and contrast are modulated. When the checks are modulated in phase (0° phase difference) no contrast is present and only the luminance is modulated. When the checks are modulated with a 90° phase difference, the second harmonic responses due to local luminance distortion are 180° out of phase and hence cancel. So only even harmonics due to contrast modulation may be found in that situation. The ERG curve (Figure 2, top) shows a clear minimum at 90° which does not differ significantly from the noise. The curve is symmetric around this point, so non-linear luminance components (0° difference) and non-linear luminance plus any contrast components from the reversal (180° difference) yielded the same response. The conclusion is that only local luminance non-linearities contributed to the second harmonic. The maximum in the simultaneously recorded EP data is found near 180° phase difference, the minimum at 0°, and an intermediate response at 90°. Therefore, since contrast stimulation increases gradually from 0° to 180°, in the EP the responses were mostly determined by the contrast modulation.

These curves can be seriously altered by the effect of stray light to the periphery. The experiment of Figure 2 was performed with a Wratten #29 (deep red) filter in front of the stimulus. This reduced the contribution of the rods to the response. When this contribution is not negligable, the curve becomes asymmetric, and the minimum differs significantly from zero. This can be observed in Figure 3, where the results of a similar experiment, this time performed with white (dotted line) or red (solid line) light, are plotted. This behaviour can largely be explained on the basis of stray light contributing to the response.

In the third set of experiments contrast reversal was produced without local luminance modulation. We used two pattern generators combined by means of a half-silvered mirror. One generator was used to produce a red (Wratten #25) and the other a green (Wratten #58) pattern. Both the generators could either produce pattern reversal or luminance stimulation. First the two sets of checks were modulated in counterphase, at a frequency of 25 Hz, with a modulation depth of 95%. In that condition the luminances of both sets were adjusted to minimize flicker perception. When this heterochromatic match was reached, we recorded the responses to pattern red-green exchange and to homogeneous red-green exchange with a modulation frequency of

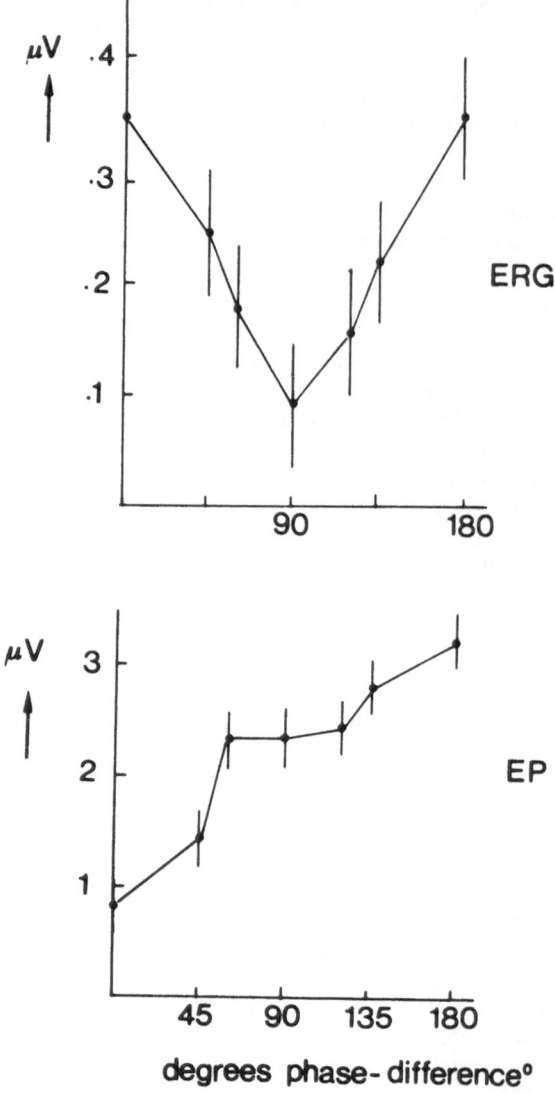

degrees phase- difference°

Fig. 2. Second harmonic amplitudes of the simultaneously recorded ERG and EP. Both sets of checks were modulated (8 Hz, 50%), with an adjustable phase difference. Check size was 60', field size 30°. A Wratten #29 filter (red) was placed in front of the stimulus, to prevent rod responses to stray light in the periphery. The background luminance (white) was as bright as the mean stimulus luminance without the red filter. When the phase difference is 0° only luminance modulation is present. When phase difference is 180° the contrast reverses twice per period, so local luminance and contrast modulation are combined in the stimulus. At the 90° phase difference, the local luminance 2nd harmonic responses are 180° apart and hence cancel. Any component at 90° would have been exclusively of contrast origin. The ERG curve shows no such component, the EP does.

260

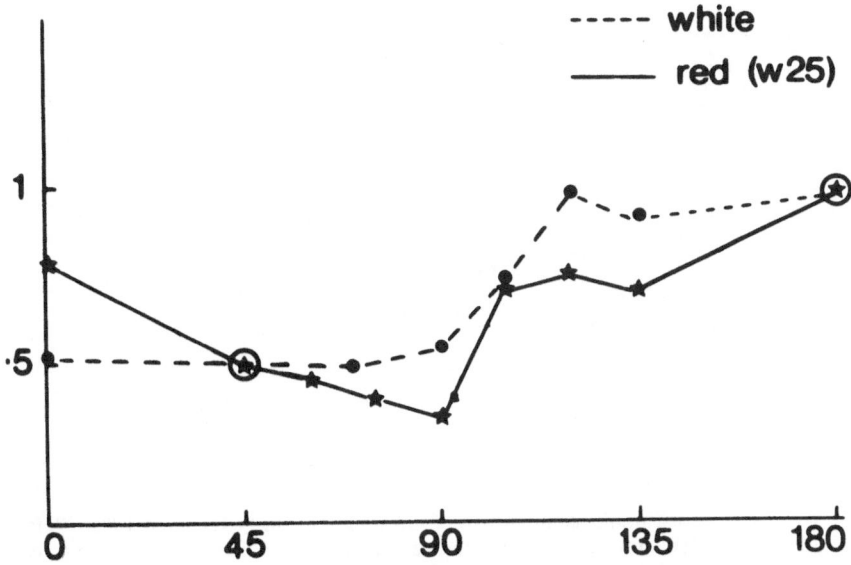

Fig. 3. Second harmonic amplitudes (normalized) of the ERG responses as a function of the phase difference. Two such experiments are plotted: with a white (dotted line) and with a red Wratten #25 stimulus (solid line). When the rods are allowed to contribute to the response a more complex curve results. This curve can be explained, however, on the basis of a combination of local luminance and stray light. When the rods are less stimulated (red light), the curve becomes more symmetric: the stray light response is reduced (see Figure 2).

4.15 Hz. Figure 4 shows the even harmonic components of the responses. While the EP recordings showed a large difference between the homogeneous and pattern red-green exchange, there was no such difference in the ERG. Therefore the ERG is determined by the local chromatic change, while the EP also contains a large pattern component.

DISCUSSION

The results of the three experiments described, all support the conclusion that the ERG recordings to pattern stimuli can be understood on the basis of the local luminance distortion only. As shown e.g. in Figure 3 conclusive experiments are only possible when good care has been taken to avoid stray light responses from the periphery. In any situation where the stimulus does contain a net luminance modulation the stray light can cause complicated interactions. The effect of stray light can also be observed in Figure 1. The modulation depth of the stray light decreases with increasing luminance of the unmodulated checks. And indeed, the responses decreased slightly with the increase of the luminance of the unmodulated checks. Note that there is still no suggestion of contrast components. Contrast would have produced a pronounced difference between e.g. the top trace and the fourth trace.

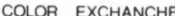

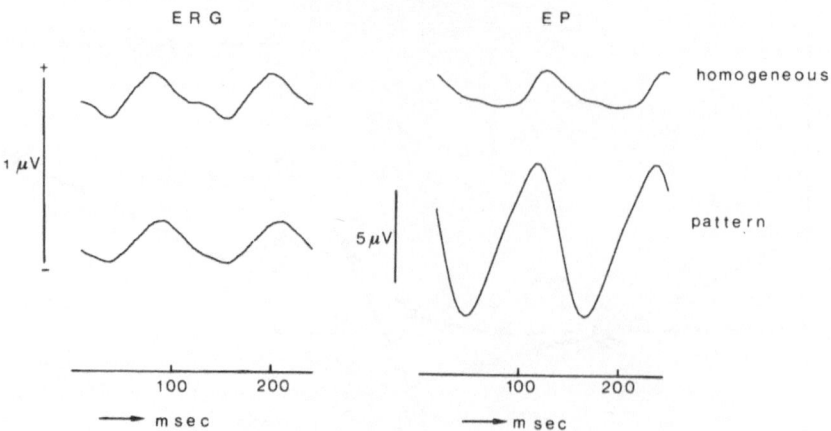

Fig. 4. The even harmonic components of the simultaneously recorded ERGs (left) and EPs (right). The top traces show the responses to homogeneous field red-green exchange, the lower traces to pattern red-green exchange. The luminances of the red and green stimuli were adjusted to obtain heterochromatic match. Checksize was 20', the field size 6°. Background luminance was equal to that of the stimulus. No significant differences to pattern and homogeneous stimuli were found in the ERG, while the EP differed substantially.

The phase difference experiment is also susceptible to stray light effects. In Figure 3 the phase difference experiment was performed with white stimulus light and with red stimulus light (Wratten #25). The net luminance modulation is maximal for the 0° phase difference (homogeneous field) and decreases gradually to zero for 180° phase difference (pattern reversal). So, the stray light modulation, and hence the accompanying complications are maximal at 0° and non-existent at 180°. This can be observed in Figure 3, where the curve became more symmetric, since the rods were less stimulated, when red light was used. The curve is symmetric when deep red light is used. Then the rods are effectively not stimulated (Figure 2). The peripheral response is dominated by the rods (Fry and Bartley, 1935). Therefore scattered light is the probable cause of the observed interaction. One has to be very cautious to reduce stray light responses in the ERG. This is not the case for the EP, where the representation of the fovea onto the cortex, favors the foveal responses.

The large stray light contribution to the ERG still seems to suggest the use of pattern reversal if one wants to study the nonlinear luminance responses of the area directly stimulated. Whenever these nonlinear components become of clinical value, coarse checks should be used, to avoid the risk that the local modulation depth is reduced by causes like internal scatter and poor focus.

From the present experiments we have concluded that the ERG to pattern reversal can be explained readily on the basis of the local luminance distortion only. Contrast components, if present at all, are smaller than the variance of the nonlinear local luminance components (i.e. less than $0.1\,\mu V$ in our conditions). That is, contrast components, if any, are of a magnitude that they can be readily confused with responses of different origin. For instance, we have observed that, in a subject who normally shows very pronounced EPs ($> 30\,\mu V$, under optimized pattern conditions), contrast components could be recorded from the eye electrode. The origin of these responses, however, proved to be non-retinal, since stimulation of the non-recorded eye, yielded the same responses. One needs only 0.3 percent of the cortical responses to obtain a measurable disturbance at the ERG electrode.

REFERENCES

Arden, G. B. (1976): The Retina – Neurophysiology. From: The Eye. Davson, H., Vol. 2A: 229-356. Academic Press, New York.

Arden, G. B., Carter, R. M., Hogg, C. R., Siegel, L. M. and Margolis, S. (1979). A gold foil electrode: Extending the horizons for clinical electroretinography. Invest. Ophthal. Visual Sci. 18: 421–426.

Arden, G. B., Vaegan, Hogg, C. R., Powell, D. J. and Carter, R. M. (1980). Pattern ERGs are abnormal in many amblyopes. Trans. Ophthal. Soc. U.K. 100: 453–460.

Arden, G. B., Vaegan and Hogg, C. R. (1982). Clinical evidence that the pattern ERG (PERG) is generated in more proximal retinal layers than the focal electroretinogram (FERG). Ann. N.Y. Acad. Sci. 388: 580–601.

Dawson, W. W., Trick, G. L. and Litzhow, C. A. (1979). Improved electrode for electro-retinography. Invest. Ophthal. Visual Sci. 18: 988–991.

Fiorentini, A., Maffei, L., Pirchio, M., Spinelli, D. and Porciatti, V. (1981). The ERG in response to alternating gratings in patients with diseases of the peripheral visual pathway. Invest. Ophthal. Visual Sci. 21: 490–493.

Fry, G. A. and Bartley, S. H. (1935). The relation of stray light in the eye to the retinal action potential. Am. J. Physiol. 111: 335–340.

Johnson, E. P., Riggs, L. A. and Schick, A. M. L. (1966). Photopic retinal potentials evoked by phase alternation of a barred pattern. From: Clinical Electroretinography. Burian, H. M. and Jacobson, J. H.: 75–91. Pergamon Press, Oxford.

Koblasz, A. J. (1978). Nonlinearities of the human ERG reflected by Wiener kernels. Biol. Cybernetics 31: 187–191.

Larkin, R. M., Klein, S., Ogden, T. E. and Fender, D. H. (1979). Nonlinear kernels of the human ERG. Biol. Cybernetics 35: 145–160.

Maffei, L. and Fiorentini, A. (1981). Electroretinographic responses to alternating gratings before and after section of the optic nerve. Science 211: 953–955.

Ogden, T. E., Larkin, R. M., Fender, D. H., Cleary, P. E. and Ryan, S. J. (1980). The use of nonlinear analysis of the primate ERG to detect retinal dysfunction. Exp. Eye Res. 31: 381–388.

Regan, D. and Spekreijse, H. (1974). Evoked potential indications of colour blindness. Vision Res. 14: 89–95.

Riggs, L. A., Johnson, E. P. and Schick, A. M. L. (1964). Electrical responses of the human eye to moving stimulus patterns. Science 144: 567.

Sherman, J. (1982). Simultaneous pattern reversal electroretinograms and visual evoked potentials in decreases of the macula and the optic nerve. Ann. N.Y. Acad. Sci. 388: 214–226.

Sokol, S. and Nadler, D. (1979). Simultaneous electroretinograms and visually evoked potentials from adult amblyopes to a pattern stimulus. Invest. Ophthal. Visual Sci. 18: 848–855.

Spekreijse, H. (1966). Analysis of EEG responses in man evoked by sine wave modu-lated light. Thesis. University of Amsterdam.

Spekreijse, H., Estevez, O. and van der Tweel, L. H. (1973). Luminance responses to pattern reversal. Doc. Ophthal. Proc. Ser. 10: 205-211.

van der Tweel, L. H. (1961). Some problems in vision regarded with respect to linearity and frequency response. Ann. N.Y. Acad. Sci. 89: 829–856.

Vaegan, Arden, G. B. and Hogg, C. R. (1982). Properties of normal electroretinograms evoked by patterned stimuli in man. Abnormalities in optic nerve diseases and amblyopia. Doc. Ophthal. Proc. Ser. 31: 111–129.

Mailing address:
The Netherlands Ophthalmic Research Institute
P.O. Box 6411
1005 EK Amsterdam, The Netherlands

HUMAN PATTERN EVOKED RETINAL RESPONSE (PERR): SPATIAL TUNING AND DEVELOPMENT

J. V. ODOM, W. W. DAWSON, P. E. ROMANO AND T. M. MAIDA

(Gainesville, Florida, U.S.A.)

ABSTRACT

Prior investigations of the PERR have noted an absence of low spatial frequency cut-off which has been interpreted to indicate an absence of lateral inhibitory processes in the retinal structures giving rise to PERR.

The results of two experiments with normal adults are presented to indicate (1) the presence of a low spatial frequency cut-off and (2) the presence of a local luminance response when high-luminance, high-contrast, low spatial frequency square wave patterns are used as stimuli. The presence of the local luminance response is used to account for the absence of spatial tuning in prior investigations. Experiment 1 using sinusoidal gratings of 20% contrast compared the spatial tuning of VECPs and PERRs. Experiment 2 used square wave gratings of 60% contrast at 86 and 43 cd/m to demonstrate greater spatial tuning at low than at high luminance. In Experiment 3, retinal responses of 3.5 month old infants and adults are compared. Infant retinal responses have the same relationship to spatial frequency as found in adults, confirming prior anatomical data that the fovea matures between 2 and 4 months postnatally.

INTRODUCTION

PERRs are inversely related in a linear manner to the log spatial frequency (Armington et al., 1971; Groneberg, 1980; Korth, 1981; Trick and Wintermeyer, 1981). The absence of reduced PERR amplitude at low spatial frequencies is interpreted as indicating (10) that PERRs lack the influence of lateral inhibition, (2) that the PERR originate in retinal layers prior to antagonistic center-surround receptive field organization (Armington et al., 1971), and (3) that the PERR is the result of retinal summation elements detecting local luminance changes (Korth, 1981) and as such does not truly represent a pattern response (Padmos et al., 1973; Spekreijse et al., 1973b). The first two experiments presented below present evidence of PERR spatial tuning. Experiment 3 compares the PERRs of infants and adults.

Doc. Ophthal. Proc. Series, Vol 37, ed. by H.E.J.W. Kolder
© 1983 Dr W. Junk Publishers, The Hague/Boston:Lancaster

EXPERIMENT 1

Methods

Subjects were two adult males corrected to 20/20 who were experienced observers. Each subject participated in two sessions consisting of one replication of all stimulus conditions.

Stimuli were photographic slides of sine wave gratings of 0.34, 0.68, 1.20, 2.22 and 3.67 cycles per degree (cpd) projected onto a 33°23' x 20° tangent screen. Mean luminance was 110 cd/m² and contrast 20%. A 0.3 ND filter served as a control. Stimuli were shifted 0.5 cycles in a square wave fashion at 1, 2, 4, 8 and 16 Hz. The PERR was recorded using the DTL fiber electrode placed under the lower eyelid and referenced to the outer canthus with a forehead ground.

Signals were amplified 10^4X. A Nicolet MED-80 acquired 50 samples. Sweep duration varied with stimulation rate consisting of two complete cycles (four reversals of the pattern). Averaged data were stored on floppy disc for subsequent analysis.

Results

Artifacts such as eye movements and luminance imbalance which may confound amplitude measurement elicit responses at approximatly the stimulation frequency, that is at the alternation rate (Armington, 1968; Johnson et al., 1966). Therefore, power at the second harmonic of the stimulation frequency (2F power) was used as the response measure. Because only the second harmonic is measured, power may be a more accurate measure of the response.

Figure 1 is the average of four replications of the stimulus conditions. Picowatts are scaled as percentage of the maximum response at that stimulation frequency. For each temporal frequency and the average across temporal frequencies, PERRs are presented as a function of log spatial frequency. Averaging across all temporal frequencies, the peak power occurs at 0.68 cpd. The response at 0.34 cpd is 26.7% less than that at 0.68 cpd and the half-power bandwidth is approximately 4 octaves.

EXPERIMENT 2

Methods

The general experimental conditions were the same as in Experiment 1. Stimuli were square wave grating with 60% contrast whose spatial frequency of the patterns varied from 0.16 to 4.50 cpd presented at 4 Hz. At a mean luminance of either of 86 cd/m² or of 43 cd/m². For each pattern size, the brighter condition was presented first then the dimmer pattern. Seventy-five sweeps of 2 cycles during (4 reversals) of the stimulus were summed for analysis.

266

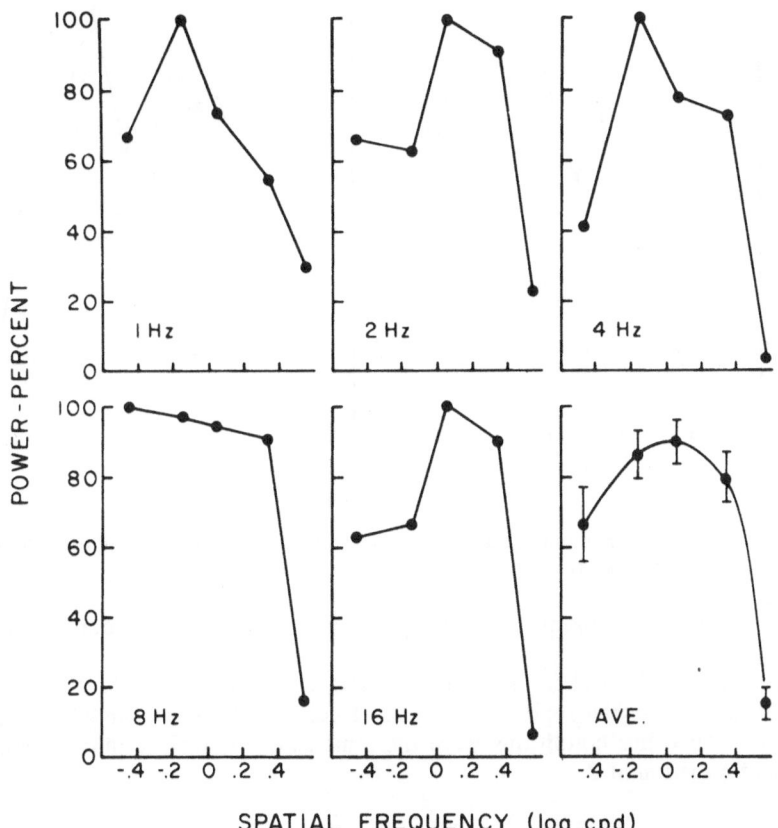

SPATIAL FREQUENCY (log cpd)

Fig. 1. Percent Power of PERRs as a function of log spatial frequency and temporal frequency. The average of all stimulation frequencies shows a peak at 0.68 cpd with a band width of 4 octaves and a low spatial frequency attenuation of 27%.

Results

Data were quantified as in experiment 1 and presented in Figure 2. To give a standard for comparison, 100% power for 43 cd/m² and 86 cd/m² conditions were 1510 and 3352 picowatts respectively. Mean luminance influenced the magnitude of the low spatial frequency attentuation as measured by 2F power, the attenuation being, 30 and 70% for the 86 and 43 cd/m² conditions, respectively.

EXPERIMENT 3

Methods

Three infants and two adults served as subjects. At the times of testing, the infants were aged 2.75 months, 3.25 months, 3.5 months and 4.5 months

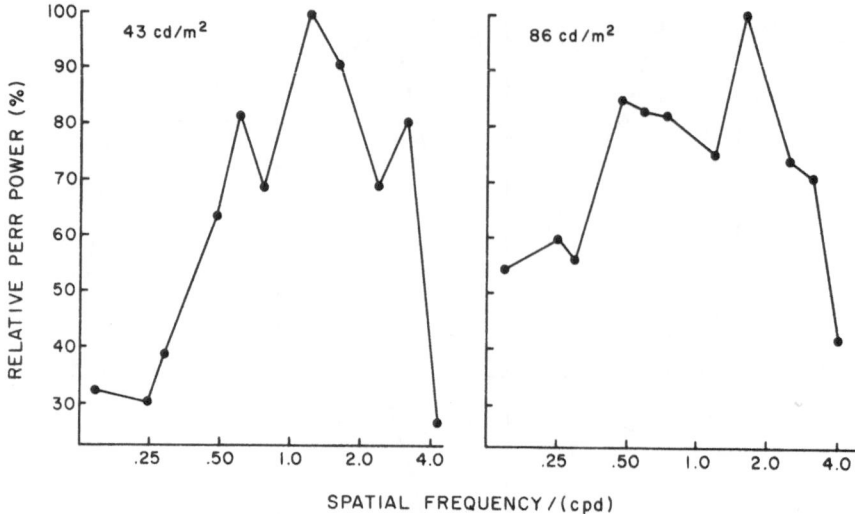

Fig. 2. Percent power and amplitude as a function of spatial frequency and mean luminance. Relative tuning is greater in the 43 cd/m² condition.

with a mean of 3.5 months; the adults were also tested for a total of four replications.

Twenty responses elicited by three square wave gratings, 1.25, 2.75, and 4.5 cycles per degree (cpd) and a 0.3 ND control alternated at 2 Hz were averaged. All other conditions were the same as in the high luminance condition of experiment 2.

Results

The percent 2F power is presented in Figure 3 for adults and infants. The maximum, non-normalized average values for the PERR are 278 and 93 picowatts for the infants and adults respectively.

DISCUSSION

The most significant single observation in the first two experiments is reduced power in the PERRS elicited by low spatial frequency patterns, indicating that the PERR arises from structures which possess an antagonistic lateral inhibitory organisation. Other investigators have failed to note a low spatial frequency attenuation (Armington et al., 1971; Groneberg, 1980; Korth, 1981; Trick and Wintermeyer, 1981). Their experiments differed from experiment 1 in several ways; they presented square wave stimuli of higher luminance and contrast, in a smaller field, and amplitude of the positive peak was the response measure. None of these differences alone can account for the discrepancy. A large field size might improve the signal to noise ratio by stimulating a larger number of ganglion cells (Armington, 1968). However, a

268

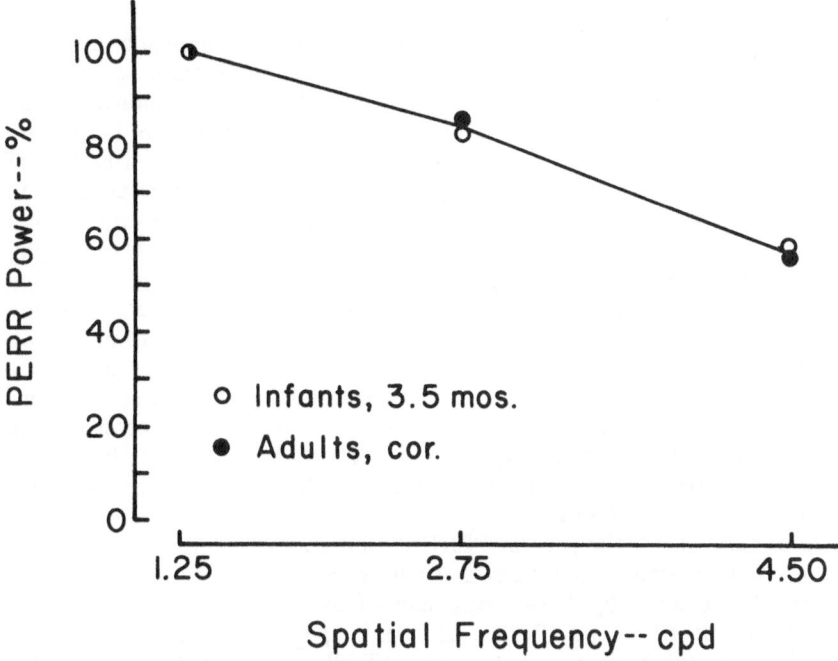

Fig. 3. Percent PERR power is plotted as a function of spatial frequency for infants 3.5 months old and adults. The relative response for pattern is very similar in the two groups.

larger field size should decrease the spatial frequency of the peak response by stimulating more peripheral ganglion cells with larger receptive fields. At 1–2 Hz stimulation rates where the responses measured by Armington and others are observable and their amplitudes are the major determinants of power. However, it has been noted that power and amplitude may yield differently shaped functions (Moskowitz and Sokol, 1980). The combination of square wave, high contrasting patterns presented at high luminance was used in experiment 2 and tuning was observed. Therefore, use of high luminance, high contrast grating cannot alone account for the differences between our results and others.

In experiment 2, there was a 30% reduction in 2F power at lower spatial frequencies at the high luminance level while at the lower luminance level there was a 70% reduction. These effects are consistent with a major local luminane response in PERR. A review of discussions of the local luminance confound in pattern reversal stimulation (Spekreijse, 1966; Regan, 1972; Spekreijse and van der Tweel, 1972; Padmos et al., 1973; Spekreijse et al., 1973a, 1973b, 1977) indicate several characteristics of the local luminance response: (1) it originates in hypothetical luminance summation fields, (2) the field have non-linear properties like asymmetric rectifiers such that their response is observed at twice the stimulation frequency, (3) the maximum response occurs when the response occurs when the pattern element size maximally stimulates the summation field.

Several predictions follow: (1) the maximum local luminance response at any adaptation level will vary with the mean luminance, so that the brighter the mean luminance, the larger the local luminance response and the smaller the low spatial frequency attenuation (2) the maximum local luminance response for a square wave stimulus would be elicited by a pattern of 100% contrast and decrease linearly with contrast, (3) at the response peak for a square wave stimulus, a sine wave stimulus of the same fundamental frequency would elicit a smaller local luminance response and (4) the magnitude of the local luminance response generally declines as spatial frequency increases; the decline need not be linear, however, for any size summation field, complete cycles yield no response as their alternation results in no luminance change while less than complete cycles result in luminance changes, the magnitude of which are proportional to the number of half cycles. Based on the prediction number one, it follows that greater relative attenuation at low spatial frequencies would occur at a lower luminance level as observed in experiment 2 indicating the large influence of local luminance responses in PERRs.

In experiment 3, the percent PERR response as a function of spatial frequency is very similar in infants and adults. Retinal acuity for infants and adults as calculated by linear regression of average PERR and log spatial frequency was 31.92 cpd (20/20) and 31.49 cpd (20/20) respectively. The similarity of the relationships between PERRs and spatial frequency for infants and adults contrasts with the large differences between adult and infant VECPs at this age (Marg et al., 1976; Sokol and Dobson, 1976).

If the PERR originates in the ganglion cell layer as some have suggested (Maffei and Fiorentini, 1981; Dawson, Maida, and Rubin, 1982), the interpretation of the results of these three experiments is more explicit. The tuning observed in experiments 1 and 2 should be closely related to the envelope defining the spatial tuning of the population of retinal cells stimulated. Exciting possibilities for future research exist in the attempt to design stimuli and analysis techniques which will permit one to analyze the function of specific ganglion cell populations.

The similarity of functions relating PERR 2F power to spatial frequency indicate a relative maturity of the infant retinal structures stimulated by pattern reversal. The ganglion cell hypothesis would imply that the very last layer of neural processing in the eye, the ganglion cells, all have the same relative ability to respond to pattern at 3–4 months as at adulthood. This interpretation is consistent with ideas of nervous system development which suggest that the final stages of maturation are completed first at lower neural centers.

ACKNOWLEDGEMENT

Research supported by NIH grants EY03781, EY04806 and an unrestricted departmental grant from Research to Prevent Blindness, Inc.

REFERENCES

Armington, J. C. (1968). The electroretinogram, the visual evoked potential and the area-luminance relation. Vision Res. 8, 263–276.

Armington, J. C., Corwin, T. R. and Marsetta, R. (1971). Simultaneously recorded retinal and cortical responses to patterned stimuli. J. Opt. Soc. Am. 61, 1514–1521.

Dawson, W. W., Maida, T. M. and Rubin, M. L. (1981). Human pattern evoked retinal responses are altered by optic atrophy. Invest. Ophthalmol. Visual Sci., in press.

Groneberg, A. (1980). Simultaneously recorded retinal and cortical potentials elicited by checkerboard stimuli. Doc. Ophthal. Proc. Ser. 23, 255–262.

Johnson, E. P., Riggs, L. A. and Schick, A. J. L. (1966). Photopic retinal potentials evoked by phase alternation of a barred pattern. In *Clinical Electroretinography* Burian, H. M. and Jacobson, J. H. (Eds.) pp. 75–91. Pergamon Press, Oxford.

Korth, M. (1981). Human fast retinal potentials and the spatial properties of a visual stimulus. Vision Res. 21, 627–630.

Maffei, L. and Fiorentini, A. (1981). Electroretinographic responses to alternating gratings before and after section of the optic nerve. Science 211, 953–955.

Mann, I. (1964). The development of the human eye. 3rd ed. New York, Grune and Stratton, 1964.

Marg, E., Freeman, D. N., Peltzman, P., and Goldstein, P. I. (1976). Visual acuity development in humans: Evoked potential measures. Invest. Ophthal., 15, 150–153.

Moskowitz, A., Sokol, S. (1980). Spatial and temporal interaction and pattern-evoked cortical potentials in human infants. Vision Res. 20, 699–707.

Padmos, P., Haaijman, J. J. and Spekreijse, H. (1973). Visually evoked cortical potentials to patterned stimuli in monkey and man. EEG Clin. Neurophysiol. 35, 153–163.

Regan, D. (1972). Evoked Potentials in Psychology, Sensory Physiology and Clinical Medicine. Chapman and Hall, London.

Spekreijse, H. (1966). *Analysis of EEG Responses in Man Evoked by Sine Wave Modulated Light.* Thesis. Junk Publishing Co., The Hague.

Spekreijse, H., Estevez, O. and Reits, D. (1977). Visual evoked potentials and the physiological analysis of Visual processes in man. In *Visual Evoked Potentials in Man: New Developments* Desmedt, J. E. (Ed.) pp. 16–89. Clarendon Press, Oxford.

Spekreijse, H., Estevez, O. and van der Tweel, L. H. (1973a). Luminance responses to pattern reversal. In: 10th ISCERG Symposium. Doc. Ophthal. Proc. Ser. Vol. 2 Pearlman, J.T. (Ed.) pp. 205–211. Junk Publishing Co., The Hague.

Spekreijse H., and van der Tweel, L. H. (1972). System analysis of linear and nonlinear processes in electrophysiology of the visual system. I. and II. *Koninklink Nederlander Academie van Wetenschappen.* Proceedings Series C, 75, 77–105.

Spekreijse, H., van der Tweel, H. and Zuidema, T. (1973b). Contrast evoked responses in man. Vision Res. 13, 1577–1601.

Trick, G. L. and Wintermeyer, D. H. (1982). Spatial and temporal tuning of pattern reversal retinal potentials. Invest. Ophthalmol. Visual Sci., 22 (Suppl.), 221.

Mailing address:
Department of Ophthalmology
West Virginia University Medical Center
Morgantown, West Virginia 26506, U.S.A.

REFERENCES

PATTERN REVERSAL ELECTRORETINOGRAMS IN SQUINT AMBLYOPIA, ARTIFICIAL ANISOMETROPIA AND SIMULATED ECCENTRIC FIXATION

H. E. PERSSON AND P. WANGER

(Stockholm, Sweden)

ABSTRACT

Pattern-reversal electroretinograms were recorded in 10 normals and 10 adult patients with squint amblyopia (visual acuity 0.3 or less). The effects of artificial anisometropia and simulated eccentric fixation were tested in normals. The pattern-reversal ERG amplitude was reduced linearly with increased defocusing. A significant amplitude reduction was observed when defocusing amounted to $+1\,D$ or more. The amplitudes were not reduced below the range of normal variability at $4°$ of simulated eccentric fixation. In amblyopic patients, refractive errors were corrected. None had eccentric fixation of more than $4°$. Yet, the pattern-reversal ERGs were lower in all amblyopic eyes compared with the opposite normal eyes. The difference in amplitude means was statistically significant. The finding supports the view that retinal function is impaired in human squint amblyopia.

INTRODUCTION

Squint and certain optical defects during early childhood may give rise to amblyopia and/or impaired binocular stereoscopic vision. It has been suggested mainly on the basis of animal experiments that these two disturbances have different pathophysiological origin and that the changes connected with amblyopia might involve retina (Ideka 1979). The present study was undertaken to test if retinal dysfunction could also be demonstrated in humans. Thus, pattern-reversal and unpatterned flash ERGs were recorded in 10 amblyopic patients and 10 controls. Two conditions were commonly associated with amblyopia, that is anisometropia and eccentric fixation. These conditions per se might influence the pattern-reversal ERG. Therefore, they were simulated and their effects tested in normals.

METHODS

When recording the pattern-reversal ERG, a black and white checkerboard pattern was presented on a standard 26 inch TV set in front of the patients at

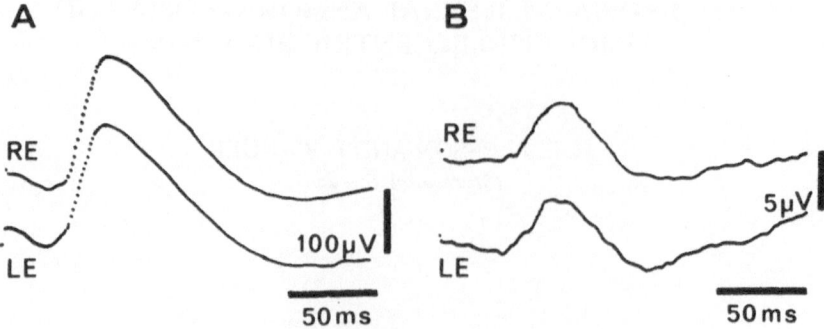

Fig. 1. Unpatterned flash(A) and pattern-reversal ERGs(B) from a normal subject.

a distance of 1.5 meter (for a detailed technical description, see Persson and Wanger, 1982). The pattern was reversed with a rate of 2 Hz. The whole stimulating field corresponded to a visual angle of 15 degrees in horizontal and 13.5 in vertical direction. Each square subtended a visual angle of 24 minutes of arc. The average luminance of the TV screen was 45 candela per square meter. Contrast setting of the pattern generator was 100%. When recording the unpatterned flash, ERG, a Grass P2 photosimulator was used and placed at a distance of ½ meter in front of the patients. Flashes were given at a rate of 1 Hz with varying relative intensities (2 and 8) of the photostimulator.

The ERGs were recorded with Arden gold foil electrodes inserted under the lower lid, not interfering with the normal optics (Arden et al., 1979). The reference electrodes were placed 2 cm posterior to the lateral canthus. Conventional averaging technique was used. Refractive errors were measured with subjective and objective methods and, when present, carefully corrected. Control pattern-reversal ERGs were recorded with positive and negative lenses added to the optimal spectacle correction. If this manoeuvre did not improve the ERG amplitude, the correction was thought to be adequate. Binocular stimulations were performed in normals and amblyopic patients without squint and sequential monocular stimulation in patients with squint.

RESULTS

10 healthy persons, 21 to 40 years of age, comprised the control group. The 2 Hz-pattern-reversal ERG from a normal person is shown in Figure 1. It is characterized by a small or absent initial negativity, dominated by a positive wave and followed by a negative after potential. The mean peak to peak amplitude of the normal group amounted to 4.9 ± 1.3 μV (Table 2). Both the pattern-reversal and the flash ERG had an interocular difference in amplitude as well as amplitude variation of less than 20% during one recording session.

Table 1 shows the clinical data of the amblyopic group. 10 patients were investigated, 16 to 39 years of age. All had a history of squint. 4 had

Table 1. Clinical data of the amblyopic group.

No	Pat	Age	Sex	Squint	Aniso-* metropia	Eccentric fixation	Visual acuity RE/LE
1	RLK	24	F	LE	–	2°	1.0/< 0.1
2	SS	29	M	RE	RE	4°	< 0.1/ 1.0
3	OB	39	M	RE	–	1°	< 0.1/ 1.0
4	JL	19	F	RE	RE	–	0.1/ 1.0
5	GA	24	F	LE	–	2°	1.0/ 0.1
6	AJ	30	M	RE	RE	–	0.2/ 1.0
7	CW	16	F	RE	–	1°	0.3/ 1.0
8	UH	18	M	RE	RE	–	0.3/ 0.8
9	KHD	32	M	RE	–	–	0.3/ 1.0
10	KL	30	F	LE	–	–	1.0/ 0.3

RE = right eye. LE = left eye.
The patients are arranged according to the degree of visual acutiy-reduction.
*Anisometropia is defined as side difference of more than 1D in spherical or cylindrical refraction.

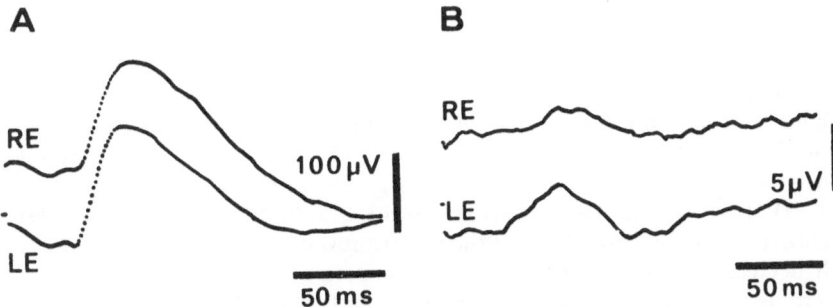

Fig. 2. Unpatterned flash(A) and pattern-reversal ERGs(B) from an amblyopic patient (No. 8). Note the reduced pattern-reversal ERG from the right, amblyopic eye(RE), but no side difference in the flash ERGs.

anisometropia which thus was corrected during registration. 5 had eccentric fixation less than 4 degrees. The visual acuity varied between less than 0.1 and 0.3.

Pattern-reversal and unpatterned flash ERGs are shown from one of the patients (Figure 2). Note the reduced pattern-reversal ERG amplitude from the right, amblyopic eye, but no side difference in flash ERGs. In 9 of the patients, the pattern-reversal ERG amplitudes from the amblyopic eyes were reduced compared with the opposite non-amblyopic eyes and below the level of normal variation.

The mean peak to peak amplitude of the pattern-reversal ERG in the amblyopic group amounted to $2.3 \pm 1.1 \mu V$ and in the opposite eyes and normal controls to $4.3 \pm 1.8 \mu V$ and $4.9 \pm 1.3 \mu V$, respectively (Table 2). This difference is statistically significant. The negative afterpotential was equal in all groups. The 5 amblyopes with eccentric fixation up to 4 degrees had pattern-reversal ERG amplitudes not statistically different from those with

Table 2. Mean amplitudes of the pattern-reversal ERGs in the different groups.

	Peak-to-peak amplitude (μV ± 1 SD)	Neg. afterpotential amplitude (μV ± 1 SD)
Normal group	4.9 ± 1.3	2.7 ± 1.3
Amblyopic group		
Normal eye:	4.3 ± 1.8	2.5 ± 1.1
Amblyopic eye:	2.3 ± 1.1	2.1 ± 1.2

Table 3. Mean amplitudes of the *a*- and *b*-waves of the flash ERGs in the different groups.

	a-wave amplitude (μV ± 1 SD)	*b*-wave amplitude (μV ± 1 SD)
Normal group	37 ± 8	154 ± 50
Amblyopic group		
Normal eye:	33 ± 9	146 ± 44
Amblyopic eye:	32 ± 13	143 ± 41

central fixation. From the data in Table 3, it is evident that no difference was observed in the flash ERGs between amblyopic eyes, opposite eyes and normal controls.

When testing the effect of artificial anisometropia, pattern-reversal stimulation was used for both eyes simultaneously. Unilateral anisometropia induced by stepwise defocusing the image to one eye with positive lenses up to + 3D. The opposite eye serving as control, the amplitude of which was set to 100. The relative amplitude of the pattern-reversal ERG decreased linearly with decreasing defocusing (Figure 3). Comparing group data, a significant amplitude reduction was already obtained at the + 1D level. The pattern-reversal ERG was also recorded when the subjects were instructed to fixate outside the center of the TV screen in nasal direction. At 4 degrees of simulated eccentricity the mean amplitude reduction amounted to 10 ± 3.5%, which was not statistically significant. At 8 degrees the amplitude reduction amounted to 34 ± 6.5%.

DISCUSSION

The present results show that the 2 Hz pattern-reversal ERG recorded from amblyopic eyes were reduced compared to those from the opposite eyes and normal controls (Persson and Wanger, 1982). All patients selected had a visual acuity of 0.3 or less. Changes in the ERG to pattern stimulation has been demonstrated by Sokol and Nadler (1979) in 3 and by Arden et al., (1980) in 10 amblyopic eyes with moderately reduced visual acuity and normal eyes, when recording bar pattern ERGs. The pattern-ERGs are therefore likely to be changed only in amblyopia with marked acuity loss.

Anisometropia and eccentric fixation are commonly associated with amblyopia. Their influence on the pattern-reversal ERG was estimated

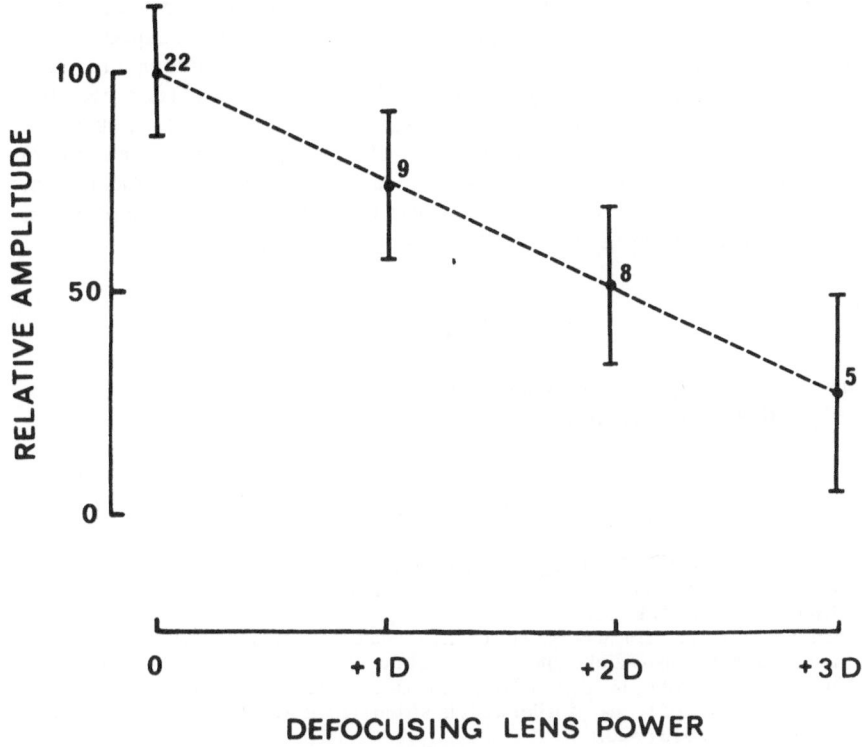

Fig. 3. Changes of the relative pattern-reversal ERG amplitude (mean ± SD) with induced refractive error in one eye. The opposite eye serving as control with its ERG amplitude referred to as 100. Numbers of recordings at each defocusing level are given.

from experiments in normals. With our technique and comparing group data, artificial anisometropia of 1D was found to significantly reduce the ERG amplitude. In all patients refractive errors were measured with subjective and objective methods and, when present, carefully corrected for the ERG recordings. Furthermore, the addition of positive and negative lenses to the spectacle correction did not increase the pattern-reversal amplitude. With simulated eccentric fixation, an amplitude reduction outside the range of normal variation was not observed until the eccentricity amounted to 8 degrees. Four patients had eccentric fixation of 2 degrees and one had 4 degrees. These 5 amblyopes had pattern-reversal ERG amplitudes not statistically different from those with central fixation. Thus, the observed difference in ERG amplitude between amblyopic and normal eyes cannot be explained by uncorrected refractive errors and eccentric fixation and is suggested to reflect impaired retinal function.

Maffei and Fiorentini (1981) reported disappearance of the pattern ERG parallelling the degeneration of retinal ganglion cells after sectioning the optic nerve in cats. It was suggested that these cells were the main source of the pattern ERG. If so, the present findings may reflect impaired function of retinal ganglion cells in human squint amblyopia. This view is supported by the demonstration of ganglion cell dysfunction in squint amblyopia in kittens (Ikeda and Tremain 1979, Chino et al., 1980). However, the pattern ERG has been argued to be a summated local luminance response and not produced by spatial contrast stimulation (Spekreijse et al., 1973, Riemslag et al., 1982) and, hence, not reflecting retinal ganglion cell activity. Whatever mechanism for the generation of the pattern ERG, the present results lend support to a retinal involvement in human squint amblyopia.

ACKNOWLEDGEMENT

This study was supported by grants from Karolinska Institute and the Swedish Medical Research Council (No. B 82–04X–062330–01).

REFERENCES

Arden, G. B., Carter, R. M., Hogg, C., Siegel, I. M. and Margolis, S. (1979): A gold foil electrode: extending the horizons for clinical electroretinography. Invest. Ophthalmol. 18: 421–426.
Arden, G. B., Vaegen, Hogg, C. R., Powell, D. J. and Carter, R. M. (1980): Pattern-ERGs are abnormal in many amblyopes. Trans. Ophthalmol. Soc. UK. 100: 453–460.
Chino, Y. M., Shansky, M. S. and Hamasaki, D. J. (1980): Development of receptive field properties of retinal ganglion cells in kittens raised with convergent squint. Exp. Brain Res. 39: 313–320.
Ikeda, H. (1979): Physiological basis of amblyopia. Trends. Neurosci. 2: 209–212.
Ikeda, H. and Tremain, K. E. (1979): Amblyopia occurs in retinal ganglion cells in cats reared with convergent squint without alternating fixation. Exp. Brain. Res. 35: 559–582.
Maffei, L. and Fiorentini, A. (1981): Electroretinographic responses to alternating gratings before and after sectioning of the optic nerve. Science. 211: 953–955.
Persson, H. E. and Wanger, P. (1982): Pattern-reversal electroretinograms in squint amblyopia, artificial anisometropia and simulated eccentric fixation. Acta. Ophthal. 60: 123–132.
Riemslag, F. C.C., Ringo, J., Spekreijse, H. and Verdyn Lunel, H. F. E. (1982): The distinction between luminance and spatial components in the pattern ERG. Doc. Ophthal. Proc. of XXth ISCEV symposium, Iowa, USA (this volume).
Sokol, S. and Nadler, D. (1979): Simultaneous electroretinograms and visual evoked potentials from adult amblyopes in response to a pattern stimulus. Invest. Ophthalmol. 18: 848–855.
Spekreijse, H., Estevez, O. and van der Tweel, L. H. (1973): Luminance responses to pattern reversal. Doc. Ophthal. Proc. of Xth ISCERG symposium. 2: 205-212.
Tuttle, D. R. (1973): Electrophysiological studies of functional amblyopia utilizing pattern reversal techniques. Masters Thesis, Univ. Louisville, USA.

Mailing address:
Departments of Neurophysiology and Ophthalmology
Karolinska Hospital
S-104 01 Stockholm
Sweden

PATTERN-REVERSAL ELECTRORETINOGRAMS IN UNILATERAL GLAUCOMA

P. WANGER AND H. E. PERSSON

(Stockholm, Sweden)

ABSTRACT

Pattern-reversal and flash electroretinograms (ERG), and oscillatory potentials (OP) were recorded from 11 patients with unilateral glaucoma. The pattern-reversal ERG amplitudes were reduced below the level of normal variation in 10 of the 11 glaucomatous eyes. The difference in amplitude means was statistically significant. No differences were observed in flash ERGs or OPs. The histopathological correlate to the visual field defects in glaucoma is retinal ganglion cell degeneration. The present electrophysiological findings support the view, based on results from animal experiments, that the pattern-reversal ERG reflects ganglion cell activity.

INTRODUCTION

Results from animal experiments and findings in patients with retinal and optic nerve disorders indicate that the electroretinogram (ERG) to pattern stimulation may be generated by the retinal ganglion cells (Maffei and Fiorentini 1981, Fiorentini et al., Dawson et al., 1982 and May et al., 1982). It is known from histopathological studies that the visual field defects in glaucoma correspond to damage of the ganglion cells and their axons (Apple and Rabb 1974, Sommer et al., 1977, Quigley et al., 1980 and Quigley et al., 1981). Consistent changes in the pattern ERG from glaucomatous eyes would support the idea that this type of ERG reflects activity in the ganglion cells.

Thus, 11 patients with unilateral glaucoma were studied, the opposite eye serving as control. In addition to the pattern-reversal ERG, unpatterned flash ERG and oscillatory potentials (OP) were recorded, since these electrical responses are considered to be generated by retinal elements other than the ganglion cells.

METHODS AND OPHTHALMOLOGICAL EXAMINATION

When recording the pattern-reversal and unpatterned flash ERGs the same techniques were used as described in Persson and Wanger (1983, this volume,

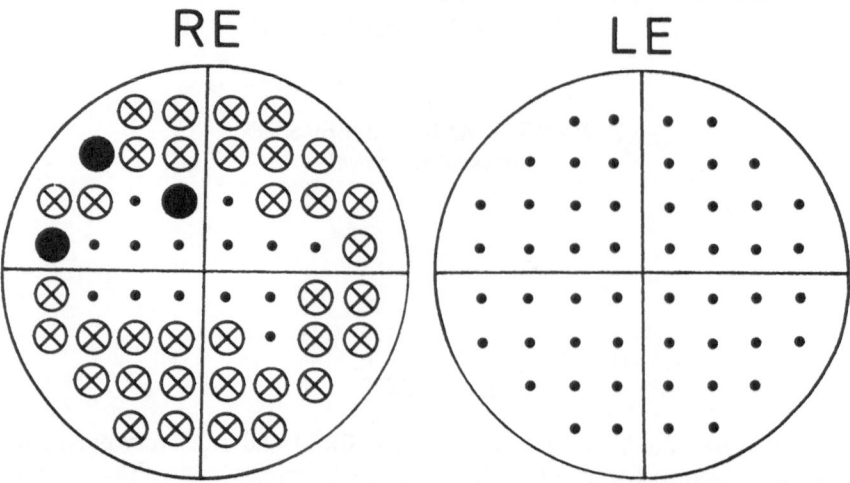

RE   LE

Fig. 1. Visual field charts (central 30 degrees) from one of the patients (no. 6). RE = right. LE = left eye. Dot = stimulus object III:1 perceived(score 0). Cross marked circle = stimulus object III: 3 perceived (score − 1). Filled circle = neither stimulus object perceived (score − 2).

for a detailed technical description, see Persson and Wanger 1982, Wanger and Persson 1983). The OPs were recorded after 10 min of dark adaptation. Stimulus flashes were given at a rate of 2 min, maximal intensity (16) on a Grass PS2 photostimulator. Special cut off frequencies (32 Hz to 320 Hz) were used in preamplifiers (Wachtmeister 1972).

The degree of glaucomatous damage was assessed by static perimetry, manually performed on a Goldmann perimeter (Haag-Streit, type 940). The results of these examination were expressed numerically as visual field scores. The test object (III:1) was presented at each of 52 locations within the central 30 degrees field. If the patient did not perceive the objects its luminance was increased by 1 log unit (III:3) and the presentation repeated. Perceiving the first dimmer object gave a score of 0, the second brighter object gave a score of − 1. Not perceiving any of the two objects at the tested location gave a score of − 2. Since 52 locations were examined the score ranged from 0 to − 104. Figure 1 illustrates the visual fields from one of the patients, representative for the group. The score from the right, glaucomatous eye was − 41 and from the opposite eye 0.

RESULTS

Table 1 presents the clinical data of the examined group. All patients had clinically manifest glaucoma in one eye. The opposite eye was normal or suffered from ocular hypertension. No abnormalities beside the glaucomatous changes were observed in the group. The visual field scores ranged from − 15 to − 104 in the glaucomatous eyes (mean − 49 SD 30) and from 0 to − 11 in the opposite eye (mean − 2 SD 3). There was a difference between eyes in

Table 1. Clinical data.

No.	Pat	Age	Sex	Glaucomatous eye	Visual acuity RE/LE	Visual field score (central 30°) RE/LE	Treatment RE	LE
1	GW	61	M	RE	HM/1.0	− 104/0	TRAB	TIM
2	TS	65	M	RE	0.3/1.0	− 104/0	TRAB	–
3	EA	68	M	LE	1.0/0.5	− 4/− 62	PILO	TRAB
4	MM	76	M	RE	0.8/1.0	− 54/− 11	TRAB	–
5	LK	67	M	RE	0.9/0.9	− 46/− 6	PILO + TIM	–
6	SL	69	M	RE	1.0/1.0	− 41/0	PILO	–
7	KF	74	F	RE	0.7/0.7	− 41/− 1	TRAB	PILO
8	JK	56	M	RE	0.9/0.9	− 36/0	PILO	–
9	ST	66	F	RE	0.5/1.0	− 22/− 2	TRAB	–
10	JB	56	F	RE	0.9/1.0	− 15/0	TIM	TIM
11	SW	58	M	RE	0.7/1.0	− 15/3	TIM	–

The patients are arranged according to the degree of defect in the 30° visual field.
RE = right eye, LE = left eye, HM = Hand movements, TRAB = Trabeculectomy, PILO = Pilocarpine treatment, TIM = Topical timolol treatment.

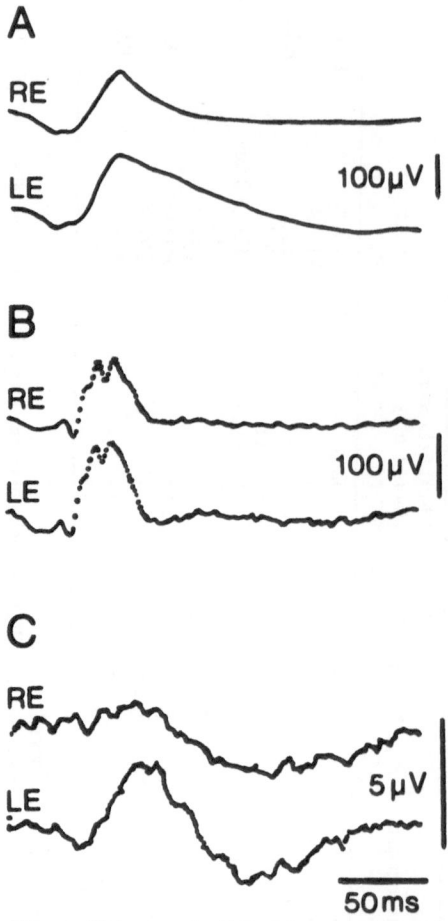

Fig. 2. Flash ERGs (A), oscillatory potentials (B) and pattern-reversal ERGs (C) from the same patient (no. 6). RE = right glaucomatous eye. LE = left eye.

surgical treatment. 6 glaucomatous eyes had been subjected to trabeculec-tomy, but none of the opposite eyes. 5 glaucomatous eyes and 4 opposite eyes were on topical treatment with eye drops.

Figure 2 shows the unpatterned flash ERG, OP and pattern-reversal ERG from the patient, whose visual fields have been presented. Note the reduced amplitude in the pattern-reversal ERG from the right, glaucomatous eye compared to the opposite eye. Flash ERGs and OPs from both eyes were identical.

There was a statistically significant difference in the mean amplitude of the pattern-reversal ERGs from glaucomatous ($1.1 \pm 0.6\,\mu$V) and opposite eyes ($2.7 \pm 0.9\,\mu$V, see Table 2). No such difference was observed regarding the a- and b-waves of the flash ERG and the OPs.

The mean amplitudes from both the surgically and the medically treated glaucomatous eyes were significantly lower than corresponding amplitudes

Table II. Mean amplitudes of the pattern-reversal and flash ERGs.

	GLAUCOMATOUS EYE (n = 11; mean ± SD μV)	OPPOSITE EYE (n = 11; mean ± SD μV)
PATTERN-REVERSAL ERG		
Peak-to-peak amplitude	1.1 ± 0.6	2.7 ± 0.9
FLASH ERG		
a-wave amplitude	32 ± 15	34 ± 11
b-wave amplitude	125 ± 52	135 ± 63

from the opposite eyes. Thus, the performed surgery can not explain the reduction in the pattern-reversal amplitude from the glaucomatous eyes. Comparing clinical and electrophysiological data a statistically significant correlation was observed between the degree of glaucomatous damage, as expressed by the visual field score, and the reduction in the pattern-reversal ERG amplitude. No correlations were noted between age or visual acuity and electrophysiological findings.

DISCUSSION

The present results show that the pattern-reversal ERGs from glaucomatous eyes were reduced in amplitude compared to those from the opposite eyes. A similar observation was reported in a recent study on the pattern-reversal ERG in one patient with glaucoma (May et al., 1982) and also mentioned in a study of patients with diseases of the peripheral visual pathways (Fiorentini et al., 1981).

The pattern-reversal ERG is likely to be influenced by factors such as age, pupil size, refractive errors, opacities of ocular media and treatment. In the present study, all patients had unilateral glaucoma and the opposite eye served as control. Pupil size was approximately equal in glaucomatous and opposite eyes. Refractive' errors were corrected. No patient showed optically significant cataracts or signs of other ocular disorder. Trabeculectomy had been performed in 6 glaucomatous eyes, but there was no difference between glaucomatous and opposite eyes regarding medical treatment. Thus, apart from the glaucoma, the performed surgery was the only factor which might influence the pattern-reversal ERG from the glaucomatous eyes though not from the opposite eyes. However, there was a statistically significant amplitude reduction also from unoperated glaucomatous eyes. Hence, the change in the pattern-reversal ERG is considered to be dependent on the glaucomatous damage. This view is further supported by the observation of a statistically significant correlation between the pattern-reversal ERG amplitude reduction and the visual field defect.

Histopathological studies have demonstrated that the ganglion cells and their axons are damaged in glaucoma (Apple and Rabb 1974, Sommer et al., 1977. Quigley et al., 1980, Quigley et al., 1981). The finding of reduced pattern-reversal ERG amplitudes from the glaucomatous eyes supports the view, based on recent animal experiments (Maffei and Fiorentini 1981), that this type of ERG reflects retinal ganglion cell activity. However, the pattern

ERG has been argued to be a summated local luminance response and not produced by spatial contrast stimulation (Spekreijse et al., 1973, Riemslag et al., 1983, this volume) and, hence, not generated by the ganglion cells. This supposition was not confirmed by Arden et al., 1980, who found that the timing, the response to frequency of stimulation, and other parameters of the pattern ERG were dissimilar from those produced by small changes of luminance. Indirect evidence that pattern ERG reflects ganglion cell activity is the present finding of unchanged flash ERGs and OPs in glaucomatous eyes, since these responses are considered to be generated by retinal elements other than the ganglion cells (Rodieck 1973).

ACKNOWLEDGEMENT

This study was supported by grants from the Karolinska Institute and from the Swedish Medical Research Council (No. B83–04X–06233–02).

REFERENCES

Apple, D. J. and Rabb, M. F. (1974): Clinicopathologic Correlation of Ocular Disease. CV Mosby Comp., St. Louis, U.S.A.

Arden, G. B., Vaegen, Hogg, C. R., Powell, D. J. and Carter, R. M. (1980): Pattern-ERGs are abnormal in many amblyopes. Trans. Ophthalmol. Soc. UK. 100: 453–460.

Dawson, W. W., Maida, T. M. and Rubin, M. L. (1982): Human pattern-evoked retinal response are altered by optic atrophy. Invest. Ophthalmol. Vis. Sci. 22: 796–803.

Fiorentini, A., Maffei, L., Pirchio, M., Spinelli, D. and Porciatti, V. (1981): The ERG in response to alternating gratings in patients with diseases of the peripheral visual pathway. Invest. Ophthalmol. Vis. Sci., 21: 490–493.

Maffei, L., and Fiorentini, A. (1981): Electroretinographic responses to alternating gratings before and after sectioning of the optic nerve. Science. 211: 953–955.

May, J. G., Ralston, J. V., Reed, B. S. and van Dyck, H. J. L. (1982): Loss of pattern-elicited electroretinograms in optic nerve dysfunction. Amer. J. Ophthal. 93: 418–422.

Persson, H. E., and Wanger, P. (1982): Pattern-reversal electroretinograms in squint amblyopia, artificial anisometropia and simulated eccentric fixation. Acta. Ophthal. 60: 123–132.

Wanger, P., and Persson, H. E. (1983): Pattern-reversal electroretinograms in unilateral glaucoma. Invest. Ophthalmol. Vis. Sci. (in press).

Persson, H. E. and Wanger, P. (1983). Pattern-reversal electroretinograms in squint amblyopia, artificial anisometropia and simulated eccentric fixation. Doc. Ophthal. Proc. of the XXth ISCEV symposium, Iowa, U.S.A., (this volume).

Riemslag, F. C. C., Ringo, J., Spekreijse, H. and Verduyn Lunel, H. F. E. (1983): The distinction between luminance and spatial components in the pattern ERG. Doc. Ophthal. Proc. of the XXth ISCEV symposium, Iowa, U.S.A. (this volume).

Rodieck, R. W. (1973): The Vertebrate Retina. Principles of structure and function. W. H. Freeman and Comp., San Francisco, U.S.A.

Sommer, A., Miller, N. R., Pollack, I. P., Maumenee, A. E. and George, T. (1977): the nerve fiber layer in the diagnosis of glaucoma. Arch. Ophthalmol. 95: 2149–2156.

Spekreijse, H., Estevez, O. and van der Tweel (1973): Luminance responses to pattern reversal. Doc. Ophthal. Proc. of the Xth ISCERG symposium. 2: 205–212.

Quigley, H. A., Miller, N. R., and George, T. (1980): Clinical evaluation of nerve fiber layer atrophy as an indicator of glaucomatous optic nerve damage. Arch. Ophthalmol. 98: 1564–1571.

Quigley, H. A., Addicks, E. M., Green, W. R. and Maumenee, A. E. (1981): Optic nerve damage in human glaucoma II. The site of injury and susceptibility to damage. Arch. Ophthalmol. 99: 635–649.

Wachtmeister, L. (1972): On the oscillatory potentials of the human electroretinogram in light and dark adaptation. Acta Ophthalmol. Suppl. 116.

Mailing address:
Departments of Ophthalmology and Clinical Neurophysiology
Karolinska Hospital
S-104 01 Stockholm
Sweden

RETROLENTAL FIBROPLASIA AND ERG

J. FRANÇOIS AND A. DE ROUCK
(Ghent, Belgium)

ABSTRACT

From the prognostic point of view, an electroretinogram is important in retrolental fibroplasia. Of the 98 personally examined cases in the last years, 65 (66%) had an extinguished ERG and belonged to the cicatricial stage grade IV or V. Thirty-two cases (34%) had some ERG response in one or both eyes (55 eyes). It may be predicted that a case with extinguished ERG has a poor prognosis and that vitrectomy with retinal attachment will not improve the function.

Reports on ERG examinations in retrolental fibroplasia (RLF) are very rare. As far as we know, only Nagata (1977) mentions that even in early stages, the potential amplitudes of the ERG are markedly subnormal and the temporal characteristics of the responses severely modified as a result of the diffuse retinal involvement. In evolved stages, the ERG is extinguished.

To classify our own cases, we used the classification of Patz and Payne (1976).

Active stages. – Stage 1A or pre RLF consists in a vasoconstriction of the retinal vessels.

Stage I or early peripheral vasoproliferative stage. – In the periphery and especially temporally, there are areas of neovascularization at the junction of the vascularized retina and the more anterior avascular zone. Moreover, at the periphery, frequently small yellowish globular bodies are seen on the retinal surface extending into the vitreous (proliferating endothelial cells).

Stage II with peripheral proliferative and posterior vascular changes, retinal hemorrhages and tortuosity of the vessels.

Stage III with further proliferation, vitreoretinal traction and vitreal hemorrhage.

Stage IV with advanced proliferation and moderate retinal detachment.

Stage V with advanced retinal detachment and proliferation.

Cicatricial stages. – Spontaneous regression may occur at any of the active stages and takes place in more or less 80% of those infants in stage I. The rate of regression decreases as the stages advance, so that stages IV and V always leave significant residue. The majority of the different phases of RLF, with the exception of grade IV and V of the cicatricial stage, are not

Table 1. Relation stage of RLF/ERG

		Cicatricial stages				Total	
		Stage 1	Stage II		Stage III	Stage IV and V	number	%
			a	b				
ERG	1	13	5	2			20	10
	2	2	10	1	5		18	9
	3		2		17		19	10
	4	1		2	5	131	139	70
Total		16(8%)	22(11%)		27(14%)	132(67%)	196	

blinding. In grade IV and V, the spontaneous regression consists only in the cessation of neovascular development and the residual abnormal fibrovascular tissue would undergo only slight atrophy. That which remains would shrink like any healing scar, causing varying degrees of retinal distortion. When the scarring involves macular distortion, the vision is poorer.

Stage I. There are only minor changes. Small areas of irregular retinal pigmentation, vitreoretinal membranes, mostly in the temporal periphery and high myopia ($> -$ 6 D) are observed.

Stage II. Disc distortion with vessels pulled to the temporal side and a small mass of opaque tissue is found. The macular is displaced temporally. We divided this group into two stages: stage IIa shows typical vascular anomalies, while stage IIb displays a diffuse retinal degenerative change.

Stage III. A retinal fold extends to a mass of opaque tissue in the temporal periphery. Retinal vessels appear to be torn-out of the nasal retina and are incorporated in the fold.

Stage IV. Incomplete retrolental mass (detached retina).

Stage V. Complete retrolental mass.

We examined electroretinographically 98 cases (196 eyes) of RLF in the cicatricial stage, the age of the children varying from 5 months to 10 years. There were 38 females (39%) and 60 males (61%). Among them we found 7 pairs of twins (7%), which is significantly higher than in the general population and demonstrates that multiple births constitute a risk factor for RLF. There is rather often a difference between the two members of a pair of twins. One may present only with a RLF of grade II, for instance, and the other with a RLF of grade V.

We first studied the relation between the stage of RLF and the ERG. As is shown by Table I, an extinguished ERG is always seen in stages IV and V, whereas the ERG is only subnormal in stages II and III and even normal in stage I.

ERG 1 (Figure 1): the amplitudes are within normal limits, when the age of the child and the conditions of examination (general anesthesia) are taken into account. The oscillating potentials may be present or not.

ERG 2: the latencies are within normal limits; the saturation amplitudes of the b-wave is higher than $150\,\mu V$.

ERG 3: the saturation amplitude of the b-wave is below $150\,\mu V$, but above $25\,\mu V$.

288

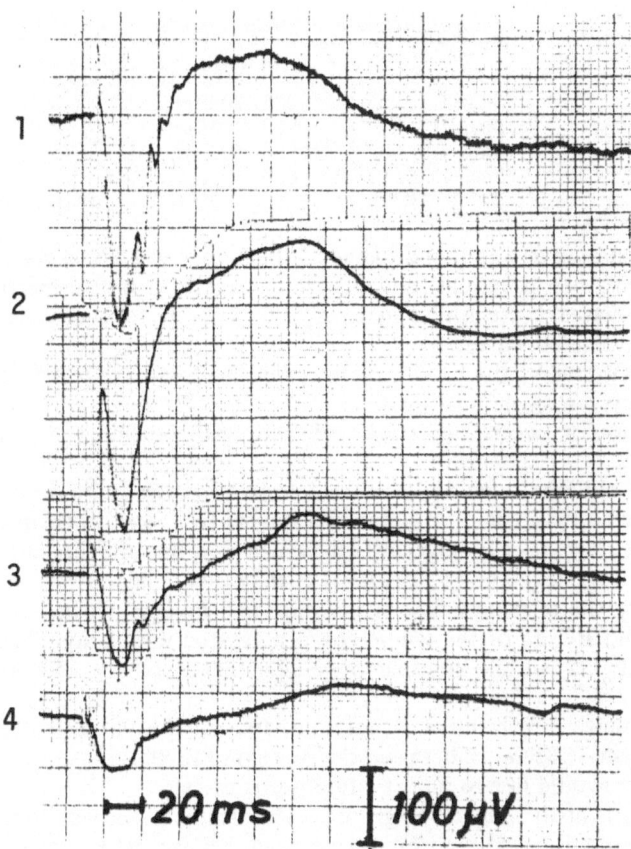

Fig. 1. Xenon stimulation 40 Joules. Four different types of response, (1) normal, (2) normal amplitude, but oscillatory potential absent, (3) reduced amplitude and (4) evolution towards extinction.

ERG 4: residual responses (less than $25\,\mu$V) or extinguished ERG.

Stage IIa shows typical vascular anomalies, while stage IIb displays diffuse retinal degenerative changes.

In stage I, the ERG is usually normal or only slightly subnormal. In 3 cases the birth weight was normal. The differential diagnosis should be made between RLF and exsudative retinopathy. In one case, however, the ERG appeared to be completely extinguished. The oscillatory potentials are mostly present, although they may be absent.

In stage II, a normal ERG can still be found and the oscillatory potentials may still be present even when there are vascular anomalies. An extinguished ERG was nevertheless found in 2 eyes with a type b retinopathy.

In stage III, no normal ERG's were found. Usually, they were markedly subnormal or even extinguished. The amplitude reduction involved all components. The b-wave was, however, more affected than the a-wave. In one

Table II. Relation Stage/Birth weight

	Birth weight
Stage I	860–3000 gr
Stage II	900–2030 gr
Stage III	1000–2020 gr
Stage IV or V	850–3000 gr

case, a normal a-wave was found, whereas the b-wave was markedly reduced. The late oscillatory potentials and off-effects remained well preserved. Off-responses (d-waves) were found in cases with severely reduced a-waves and nearly extinguished b-waves.

In stages IV and V, the ERG was always extinguished. No responses could be obtained even with summation.

The relation between the stage and the birth weight is not obvious (Table II).

We saw 3 children, who had a normal gestational age and a normal birth weight, but who nevertheless developed a typical RLF. One of them received oxygen (RE, stage II, LE stage IV), the other two not (RE and LE of one child stage V, RE stage I and LE stage III in the other child).

Concerning the relation between the stage and myopia, we had 65 eyes in stages I, II and III: 21 of the whole group presented with a myopia of more than -5 D and 2 with a myopia of -2 D, that is to say 35% displayed myopia.

An asymmetric involvement is not rare. Among the 98 cases, 19 (19%) showed a marked difference between the two eyes (Table III).

Finally, we should like to report 4 interesting cases:

Case I (Gr.): birth weight 860 gr, one twin brother died, was 2 months in incubator, normal psycho-motor development, R.E.: RLF stage V with extinguished ERG, but L.E.: RLF stage I with normal ERG and without myopia.

Case II (G.E.): birth weight 1700 gr, was 2 weeks in incubator. RLF stage II (diffuse dystrophy of the retina with pigment clumps and small atrophic spots, atropic focus at the macula, disc and retinal vessels normal), ERG normal.

Case III (C.S.): birth weight 900 gr, was 4 months in incubator. R.E.: stage II (diffuse dystrophy with depigmented areas), extinguished ERG. L.E.: stage I (albinoid fundus) extinguished ERG.

Case IV (V.P.): birth weight 800 gr, was 2 months in incubator. R.E.: stage III, very subnormal ERG, but normal off-effect.

CONCLUSION AND SUMMARY

From the prognostic point of view, an electroretinogram is important in retrolental fibroplasia. With only 8 exceptions, all the positive ERG's (57) belonged to the cicatricial stages I, II or III. On the other hand, the more preserved the ERG, the milder the retinopathy. It may be predicted that a

Table III. Asymmetric Involvement

one eye	fellow eye	No. of cases
stage I	stage II	5
stage I	stage III	3
stage I	stage V	2
stage II	stage IV or V	5
stage III	stage V	4

case with extinguished ERG has a poor prognosis and that a vitrectomy with retinal reattachment will give no functional improvement. Cases with a recordable ERG will have some and perhaps good vision even without any intraocular operation.

REFERENCES

Francois, J.: Risk factors in retrolental fibroplasia. Presented at the Club Gonin Meeting, Cordoba (Argentina), 31st March, 1982.
Nagata, M.: Treatment of acute proliferative retrolental fibroplasia with xenon-arc photocoagulation. Jap. J. Ophthalmol., 21, 436–459, 1977.
Patz, A. and Payne, J. W.: Retrolental fibroplasia. In: Clinical Ophthalmology (Th. D. Duane, ed.), Harper and Row, Vol. 3, Chapter 20, 1976.

Mailing address:
University of Ghent
Place de Smet De Nayer 15
B-8700 Ghent, Belgium

ON THE RECOVERY OF THE ELECTRORETINOGRAM OF INTRAVITREAL IRON PARTICLES

J. G. H. SCHMIDT AND M. S. J. WASSERSCHAFF

(Cologne, West Germany)

ABSTRACT

Based on clinical findings and animal experiments, the recovery of the ERG after extraction of intravitreal iron wires is reported. The following results are emphasized:
(1) Under the given experimental conditions, it appears that after the removal of iron splinters a recovery from the metal toxicity takes place, however, to a very limited degree only.
(2) Spontaneous arrest of the metallosis can occur.
(3) Experiments with equally-sized glass splinters show that the penetration of the foreign body alone or the manipulation during its removal can influence the a- and b-wave amplitudes significantly. These changes are reversible as long as the tissue damage is limited.
(4) The relevance of the electroretinographic findings and the influence of other prognostic factors are discussed.

INTRODUCTION

The primary aim of the operative removal of metallic foreign bodies is the avoidance of the progression of the metallosis. Only in special cases is the operative procedure on eyes with retained intraocular particles restriced to repairing the mechanical damage without removal of the splinter. This is the case with very small or inert materials and when encapsulation makes particles difficult to access. Furthermore, removal of the metal splinter should reverse the metallosis. On the basis of animal experiments we intend to answer the question whether or not we can expect a recovery of the ERG after removal of intravitreal iron wires. It appears that our results are not only affected by the metal toxicity but also to a considerable degree by the surgical trauma and other factors.

METHODS

Albino rats (Wistar), ranging in weight between 150 and 240 grams, were anesthetized with Halothan 'Hoechst': $O_2 : N_2O$ as 2 to 3 l/min containing

3.7% Halothan at the beginning. O_2 :N_2O as 0.4 to 0.8 l/min containing 2.0% Halothan during the following 20—30 min. Iron wire was obtained from Koch & Light Laboratories Ltd., Colnbrook, Bucks, England, Nr. 8954—00. Contaminations (ppm): Cu less than 1; Mg 1; Mn 2; Ni 5; Si 2; Ag less than 1. The wire was implanted near the ciliary body far enough into the vitreous body so that a surface of 1.3 mm^2 was exposed. A loop on the end of the wire enabled us to extract the splinter later without much manipulation. The loop was covered by conjunctiva which was closed with a suture. The ERG was recorded by placing one electrode into the lid, another one into the skin between the ears and a cotton electrode on the cornea. The fast components of the ERG were recorded with a push-pull amplifier (Dr. Ing.J.F. Tönnies, 78 Freiburg/Breisgau, FRG) Nr. 0—353 having a time constant of 2 seconds and photographed from the oscilloscope. The light source was a set of fluorescent tubes (Osram-L 20 W 15) which produced an intensity of up to 1600 Lux at the cornea. The flash duration was 5 msec.

RESULTS

(A) Clinical findings.

34 year old man — While hammering a metal ring on March 16, 1978 a 2 mm long foreign body perforated the cornea of the right eye and penetrated into the retina close to the optic disc and the macula. This caused a preretinal hemorrhage and a sector-like visual field loss. Visual acuity was OD 0.1, OS 0.9 — laser coagulation of this area. The corneal laceration was self sealing. ERG (March 29, 1978) showed OD minimal amplitudes; OS normal a- and b-wave amplitudes. EOG: L/D ratio OD pathological; OS normal. August 11, 1978. Partial absorption of hemorrage. Visual acuity OD 0.6. ERG: normal a- and b-waves OU. September 2, 1982. ERG: normal a- and b-waves OU. EOG: L/D ratio normal OU. However, the absolute values of the injured eye were still lower (OD: 150/75 mV; OS 325/150 mV). No improvement of the visual field loss. Foreigh body covered by scar tissue.

(B) Animal Experiments.

(i) Intact fellow eyes. The a- and b-wave amplitudes of the intact eyes are given as average values of 3 groups with 15 rats each in Figure 1. The amplitudes are constant for the first 3 weeks of observation. Thereafter the amplitudes decrease slightly.

(ii) The effect of the mechanical trauma on the ERG. One day after the implantation of a glass peg, the same size as the iron wires, a- and b-wave amplitudes decreased to 74% and 76% respectively compared to the intact eye. Within 10 days a recovery to 90% and 87% respectively occurred. The foreign body extraction caused a second amplitude decrease to 72% and 70% respectively. A fast recovery in the next two weeks and a slow increase in the subsequent month followed. After 150 days the a-wave amplitude reached 100% and the b-wave 90% of the initial value.

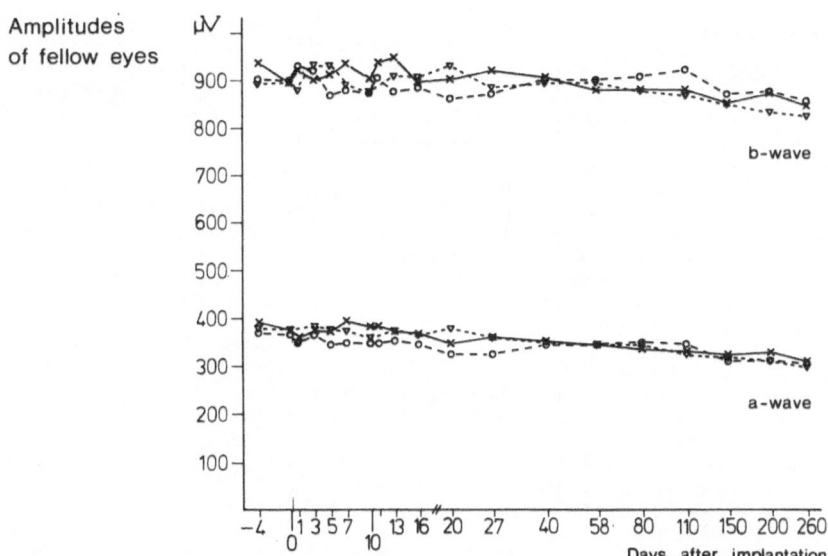

Fig. 1. ERG amplitudes of normal eyes of rats.

(iii) The effect of the metallosis on the ERG. After implantation of an iron wire into the vitreous body, the amplitudes of the a- and b-wave decrease to 33% respectively within 24 hrs (Figure 2a and b). This loss of approximately 70% of the initial activity includes the sum of the traumatic and metal-toxic damages. The extent of this total damage does not change during the following 10 days. The absence of recovery during this period, such as in cases of glass particles, indicates progression of the metallosis within these 10 days. One day after the extraction of the iron wire we found a further a- and b-wave decline. After the considerable amplitude changes due to implantation and extraction of the foreign bodies, the amplitudes change only slightly later. It has to be noticed that a- and b-wave amplitudes of eyes from which the iron has been removed are only slightly higher than those of eyes remaining further exposed to iron. The difference amounts to 4%–8% for the a-wave and to 2%–5% for the b-wave, depending on the time of observation (Figure 3).

DISCUSSION

Our findings in cases of intraocular foreign bodies elucidate the rationale for therapeutic procedures. The clinical assessment is already complicated by the difficulty of estimating the effects of the particular factors that determine the degree of the metallosis (Schmidt, Stute & Weber 1972; Schmidt, Mićović & Stute 1977). Furthermore, mechanical trauma, hemorrhages with their chemical implications and other factors are to be included in our considerations. Besides, it is possible that our therapeutic interventions lead to a

295

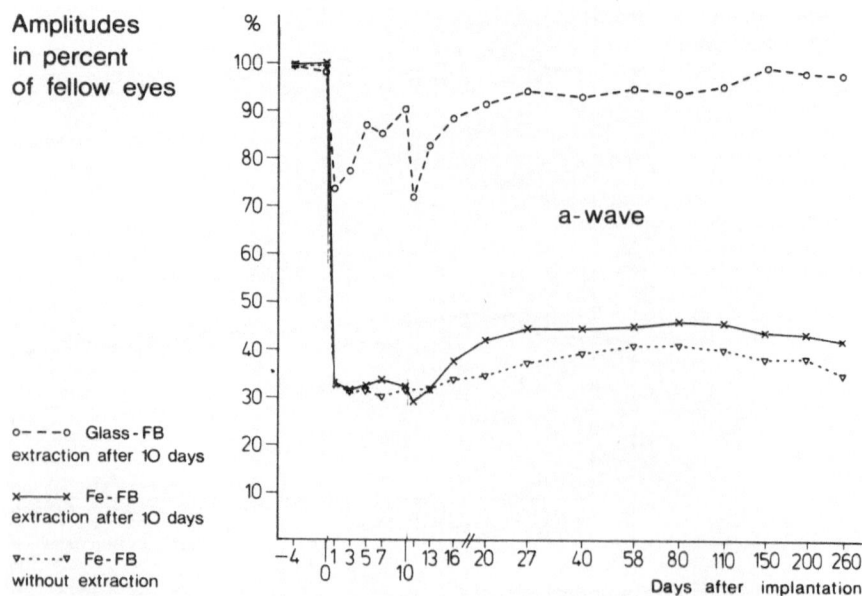

Fig. 2a. ERG a-wave from rat eyes following implantation of a glass splinter or an iron foreign body with and without surgical removal.

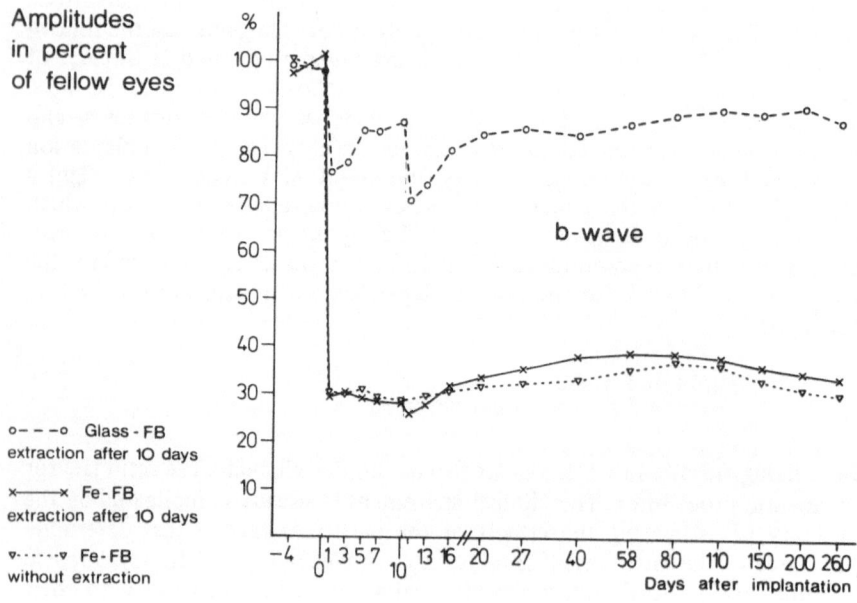

Fig. 2b. ERG b-wave from rat eyes following implantation of a glass splinter or an iron foreign body with and without surgical removal.

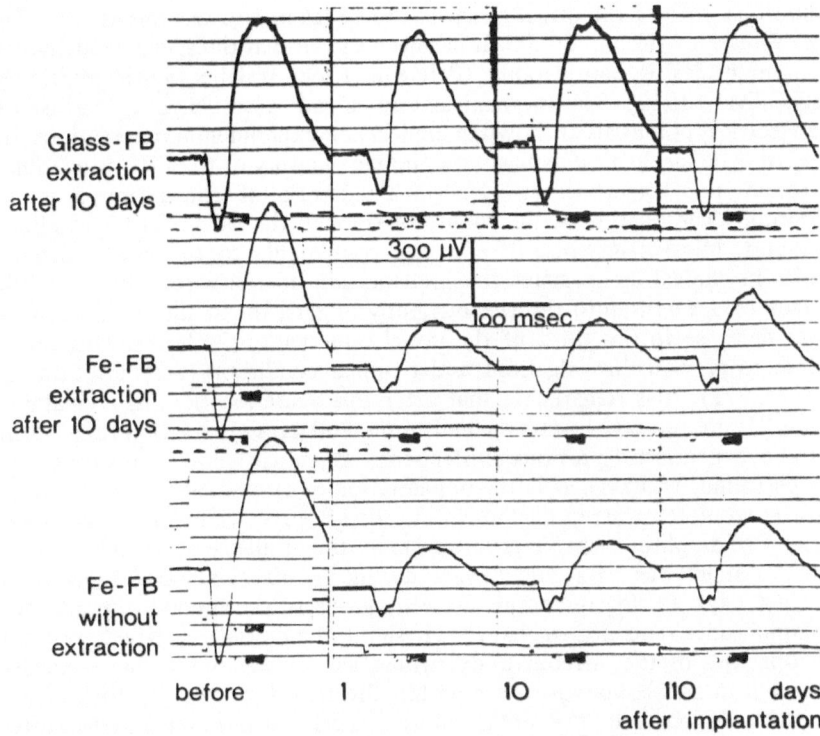

Fig. 3. Original ERG tracing before and after extraction of an intraocular foreign body.

change of the condition. Light- and laser coagulations close to the foreign body can cause a decrease of oxygen tension in the adjacent tissue and thereby a reduction of ionization of the metal. Encapsulation can have the same effect.

Because of the multiplicity of the damage-factors and their variability, no quantitative assessment can be made, despite extensive clinical studies. Therefore, animal experiments were performed in order to make a statement about the recovery from mechanical damage and from metal toxicity.

For the valuation of electrophysiological findings, often the potential of the affected eye is brought in relation with the data of the intact eye. Summarizing the average values of the 3 groups of fellow eyes (Figure 1), a constant potential is shown within the first 3 weeks. Thereafter, the potentials decline slightly. When representing the time in log units the decrease in amplitude is linear. An influence of anesthesia is not likely, since no significant decline was observed during 10 anesthesias over a short time. A decrease appeared only during the following anesthesias which were taken in increasingly longer intervals. Also, including previous results (Stute, Schmidt & Weber 1977), we may proceed on in the assumption that halothan[R] influences the electroretinographical potentials only negligibly under our test conditions. Instead the effect of age has to be taken into account as cause for the decrease of the amplitudes. It has been shown that the age-dependence of the amplitudes is considerable (Peterson 1968; Weleber 1981; Martin & Heckenlively 1982). The mechanical trauma can cause a drastic decrease of the electrical potentials as shown in clinical and experimental observations. In cases of little mechanical damage, a complete recovery of the ERG is possible.

Under our experimental conditions siderosis of the retina is most important. The relation of the splinter surface to the weight of the eye bulb (Schmidt, Mićović & Stute 1977), was comparable to the largest foreign bodies in clinical cases. After the implantation of iron wires with an active surface of $1.3\,mm^2$ into the vitreous body of rats, the a- and b-wave amplitudes decrease to one-third of the initial value within 24 hours. This corresponds to previous investigations under similar conditions (Schmidt, Stute & Weber 1971). It is remarkable that after this acute reaction, the remaining potentials are preserved until the end of the 260 days observation time. As in our above-mentioned previous experiments, a gradual recovery of about 10% can be found. Likewise, after the implantation of other metal wires of similar surface, we noted a steep decline within 2 to 3 days, while later only minor changes of amplitude were registered. Under the influence of intravitreal lead particles there was an a- and b-wave decline to 30% and 40% respectively within 4 days. During the entire succeeding observation period of 6 months, the amplitudes remained unchanged. It should be considered whether or not the opacities of the vitreous body, which we can see ophthalmoscopically around iron and copper particles within the first 1 or 2 days, stop further spreading of ions into the retina. Those opacities were never observed after implantation of lead splinters. Copper wires, on the other hand, caused a total ERG extinction within 24 hours despite intensive opacities.

Thus, the question arises whether the generators for the ERG potentials have a different susceptibility to different metals. Previous experiments have shown that e.g. the scotopic and photopic potentials can be damaged to various degrees by the same foreign body (Schmidt 1977). Only a few data are published about the recovery of the ERG after removal of intraocular metal particles. In 1975 we reported in Sarasota about our findings regarding copper splinters. We found that the recovery of the ERG of rats is more complete the sooner the extraction is performed. Declercq and Meredith have shown, in experimental siderosis in the rabbit, that removal of the foreign body does not improve the ERG nor prevent its further deterioration.

From these results a series of conclusions can be derived for our clinical situations. The electroretinography as an objective method has a particular value, especially in the comparatively frequent cases of children with non-magnetic intraocular foreign bodies. Electrodiagnostic findings have to be used in connection with the other tests of retinal function.

ACKNOWLEDGEMENT

We are grateful to Mrs. Doris Hartkopf and Miss Angela Peters for their technical assistance.

298

REFERENCES

Declercq, S. S. & P. C. A. Meredith: Electrophysiology in experimental siderosis: a follow-up study after removal of intraocular foreign body. Doc. Ophthal. Proc. Ser. 15th I.S.C.E.V. symposium, Ghent, 1977, 69–72.

Martin, D. A. & J. R. Heckenlively. The normal electroretinogram. Doc. Ophtal. Proc. Ser. 31. Dr. W. Junk Publ., The Hague 1982, 135–144.

Peterson, H.: The normal b-Potential in the single-flash clinical Electroretinogram. Acta. Ophthalmologica, Suppl. 99, Copenhagen 1968.

Schmidt, J. G. H., A. Stute & E. Weber.: Elektroretinographische und ophthalmoskopische Befunde bei intraocularen Metallfremdkörpern der Ratte. Ber. Dtsch. Ophthal. Ges. (Heidelberg) 71, 391–396 (1971).

Schmidt, J. G. H. & A. Stute.: Electroretinogram and ophthalmoscopic findings in intravitreous iron, copper and lead particles. Doc. Ophthal. Proc. Ser. Xth I.S.C.E.R.G. Symposium, Los Angeles. Dr. W. Junk Publ., The Hague 1973, 85–90.

Schmidt, J. G. H., V. Mićović & A. Stute.: Surface area sizes of intravitreal copper particles: their effects on the ERG of rabbits and rats. Doc. Ophthal. Proc. Ser. Vol. 15, 63–67. Dr. W. Junk Publ., The Hague, 1977.

Schmidt, J. G. H.: Metallosis retinae – Pathophysiologie und Klinik. Ber. Dtsch. Ophthal. Ges. (Heidelberg) 75, 670–674 (1977).

Stute, A., J. G. H. Schmidt & E. Weber.' On the effect of urethane and Halothane[®] on the ERG of rats. Doc. Ophthal. Proc. Ser. Vol. 15, 13–19. Dr. W. Junk Publ., The Hague, 1977.

Weleber, R. G.: The effect of age on human cone and rod ganzfeld electroretinograms. Invest. Ophtal. 80, 392–399 (1981).

Mailing address:
Univ.–Augenklinik
D-5000 Köln 41, F.R.G.

ELECTROPHYSIOLOGICAL AND CLINICAL FINDINGS AFTER ACUTE CHLOROQUINE POISONING

J. G. H. SCHMIDT, W. BÖTTCHER AND G. HEINMANN

(Cologne, West Germany)

ABSTRACT

The report deals with medical and ophthalmological findings of a sixteen-year-old girl, who had taken 50 tablets Resochin$^{(R)}$ (7.5 g chloroquine base) with the intention to commit suicide. The shock symptoms and the asystole beginning at the end of the first hour after ingestion were treated with gastric lavages, resuscitation and plasmapheresis. After that a pronounced decrease of the chloroquine level in the blood serum was measured. On the 4th and the 26th day after intoxication no morphological or functional ocular changes were observed. The ERG and both the absolute and relative values of the EOG were normal.

INTRODUCTION

Since the introduction of chloroquine in 1946 this pharmacological agent has been applied on a large scale predominantly in cases of rheumatoid arthritis, various kinds of skin diseases as well as for prophylaxis and therapy of malaria. For the treatment of all these diseases it has proved to be the most effective drug. During long term treatment peculiar opacities in the corneal epithelium have repeatedly been noticed, which, however, spontaneously cleared within several months after discontinuing the drug. From a prognostic point of view the side effects on the pigment epithelium and the retina are much more serious and similar to retinitis pigmentosa. These effects can be detected by means of the electroretinogram (ERG) and the electrooculogram (EOG).

In contrast to the known side effects during long term treatment a few reports concern acute chloroquine intoxications. We report on a sixteen-year-old girl who took 7.5 g of chloroquine base with the intention to commit suicide.

RESULTS

Medical findings are listed in Figure 1.

About 40 minutes after taking 50 tables of Resochin$^{(R)}$ (7.5 g chloroquine

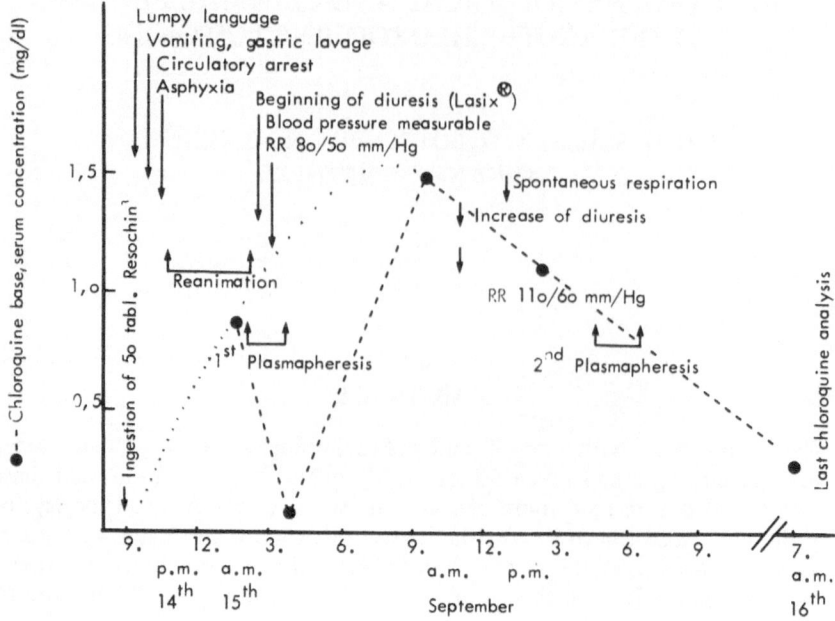

Fig. 1. Time course of the symptoms and therapeutic procedures following ingestion of
7.5 g of chloroquine

base) the patient was admitted to the Vincenz-Palotti-Hospital in 5060
Bergisch-Gladbach 1 (West Germany). At the time of admission the patient
showed slurred speech and vomited twice spontaneously. Sixty minutes
after taking the tablets respiratory arrest and a fall in blood pressure
occurred. Immediate steps were initiated for resuscitation (extracorporal
heart massage, intubation and artificial respiration). Catecholamines
(Dubutrex[R], Dopamin[R], alkalizing measures (Tutofusin[R], Tris[R]),
and gastric lavages were continued for more than four hours; however,
the blood pressure could not be registered. The heart rate remained regular
and the EKG did not show enlarged QRS-complexes, only marked disorders
in repolarization. During resuscitation 2.5 l of electrolytic solution were
infused; however, no diuresis was observed. Five hours after the ingestion
of the drug a plasmapheresis was started while resuscitation efforts continued. The haemoprocessor by Fresenius, D-638 Bad Homburg v.d.H., and
a plasmaseparator with the model designation 'plasma-flow H I 05' by Asahi
were used. At the end of the first plasmapheresis the blood pressure was
measurable for the first time, diuresis began and the patient was breathing
spontaneously and awoke. For a second treatment with plasmapheresis the
patient was transferred to the 1. Medical Clinic of the Municipal Hospital in
Köln-Merheim. After a few days here cerebral functions had normalized.
Chloroquine in blood and eluate was determined by Clarke's method.

302

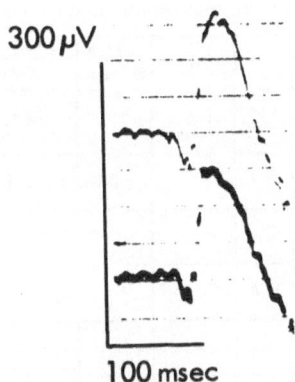

300 μV

100 msec

Fig. 2. ERG four days after Resochin[R] intoxication. Heavy line right eye, thin line left eye. 1600 lux at the cornea, flush duration 1 msec.

OPHTHALMOLOGICAL FINDINGS

Fourth day after intoxication (18 Sept. 1981). Patient is not yet capable of full cooperation.
Visual acuity OD: 0.4, glasses do not improve
OS: 0.3 with − 1.0 sph = 0.5
ERG: bilaterally scotopically normal (Figure 2).
Slit lamp and fundus findings normal

Twenty-second day after intoxication. Full cooperation of patient.
Visual acuity OU: 1.0
Color sense:
  1. Ishihara plates (24 plates, 1973): both left and right correctly identified
  2. 28 Hue de Roth-test according to Farnsworth-Munsell: No error OU
  3. Nagel anomaloscope (model 1)
      (a) normal equation: orange/orange
      (b) extreme equation: Lithium 0: green/brown
                              Lithium 73: red/orange
      (c) Rayleigh equation: OD 0.85−1.0; OS 0.89−0.95
Visual fields (Goldmann Perimeter): bilaterally full to I:2, I:3 and I:4 isopters OU
ERG: Scotopically and photopically normal OU
EOG: Absolute and relative values normal OU
Slit lamp and fundus findings normal OU

DISCUSSSION

Toxic doses of chloroquine induce − approximately 30 minutes after oral intake − shock, confusion, unconsciousness, and convulsions. In severe cases respiratory arrest and cardiac asystole occur within the first two hours. Apart

303

Table 1. Published tissue levels of chloroquine in man. chloroquine base mg/100 g.

	Prouty & Kuroda		Irey	Kiel	Klug & Schneider	Robinson et al		Sarvesvaran		Ifftsits-Simon			
	8 Non Suicides	2 Suicides	Mean Values 15 Pat.	12 Suicides		Case 1	2	Case 1 - 2		Case 1	2	3	4
Blood periph.			4,7		2,0	1,6	1,2	6,6	4,5	2,4		5,1	3,1
Liver blood						9,0	4,4	5,1	12,5				
Liver	0,43-4,8	90,0	30,8	20,0-75,0	43	17,5	34,4			23	28	14	
Kidneys	0,06-0,6	47,0	20,6	11,0-64,0		7,0	30,0	86,4		16	18	3	16
Heart	0,41-2,0	8,4		4,0		5,7							
Brain	0,07-0,7	1,1	1,1							4,2	1,1	0,1	2,4

from convulsions all these symptoms were found in the case described. Different doses were reported for chloroquine being lethal or survivable (N. S. Irey, 1974). Two hundred fifty mg of Resochin[R] (chloroquindi-phosphate) are equivalent to 150 mg of effective chloroquine base. Tabbara (1962) considered 1−1.5 g and Larribaud et al., (1961) 2 g to be the minimal lethal dose for adults. On the other hand, it has been reported that an adult survived 6 g of Resochin[R] and a two-year-old child recovered from a dose of 2.5 g with intensive treatment by gastric lavages and air insufflation beginning approximately 45 minutes after swallowing the tablets (Markowitz et al., 1964).

Cann and Verhust (1961) reported three other children, 14 months, two and three years old, who (when unattended) had taken approximately 1 g, 1−2 g and 3.5 g of chloroquine phosphate respectively. All patients died within 2 and $2\frac{1}{2}$ hours after swallowing the tablets, even though − besides other therapeutic measures − a gastric lavage was performed 45 and 60 minutes after taking the tablets. Considering the data above the question arose why our patient survived the ingestion of 7.5 g of chloroquine base. It can be assumed that both the vomiting and the early initiation of gastric lavage eliminated a considerable amount of the drug.

In addition, the measured concentration of chloroquine in plasma has to be taken into consideration. After therapeutic doses, the chloroquine blood level varies around 0.01 mg/dl. Concentrations higher than 1 mg/dl might lead to death (Table 1). The observed plasma drug level of 0.9 mg/dl in our patient, $4\frac{1}{2}$ hours after taking the tablets, is within the lower limits of a lethal dose indicating that a considerable amount of the drug had not been absorbed.

The following rough calculations confirm this: from the total ingested dose (7.5 g) a concentration of 125 mg/Kg bodyweight results. A plasma concentration of chloroquine between 3−3.6 mg/dl should have been obtained in blood assuming complete absorption. By only 0.9 mg/dl was measured. Furthermore the question has to be answered whether the plasma-pheresis and other factors were involved in the elimination of the drug.

Immediately after the first determination of chloroquine in plasma the pheresis was initiated. At the end of this procedure the lowest chloroquine level was determined. Diuresis began soon after treatment with Furosemide. This may have also eliminated some chloroquine. But the amount of drug eliminated cannot be high at this time considering the enormous rise of the chloroquine concentration in blood. During the following hours blood pressure and respiration returned to normal. It might be assumed that these were decisive factors for the increased chloroquine elimination. Since only small amounts of chloroquine were determined in the eluate during the second plasmapheresis the elimination via kidneys and intestine of free – not tissue bound – drug may be the most important mechanism. The last concentration of chloroquine measured on September 16th at 7 a.m. suggests a considerable back diffusion of the drug from tissue into the blood. Such a back diffusion, however, is likely while the concentration of chloroquine in the plasma decreased enormously during the first plasmapheresis. Plamapheresis may have also helped to overcome the renal shutdown. These speculations illustrate the general problem of a kinetic description and interpretation for a drug with high tissue-binding affinity using a concentration time course in blood or plasma. The concentrations can only give valid information if a distribution equilibrium of the drug in the body has taken place. For an anticonvulsive drug 1–2 weeks are necessary to reach such a distribution equilibrium. For chloroquine it should be considerably longer considering its high tissue affinity and distribution.

Prouty and Kuroda investigated people using chloroquine prophylactically for long periods. Two cases of suicide were involved in this study. The results can be compared to those of other authors (Table 1). The different data for one organ may be explained by different intervals between ingestion and the removal of tissue samples as well as by different procedures of extraction (Ifftsits-Simon, 1968). Usually liver and kidneys contain the highest levels of chloroquine. The concentrations determined in the brain are considerably lower. Bernstein et al., (1963) showed that – based on animal experiments – iris and choroid absorb significantly higher amounts of chloroquine than other tissues. For the retina as a part of the brain, however, one might assume a lower affinity for chloroquine. If the concentration in blood is high at the beginning of chloroquine therapy a toxic accumulation of the drug may not yet take place in the retina.

The research of several authors demonstrated that chloroquine influences – among other things – the composition of DNA and RNA (Schellenberg and Coatney, 1960; Allison et al., 1965; Cohen and Yielding, 1965; Allison et al., 1966) and combines with mitochondria easily (Magnussen and de Fine Olivarius, 1977). Consequently, myopathies were observed repeatedly during long treatment (Eadie and Ferrier, 1966; Ebringer, 1971; Gerard, 1973). The pronounced effect of chloroquine on the myocardium can be explained by the high concentration of mitochondria in this muscle. Alterations of the myocardium after acute chloroquine intoxications were observed only in a few sporadic cases (Sanghvi and Mathur, 1965; Don Michael and Aiwazza, 1970). Mitochondria are also plentiful in the pigment epithelium. The ophthalmological symptoms from chronic intoxications with chloroquine is similar to those of diffuse tapetoretinal dystrophies. Acute intoxications with chloroquine have so far not shown similar symptoms.

ACKNOWLEDGEMENT

We are grateful to Doris Hartkopf and Angela Peters for their technical assistance.

REFERENCES

Allison, J. L., R. L. O'Brien and F. E. Hahn. DNA: reaction with chloroquine. Science 149, 1111–1113 (1965).

Bäumler, J. und M. Lüdin. Tödliche suizidale Vergiftung mit Chloroquine. Arch. Toxikol. 20, 96–101 (1963).

Bernstein, H. N., N. J. Svaifler, M. Rubin and A. M. Mausour. The ocular deposition of chloroquine. Invest. Ophthal. Visual Sci. 2, 384–392 (1963).

Bourrelier, J., R. Lebreton. Suicide par la Nivaquine. Ann. Med. Leg. 35, 221–229 (1935).

Clarke, E. G. C. Nature, Lond. 181, 1152 (1958).

Cann, H. M. and H. L. Verhulst. Fatal acute chloroquine poisoning in children. Pediatrics 27, 95–102 (1961).

Cohen, S. N. and K. L. Yielding. Inhibition of DNA and RNA polymerase reaktions by chloroquine. Prac. Natl. Acad. Sci. USA 54, 521–527 (1965).

Don Michael, T. A. and Aiwazzadeh, S.: The effects of acute chloroquine poisoning with special reference to the heart. Am. Heart J. 79, 831–842 (1970).

Eadie, M. J. and T. M. Ferrier. Chlorquine myopathy. J. Neurolog. Neurosurg. Psychiatry 29, 331–336 (1966).

Ebringer, A., Chloroquine myopathy. Brit. Med. J. 2, 770–774 (1971).

Gerard, J. M., N. Stoupel, A. Collier and J. Flament-Durand. Morphologic study of a neuromyopathy caused by prolonged chloroquine treatment. Eur. Neurol. 9, 363–368 (1973).

Good, M. I. and R. I. Shader. Behavioral Toxicity and Equivocal Suicide Associated with Chloroquine and Its Derivatives. Am. J. Psychiatry 143, 798–801 (1977).

Iffsits-Simon, C., Fatal suicidal Chloroquine Poisonings. Arch. Toxikol. 23, 204–208 (1968).

Irey, N. S., Blood and Tissue concentrations of Drugs Associated with Fatalities. Med. Clin. North Amer. 58, 1093–1102 (1974).

Kiel, F. W., Chloroquine Suicide. JAMA 26, 398–400 (1964).

Klug, E. and V. Schneider. Tödliche Vergiftung durch Chloroquin. Arch. Toxikol. 26, 176–178 (1970).

Larribaud, J., P. Colonna, M. Chevrel, J. Romani, J. Roux, A. Pidoux, R. Renouf, R.-Y. Levebre. Intoxication aigue par la Chloroquine absorbée par voie orale. A propos de deux observations. Presse Med. 69, 2193–2196 (1961).

Magnussen, I. and B. de Fine Olivarius. Cardiomyopathy after chloroquine treatment. Acta Med. Scand. 202, 429–431 (1977).

Markowitz, H. A. and J. M. McGinley. Chloroquine Poisoning in a child. JAMA 26, 950–951, (1964).

Prouty, R. W. and K. Kuroda. Spectrophotometric Determination and Distribution of Chloroquine in Human Tissues. J. Lab. Clin. Med. 477–480 (1958).

Robinson, A. E., A. I. Coffer and F. E. Camos. The distribution of chloroquine in man after fatal poisoning. J. Pharm. Pharmac. 22, 701–703 (1970).

Sarvesvaran, R., Chloroquine Poisoning: Two Fatal Cases, Med. Sci. Law 19, 265–267, (1979).

306

Sanghri, L. and B. B. Mathur. Electrocardiogram after chloroquine and emetine. Circulation 32, 281–285 (1965).

Schentag, J. J., W. J. Jusko, J. W. Vance, T. J. Cumbo, E. Abrutyn, M. DeLattre and L. M. Gerbracht. Gentamicin Disposition and Tissue Accumulation on Multiple Dosing. J. Pharmacokinetics and Biopharmac. 5, 559–577 (1977).

Tabbara, W., J. Proteau, R. Le Breton L. Dérobert. Trois intoxications mortelles par la nivaquine dues à des lentatives d'avoutement criminel. Ann. Méd. Lég. 42, 148–152 (1962).

Mailing address:
Univ.-Augenklinik
D-5000 Köln 41, F.R.G.

SYNCHRONIZATION OF ERG SIGNS OF RETINAL ISCHEMIA

J. R. BRUNETTE AND G. LAFOND

(Sherbrooke, Quebec, Canada)

ABSTRACT

Ischemia was induced in rabbits in order to study its effect on time and amplitude of the oscillatory potentials (OP) of the ERG. Ischemia was obtained by clamping the retrobulbar vascular supply. The system provided incremental increases of clamping from control level to total ischemia and ERG extinction. The method is valid and has been compared to other techniques. Results show that delays increase and amplitudes decrease probably simultaneously, with increasing levels of ischemia, amplitude changes showing slightly earlier. However delays are not statistically significant until high levels of ischemia are attained at which amplitude loss has already become evident. It is our impression that although time and amplitude of the OP's are modified simultaneously by ischemia, amplitude loss is the significant parameter.

INTRODUCTION

Electroretinographic (ERG) monitoring of retinal ischemia both in clinical and in animal experimentation has provided us with a number of electrophysiological signs to observe. B-waves have been shown to loose amplitude or become hypernormal, and oscillatory potentials (OP) decrease in amplitude and number (1–10). B-waves and OPs show delays in timing of the response (2, 3, 7–10). All of these signs have been adequately described. Often however apparent contradictions seem to exist in the literature. It is the aim of this paper to describe the synchronisation of these ERG signs and correlate them to variations in the level of ischemia that causes them.

MATERIAL AND METHODS

The present contribution consists in the evaluation of b-waves and OPs of six adult albino rabbits weighing approximately 3 kgs. Ischemia was produced by clamping of the retrobulbar neurovascular pedicle. The level of clamping could be incrementally and remotely controlled. All ERGs were collected in full dark adaptation. OPs were recorded using maximal intensity of stimulation and passbands of 80–250 Hertz, b-waves with 3.5 log units attenuation and at 0.8–50 Hertz. Intensity of stimulation was kept constant and full intensity produced at 1.8 lumen ft^2. The level of clamping is described as percent of pressure needed in the system to extinguish the ERG and ophthalmoscopically collapse the retinal circulation. Methods are fully described elsewhere.

RESULTS

Samples of OP recordings are shown in Figure 1. Results for b-waves are essentially similar to those already published and waveforms, detailed analysis and statistics are not presented here (1–2).

Figure 2 shows results of b-wave and OP amplitude during incremental increases of the level of ischemia. The b-wave amplitude rises rapidly and progressively up to a peak, at the 50% level of ischemia and then rapidly decreases down to extinction at the 100% ischemia level (Table 1). OPs show practically no loss of amplitude until after the b-wave peak but then rapidly and progressively also collapse down to extinction (Table II).

Figure 3 shows the results of b-wave and OP implicit time values under the same experimental conditions. Both OPs and b-wave show progressively increasing delays of response. B-wave delays are more apparent and appear earlier than those of OPs, these last becoming significant only after the 50% level of ischemia.

DISCUSSION

Four ERG parameters which are affected by ischemia are discussed here: amplitude and delay for b-waves and OPs. These show independent variations which vary widely with the level of ischemia. Only markedly significant changes will be taken into account for the following discussion in order to extract clearcut conclusions. Let us recall that early signs of ischemia are in fact due to moderate circulatory disturbances. All reports in the literature dealing with losses of b-wave amplitude deal only with the last part of our curves, when b-waves start loosing amplitude. Furthermore, these are results obtained using rabbits, an animal in which retinal vascularisation is mainly choroidal and should not be freely applied to results obtained from clinical material (11).

The present experimental results suggest a synchronisation of ERG signs according to the level of ischemia. These are shown in Table III. The very first sign of ischemia is a b-wave hyper-response (level 1) followed rapidly by a delay of the b-wave (level 2). Then only do OP signs become significant: The amplitude of P_3, the first significant clinical OP, decreases (level 3). It is noteworthy that OPs and b-wave amplitude are modified separately and differently by ischemia: no OP hyperpolarization was observed and the loss of b-wave amplitude does not follow the same pattern as that of the OPs.

% ISCHEMIA

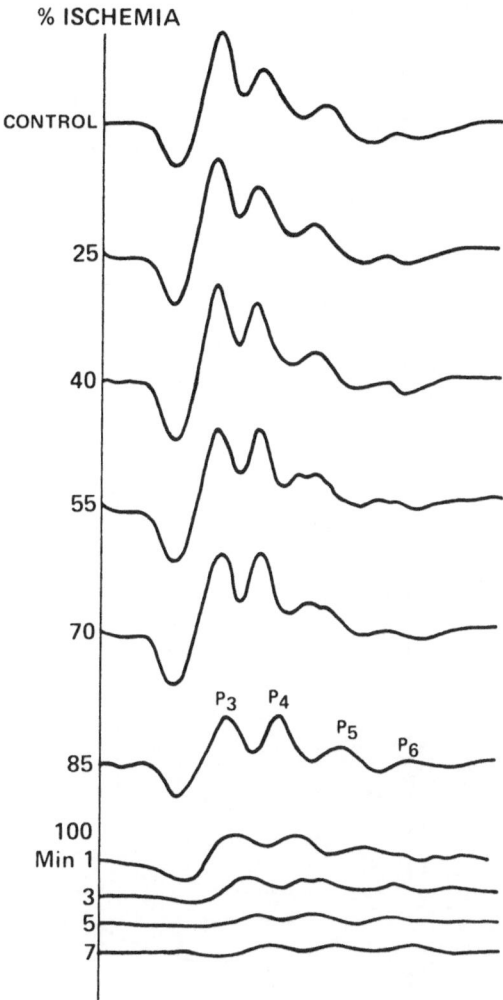

Fig. 1. Original tracing of oscillatory potentials of rabbits depending on degree of ischemia.

At the level 4 ischemia the b-wave is delayed and loses amplitude, while some delay of OPs dominate. It is important to observe that the b-wave is practically nonexistent.

This is extremely important for discussing ERG signs of ischemia. However labelled the level of ischemia is described in a given publication, if a loss of b-wave amplitude is present the ischemia is definitely severe. From level 5 on, amplitudes decrease progressively down to extinction while delays increase considerably for both b-waves and OPs.

However difficult the comparison of material such as the present with clinical experience one can not help but observe that they appear to correlate.

311

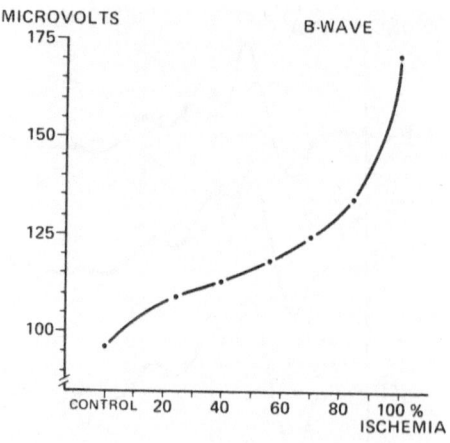

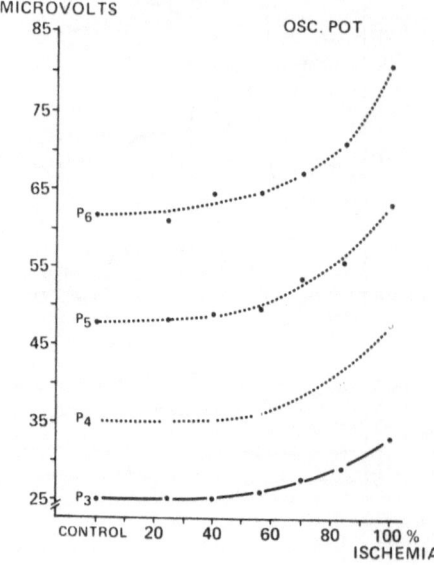

Fig. 2. ERG b-wave amplitude and oscillatory potentials amplitude depending on degree of ischemia.

Although we do not have at hand published results correlating b-waves and OPs signs in clinical ischemia as such we do have a comparison of amplitude and delay of OPs in diabetics, a presumed ischemic condition. These show that OPs amplitudes are more sensitive to identify pre-retinopathic diabetics than delay, which conforms to the present results (12). Yet more recent results show that b-wave hypernormality would be the most sensitive sign of early retinal ischemia. Thus, clinical results appear to follow the same pattern as those presented here.

Table 1. Mean and standard deviation of amplitude (microvolts) and implicit times of b-waves at incremental increases of ischemia from control values in rabbits.

LEVEL OF ISCHEMIA	AMPLITUDE	IMPLICIT TIME
CONTROL	68.6 ± 38.2	93.1 ± 7.5
25%	142.1 ± 73.9	109.2 ± 7.3
40%	199.0 ± 87.5	113.0 ± 10.3
55%	259.5 ± 125.8	117.5 ± 9.3
70%	242.2 ± 148.4	124.5 ± 10.3
85%	120.9 ± 95.2	133.6 ± 8.3
*100%	30.4 ± 6.5	170.9 ± 13.7

*Immediately after clamping, before extinction of response.

Table II. Mean and standard deviation of amplitudes (microvolts) and implicit times (milliseconds) of oscillatory potential at incremental increases of ischemia from control values, in rabbits.

LEVEL OF ISCHEMIA	P3		P4		P5		P6	
	AMP.	DELAY	AMP.	DELAY	AMP.	DELAY	AMP.	DELAY
CONTROL	36.3 ± 15.3	25.1 ± 1.4	22.5 ± 9.3	35.5 ± 2.3	10.8 ± 2.0	47.8 ± 2.9	7.5 ± 2.7	62.0 ± 4.2
25%	34.1 ± 16.2	25.1 ± 1.4	25.0 ± 11.4	35.5 ± 1.9	10.0 ± 5.4	48.0 ± 2.9	4.0 ± 1.5	61.1 ± 1.5
40%	30.8 ± 14.2	25.1 ± 1.4	22.5 ± 11.2	35.5 ± 2.8	8.3 ± 2.5	48.6 ± 2.6	4.0 ± 1.5	64.3 ± 3.2
55%	28.3 ± 13.6	26.1 ± 1.7	23.3 ± 10.3	36.3 ± 2.7	10.0 ± 3.1	49.8 ± 3.7	4.0 ± 1.5	64.5 ± 3.3
70%	27.5 ± 11.7	27.6 ± 2.5	21.6 ± 10.3	39.6 ± 5.4	6.1 ± 3.1	53.0 ± 5.4	3.0 ± 1.0	67.1 ± 5.0
85%	17.5 ± 6.1	28.5 ± 2.6	16.1 ± 6.8	40.0 ± 3.8	5.8 ± 3.3	55.3 ± 3.2	3.1 ± 1.3	71.1 ± 5.0
100%*	5.1 ± 2.6	32.6 ± 2.6	4.0 ± 1.5	47.6 ± 3.8	2.8 ± 1.3	63.8 ± 5.3	2.3 ± 0.8	81.1 ± 5.7

*Immediately after clamping, before extinction.

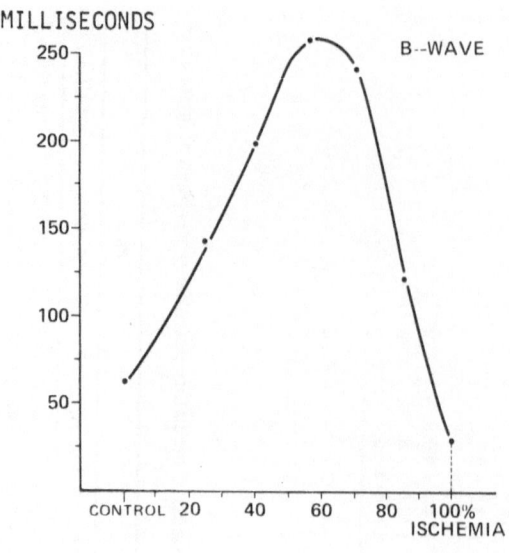

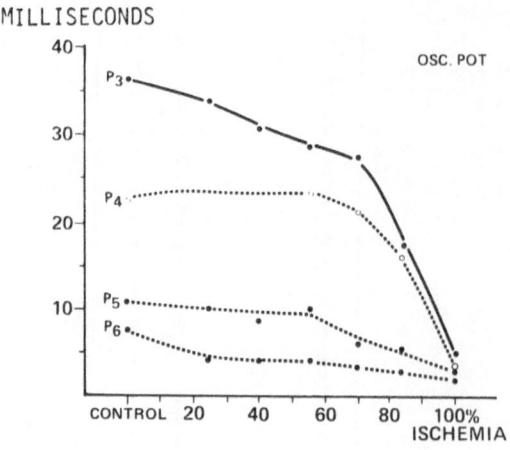

Fig. 3. ERG b-wave implicit time and oscillatory potentials peak time depending on degree of ischemia.

ACKNOWLEDGEMENT

This work was done under the MRC grant 2593.

REFERENCES

1. Brunette, J. R., Desrochers, R.: Oscillatory potentials: a clinical study in diabetics. Can. J. Ophthalmol., 5: 373–80, 1970.
2. Brunette, J. R., Olivier, P., Galeano, C. and Lafond, G.: Hyper-responsive and delayed ERG of acute ischemia. Can. J. Ophthalmol. in press.

Table III. Synchronisation of ERG signs of incremental ischemia in rabbits.

INCREMENTAL INCREASE IN LEVEL OF ISCHEMIA	B-WAVE		OSC.POT.	
	AMPLITUDE	DELAY	AMPLITUDE	DELAY
1	HYPER			
2	HYPER	DELAY		
3	HYPER	DELAY	LOSS	
4	'NORMAL'	DELAY	LOSS	DELAY
5	LOSS	DELAY	LOSS	DELAY
6	EXTINCT ERG.			

3. Brunette, J. R., Olivier, P., Galeano, C. and Lafond, G.: Intensity related ERG signs of acute ischemia. Can. J. Ophthalmol. in press.
4. Frost-Larsen, K., Larsen, H. W., Simonsen, S. E.: Oscillatory potential and nyctometry in insulin-dependent diabetics. Acta. Ophthal. (Copenh) 58: 6, 878–888, 1980.
5. Simonsen, S. E.: The value of the oscillatory potential in selecting juvenile diabetics at risk of developing proliferative retinopathy. Acta. Ophthal. (Copenh) 58: 6, 865–78, 1980.
6. Gjotterberg, M.: The electroretinogram in diabetic retinopathy. Acta. Ophthal. (Copenh.) 53: 521–33, 1974.
7. Yonemura, D., Kawasaki, K.: Electrophysiological study on activities of neuronal and non-neuronal retinal elements in man with reference to its clinical application. Jpn. J. Ophthalmol. 22: 195–213, 1977.
8. Yonemura, D., Kawasaki, K., Okumura, T., Tanabe, J., Nakagawa, H., Yamamoto, S.: Electrophysiological analysis of retinal disorders in diabetes mellitus. Scientific exhibition. The 23rd International congress of Ophthalmology, Kyoto, May 14–19, (1978a).
9. Yonemura, D.: Study of the human electroretinogram: new approaches to ophthalmic electrodiagnosis. Proceedings of the XVIth symposium of the ISCEV. Morioka, 1978. Tazawa edit. Suppl. Jap. J. Ophthalmol. Tokyo, 1979, pp. 1–13.
10. Harnois, C., Brunette, J. R.: ERG signs of experimental chronic ischemia of the retina. Can. J. Neurol. Sc. in press.
11. François, J., Neetens, A.: Comparative anatomy of the vascular supply of the eye in vertebrates. The Eye, 5: 1–70, H. Davson and L. T. Graham Jr. Editors. Academic Press. New York, 1974.
12. Brunette, J. R.: ERG evaluation of diabetic retinopathy: oscillatory potentials amplitudes or delays. Can. J. Ophthalmol. in press.

Mailing address:
Department of Ophthalmology
University of Sherbrooke
Sherbrooke, Quebec JIH 5N4, Canada

THE ACTION OF OPIATES ON THE OSCILLATORY POTENTIALS OF THE ELECTRORETINOGRAM (ERG)

L. WACHTMEISTER

(Huddinge, Sweden)

ABSTRACT

The neurochemical effects of the opiates, methadone and morphine, and their blocking agent, naloxone, were tested on the mudpuppy retina. A low concentration of methadone selectively and differentially decreased the intermediate oscillatory potentials (OPs) of the electroretinogram. There was no appreciable change of the threshold sensitivity and the stimulus response curves of the a- and b-waves. Higher concentrations further decreased the intermediate OPs, reduced the rest of the OPs and diminished the suprathreshold b-wave about 70%. Morphine in corresponding concentrations had similar effects. A concurrent application of naloxone and opiates showed that the depressive action of the opiates was blocked.

The results indicate that there are probably opiate receptors in the mudpuppy retina and that the intermediate oscillatory potentials probably reflect activity in neuronal synapses which are modulated by opiates.

INTRODUCTION

Information bearing on the origins of the oscillatory potentials (OPs) of the electroretinogram (ERG) has been mainly contributed by animal studies. In the mudpuppy retina there is now evidence that chemically different synaptic activities might underlie the individual peaks of the oscillatory potentials. The earlier OPs seem to reflect GABA-ergic neuronal activity whereas the later OPs seem to be generated by glycinergic pathways and are perhaps related to the off-effect (Wachtmeister & Dowling 1978, Kojima & Zrenner 1978, Wachtmeister 1980, 1981 a, b).

Opiates have been described to affect visual performance (Rothenberg et al., 1979), opiate binding sites have been identified in the homogenized retina of several species (Medziradsky 1976, Howells et al., 1980) and high affinity binding to retinal membrane preparations (similar to those reported in the whole brain) has also been reported for naloxone an opiate blocking agent (Howells et al., 1980). However, the effect of opioid activity on the retina an extension part of the brain is unknown.

Thus, in the present study the action of the opiates, methadone and

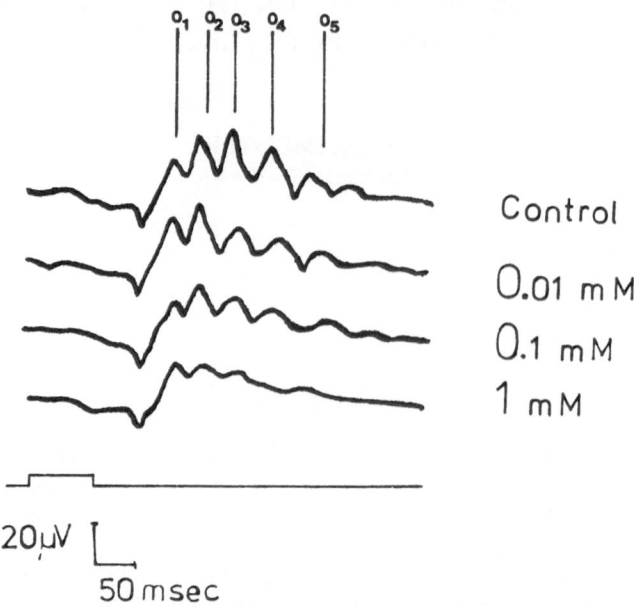

O_1 O_2 O_3 O_4 O_5

Control

0.01 mM

0.1 mM

1 mM

20μV

50 msec

Fig. 1. Effects of different concentrations of methadone on the OPs of the ERG. The ERG was recorded with a short time constant (15 msec) and in response to stimulus light of 75 msec duration and an intensity of log - 2.00 delivered at an interval of 30 sec. The effects appeared within 1 min after the drug was added and gradually increased reaching a maximum at about 2–5 min when these recordings were taken.

morphine, and their blocking agent naloxone, on the OPs of the electroretinogram were studied. An effect of opiates on retinal function would indicate the presence of opiate receptors in the retinal neuronal network and also allow further analysis of the origin of the OPs.

MATERIAL AND METHODS

The methods employed here are essentially the same as described elsewhere (Wachtmeister 1980). The light source was a tungsten ribbon filament lamp (Zeiss 6V/15W) and the maximum output was 8.7×10^{18} photons/cm^2 sec measured by a Hagner Universal Photmeter. The ERG was recorded in response to flashes of 75 msec duration delivered at a constant interval of 30 seconds. The active electrode was placed in the vitreous and the indifferent electrode behind the eye. Drops of about 4 μl solution containing the different drugs were applied to the open eye-cup. The amplitudes of the a- and b-waves and the OPs were measured as previously described (Wachtmeister 1980). Observations were made from 22 retinas of the mudpuppy.

RESULTS

Figure 1 depicts the transretinal ERG recorded with a short time constant and evoked with full-field flashes 4 log units above b-wave threshold at an

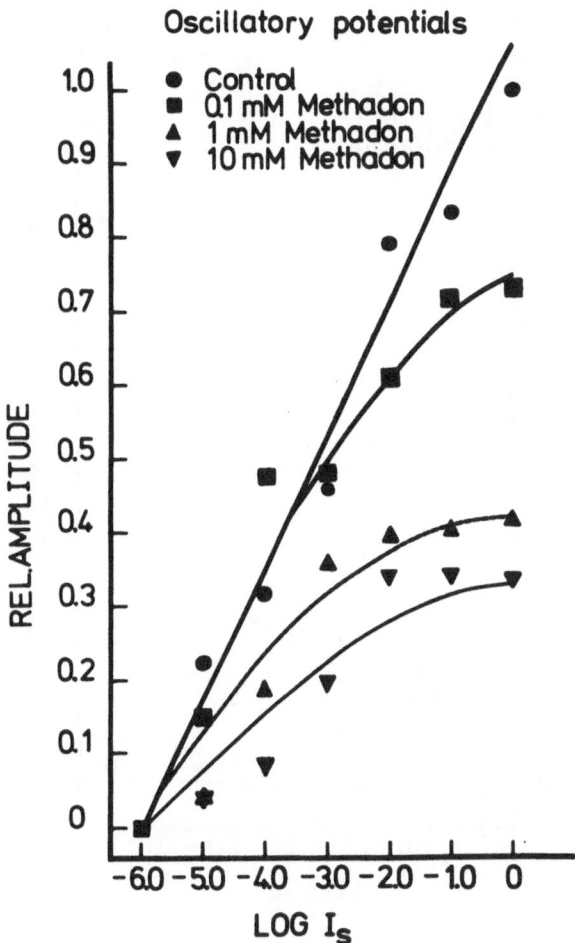

Fig. 2. Stimulus response curves of the OPs, a- and b-waves before and after the application of methadone. A. Relative summed aplitudes of the OPs.

interstimulus interval of 30 seconds. Usually five to seven OPs can be identified superimposed on the b-wave. The first five were prominent in most recordings and therefore the attention was focused particularly on these waves.

About two minutes after a low concentration (0.1 mM) of methadone was applied to the open eye cup a differential and selective attenuation of the third and fourth potential occurred. Higher concentrations (1 mM and 10 mM) further decreased the amplitudes of the third and fourth peak and also reduced the rest of the oscillations.

Figure 2 shows that low concentrations of methadone (0.1 mM) reduced the stimulus response function of the OPs whereas the threshold sensitivity and suprathreshold amplitudes of the a- and b-waves were virtually unaltered. Higher doses of methadone (1 mM and 10 mM) further decreased the

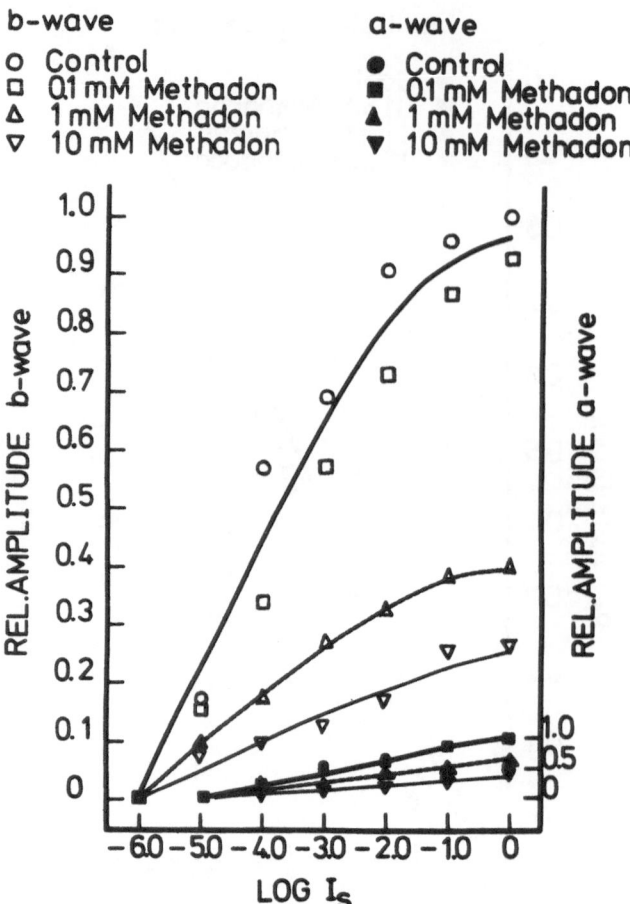

b-wave
o Control
□ 0.1 mM Methadon
△ 1 mM Methadon
▽ 10 mM Methadon

a-wave
● Control
■ 0.1 mM Methadon
▲ 1 mM Methadon
▼ 10 mM Methadon

Fig. 2. Stimulus response curves of the OPs, a- and b-waves before and after the application of methadone. B. Relative amplitudes of the a- and b-waves.

amplitudes of the OPs and also diminished the suprathreshold a- and b-waves about 60–70%. No appreciable change of the peak latencies of the a- and b-waves was noted. Application of morphine in corresponding concentrations had similar effects as methadone.

When the retina was exposed to a low concentration (0.01 mM) of the opiate antagonist, naloxone, a selective and differential reduction of the OPs occurred which is illustrated in Figure 3. Again, the third and fourth OPs were more sensitive to the drug than the rest and were reduced about 40%. Higher doses caused a further decrease of the third and fourth OP, and diminished the rest of the OPs.

Low concentrations of naloxone depressed the stimulus response curve of the OPs whereas no appreciable effect on the stimulus response functions of the a- and b-waves was noticed (Figure 4). When the highest dose of naloxone

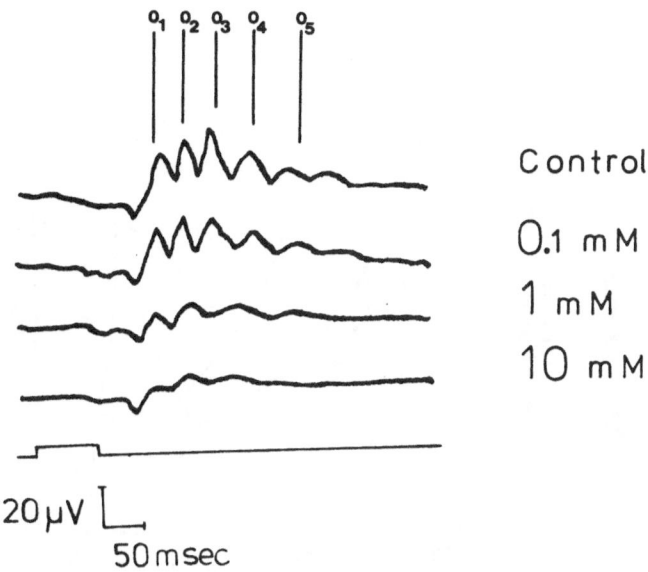

Fig. 3. The effects of different concentrations of naloxone on the OPs of the ERG. The same recording conditions as in Figure 1. The effects appeared and the recording times were the same as in Figure 1.

was used there was a decrease of the suprathreshold a- and b-waves of about 30%. The peak latencies of the a- and b-waves were not noticeably altered.

Figure 5 shows that when the agonist and antagonist were concurrently applied the depressive action of methadone was blocked.

Control experiments showed that application of Ringer's solution alone produced no apparent effect on the ERG.

To summarize, the present experiments demonstrated that the OPs of the ERG are sensitive to opiates and that these effects can be blocked by simultaneous application of an opiate antagonist, naloxone.

In conclusion these findings support previous pharmacological studies and suggest that:

1. Firstly, the OPs reflect activity in inhibitory neuronal pathways.

2. Secondly, the individual oscillatory peaks seem to have different origins and the intermediate OPs reflect activity in neuronal synapses which can be modulated by opiates.

3. Thirdly, there is a role for opiates also in the pheripheral part of the visual system, the retina.

ACKNOWLEDGEMENT

This investigation was supported in part by a grant from the Swedish Medical Research Council (project no. 04X–05411). Naloxone was kindly provided by Endo Laboratories, Inc., U.S.A.

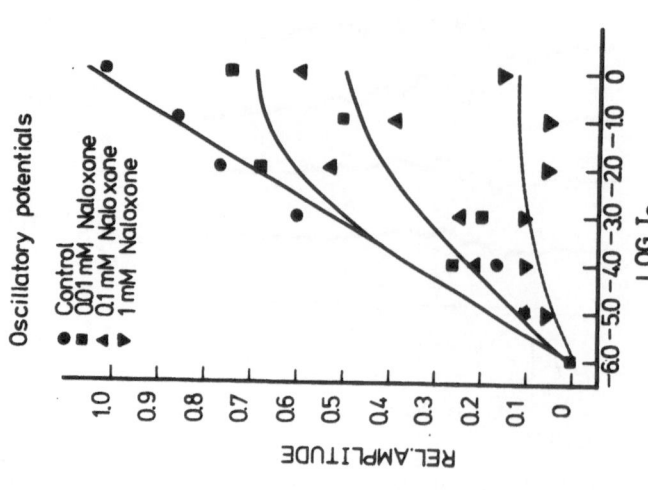

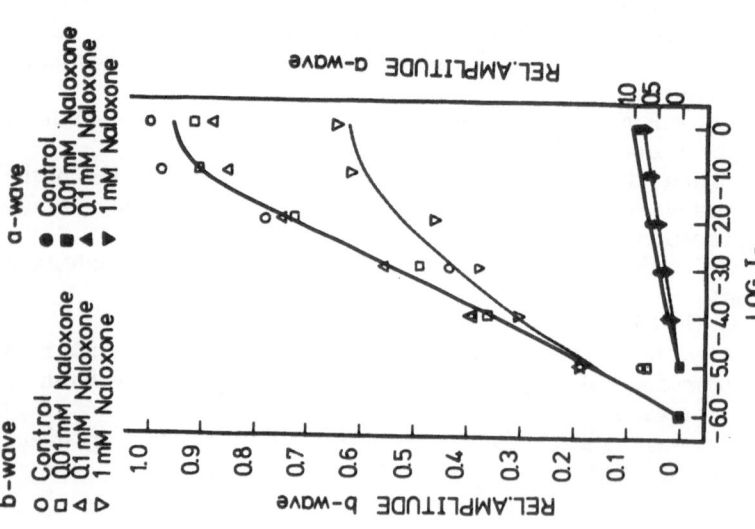

Fig. 4. Stimulus response curves of the OPs, a- and b-waves before and after the application of naloxone. A. Relative summed amplitudes of the OPs. B. Relative amplitudes of the a- and b-waves.

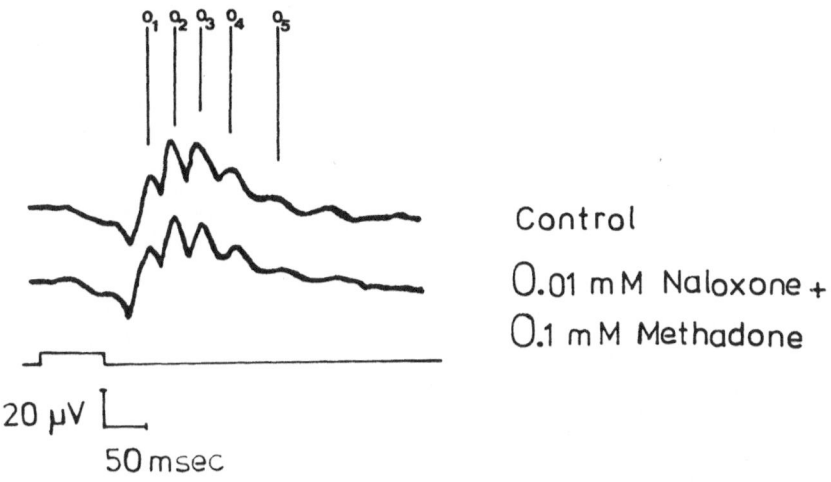

Control

0.01 mM Naloxone +

0.1 mM Methadone

20 μV

50 msec

Fig. 5. The effects of concurrent application of an agonist methadone and an antagonist, naloxone on the OPs of the ERG. The same recording conditions as in Figure 1.

REFERENCES

Howells, R. D., Groth, J., Miller, J. M. & Simon, E. J. (1980). Opiate binding sites in the retina. Properties and distribution. J. Pharmacol. Exp. Ther. 215: 60–64.

Kojima, M. & Zrenner, E. (1978). Off-components in response to brief light flashes in the oscillatory potentials of the human electroretinogram. Alb Graefes Arch. klin. exp. Ophthalm. 206: 107–120.

Medzihradsky, F. (1976). Stereospecific binding of etorphine in isolated neural cells and in retina, determined by sensitive microassay. Brain. Res. 108: 212–219.

Rothenberg, S., Peck, E. A., Schottenfeld, G. E., Betley, G. E. & Altman, J. L. (1979). Methadone Depression of Visual Signal Detection Performance. Pharmac. Biochem. / Behav. II, 521–527.

Wachtmeister, L. & Dowling, J. D. E. (1978). The oscillatory potentials of the mudpuppy retina. Invest. Ophthalmol. 17: 1176–1188.

Wachtmeister, L. (1980). Further studies of the chemical sensitivity of the oscillatory potentials of the electroretinogram (ERG) I GABA- and glycine antagonist. Acta. ophthalmol. 58: 712–725.

Wachtmeister, L. (1981a). Further studies of the chemical sensitivity of the oscillatory potentials of the electroretinogram (ERG) II. Glutamate-aspartate and dopamine antagonists. Acta. Ophthalmol. 59: 247–258.

Wachtmeister, L. (1981b). Further studies of the chemical sensitivity of the oscillatory potentials of the electroretinogram (ERG) III. Some Ω aminoacids and ethanol. Acta. Ophthalmol. 59: 609–619.

Mailing address:
Department of Ophthalmology
Karolinska Inst./Huddinge Univ. Hospital
Huddinge, Sweden 14186

ERG 'C'-WAVE AS ELICITED USING FAST RANDOM STIMULI

D. V. SCHOON AND M. P. HARRIS

(Irvine, California, U.S.A.)

ABSTRACT

Microprocessors allow the evaluation of responses to fast random stimuli and make such applications as were used in this study feasible for clinical use. Fast random light flashes of near constant intensity were used in eliciting ERG's from each eye of 20 subjects. One eye of each subject was then dilated using Cyclogel 1%. The major positive wave following the b-wave was evaluated before and after dilation. This wave which we have called the 'C'-wave showed a significant decrease in implicit time after dilation and a small increase in amplitude. The ERG's of two patients having been diagnosed as having retinitis pigmentosa are shown. In one, the 'C'-wave was nearly flat and in the other the 'C'-wave was present but the negative wave after the b-wave was very small.

INTRODUCTION

Several investigators using slow regular stimuli have stated that the c-wave of the human ERG flattens out when the pupil is pharmacologically dilated (Pearlman 1962; Riggs & Johnson 1949). Several artifacts such as the pupillary reflex and blink reflex apparently contribute to the potential changes coming in the ERG after 100 msec. Several laboratories have used long stimuli 1 to 10 sec (Marmor 1982; Skoog & Nilsson 1974; Röver et al., 1982; Takahashi et al., 1979) together with DC amplifiers and nonpolarizable electrodes to obtain the c-wave. Because we are measuring responses to very short stimuli, we may not be measuring a potential change which is analogous to these c-waves; we shall refer to the positive wave we obtain as the 'C'-wave.

We have used a microprocessor computer to trigger fast random stimuli and to process the information obtained. In this way responses that are time locked to the stimulus but which are much slower than the retinal response are essentially eliminated. Thus, the pupillary reflex, the blink reflex and the facial muscle potentials are not a significant part of the response obtained. Also, ambient electrical noise does not significantly contribute to the response as it cannot stay time locked to the stimulus.

METHOD

ERG's were obtained from each eye of 20 subjects. These subjects were between 23 and 64 years of age. There were 7 males and 13 females. In none of the subjects was there a family history of retinal dystrophy. One subject had an amblyopia in one eye (visual acuity 20/200), diagnosed as being related to a congenital esotropia and one subject had a unilateral maculo-pathy (visual acuity in that eye was 20/200), diagnosed as being related to histoplasmosis. The remaining 38 eyes were normal, having corrected visual acuities of at least 20/25 and no ophthalmoscopically visible retinopathy.

The visual stimulus was obtained from a pulsed xenon source (Chadwick-Helmuth Strobex Point Source Model 136). This has a constant output of 0.15 joules per 20 microsecond flash with less than 2% variation of intensity between flashes (manufacturer's specification). The source was housed in a box lined with black felt and was positioned 53 cm from the patient's eyes. A circular aperture subtending $15°$ in diameter was located between the light source and the patient. A diffuser covering the aperture attenuated the flash by 0.45 log units. The subject viewed the stimulus monocularly through a window at one end of the box.

A gold electrode was used on the lower lid of the eye being evaluated. One gold clip electrode was placed on an ear lobe as reference and another gold clip electrode on the other ear lobe served as ground. The responses were fed through Isoswitches into a high Z probe.

A Grass Model P511 H preamplifier was used with half-amplitude filters set at 1 Hz (low) and 300 Hz (high). A 60 Hz line filter was used.

The flash was triggered in a rapid random binary fashion as described by Larkin et al., (1979). Time bins of 16 milliseconds were used in which there was a flash triggered with a probability of $\frac{1}{2}$. Each line graph obtained represented responses obtained from 60 seconds of stimulation or summed responses from approximately 1875 stimuli.

The microprocessor computer was hard wired to weight the potential changes following a time bin in which a stimulus was given with a factor of $+1$. The potential changes following a time bin in which no stimulus occurred were given a weighting factor of -1. This allowed the overall background noise to tend toward 0. Potential measurements were taken each msec and the above cross correlation weighting and summing of the cross correlations was done by the computer. Two hundred fifty-six data bins of 1 msec width were evaluated after the start of each stimulus time bin.

A Hewlet Packard X–Y Plotter model 7015–B was used to obtain a hard copy of the summed ERG's obtained on the display screen. Two sixty second testing runs were obtained on each eye prior to dilation. One eye of each subject was then dilated using 1% Cyclogel. Two ERG testing runs were then obtained from the dilated eye.

RESULTS

Because our computer recorded potential changes only to 256 msec after a stimulus time bin, we found that the peak of the 'C'-wave did not appear to

326

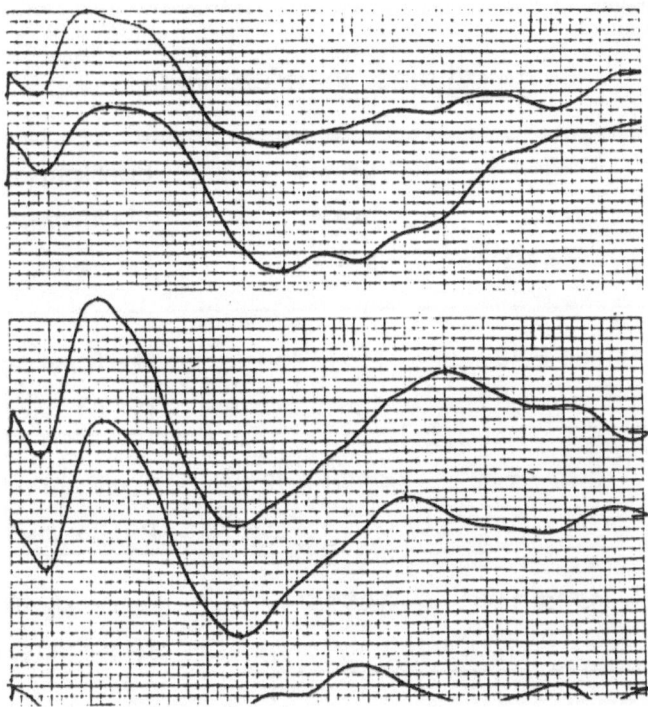

Fig. 1. The top two ERG's were obtained from a normal subject's left eye. The lower two ERG's were obtained from the same eye after dilatation. Each vertical division represents approximately 0.36 microvolts and each horizontal division represents 4 milliseconds.

have been reached in some of our subjects. In the undilated eyes, of the 80 ERG's obtained, 44 appeared to show that the 'C'-wave had reached a maximum. For purposes of calculation, those that had not reached a maximum were considered as having a maximum amplitude at the amplitude reached at 256 msec. Using this approximation, the true mean value of the implicit time and the amplitude would in fact be larger than we calculated.

In 38 of the 40 ERG's obtained from the eyes dilated with Cyclogel, the 'C'-wave appeared to have reached its maximum before 256 msec.

A typical ERG which had not reached the 'C'-wave maximum before dilation and which after dilation with 1% Cyclogel did reach its maximum, is seen in Figure 1.

Table 1 tabulates the means and standard deviations of the amplitudes of the various waves obtained from the undilated and dilated eyes. We have taken the liberty of giving the name 'F-wave' to the major negative deflection following the b-wave and preceding the 'C'-wave. We have used the lowest point of the negative trough between the b-wave and 'C'-wave as the implicit time for this wave, and we have taken the potential difference between the

Table 1. Amplitudes of ERG components evokes by random stimuli is undilated and mydriatic human eyes.

Amplitudes in micro volts

	Undilated N=40 $\bar{X}\pm$ SD	Dilated N=20 $\bar{X}\pm$ SD	Significance of difference of means
A wave	.93 ± .43	1.22 ± .45	Significant at P<.01 level
B wave	3.49 ± 1.42	4.35 ± 1.12	Significant at P<.05 level
F wave	4.71 ± 1.93	6.96 ± 2.49	Highly significant at P<.001 level
"C" wave	4.72 ± 1.94	5.63 ± 1.93	Not significant

peak of the b-wave and deepest dip of this trough as the amplitude of the F-wave. In this table, we have also tabulated the significance of the difference of the means obtained for the undilated eye and those obtained for the dilated eye. A difference is listed as being 'highly significant' if $P < 0.001$. The small magnitude of the voltages is related to the fact that under our conditions of testing we have essentially used a weak stimulus on a strong background.

Table 2 tabulates the means and standard deviations of the implicit times of the various waves obtained from the undilated and dilated eyes. We again call the major negative wave between the b-wave and the 'C'-wave the F-wave. The significance of the difference of the two means for the dilated and undilated groups is tabulated.

Figures 2 is a line graph showing the relation of the mean values of the implicit times and amplitudes for the ERG's of the undilated and dilated eyes. A scattergram, Figure 3, is presented to show the distribution of the values of the amplitudes and implicit times of the 'C'-wave of ERG's done on each of the 40 eyes prior to dilation, and on the 20 eyes which were dilated. These tend to show that the peak of the 'C'-wave comes earlier when the pupil is dilated with Cyclogel. No decrease in amplitude of the 'C'-wave is seen after dilation. Although a significant increase in the amplitude of the 'C'-wave after dilation of the pupil could not be demonstrated.

328

Table 2. Implicit time of ERG components evoked by random stimuli in undilated and mydriatic human eye.

Implicit times in msec.

	Undilated N = 40 $\overline{X} \pm$ SD	Dilated N = 20 $\overline{X} \pm$ SD	Signiifcance of difference of means
A wave	12.71 ± 1.71	12.45 ± 1.58	Not significant
B wave	52.69 ± 9.37	44.31 ± 6.92	Highly significant (P < .001)
F wave	122.96 ± 12.14	101.48 ± 12.23	Highly significant (P < .001)
'C' wave	240.46 ± 20.51	204.25 ± 27.23	Highly significant (P < .001)

DISCUSSION

Rapid random stimuli used with a cross correlation weighting of the potential changes is feasible using computers. The late portion of the ERG can be evaluated. The 'C'-wave obtained does not flatten after pupillary dilation. The 'C'-wave after dilation of the pupil has a significantly shorter implicit time than it has prior to dilation.

We have had one patient having diagnosed retinitis pigmentosa showing a flat 'C'-wave (see Figure 4). He was adopted and did not know his family history. Unlike the several other patients with retinitis pigmentosa we have examined, who were tested early enough to have a recognizable ERG, this man appears to have a relatively good b-wave but an essentially flat 'C'-wave. The ERG of a young patient with diagnosed retinal dystrophy not showing a low 'C'-wave is also shown, Figure 5.

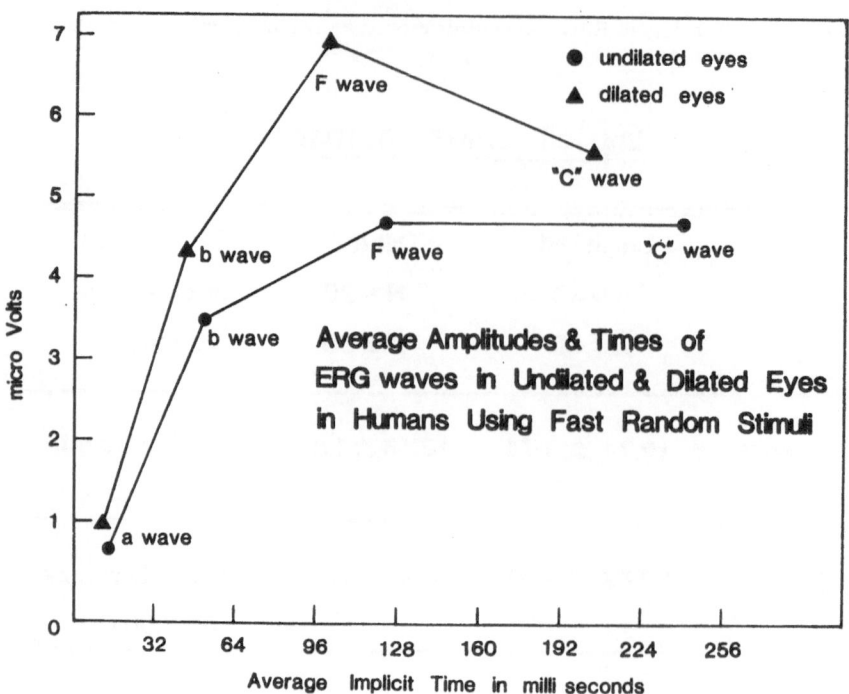

Fig. 2. Line graph of average values of ERG waves.

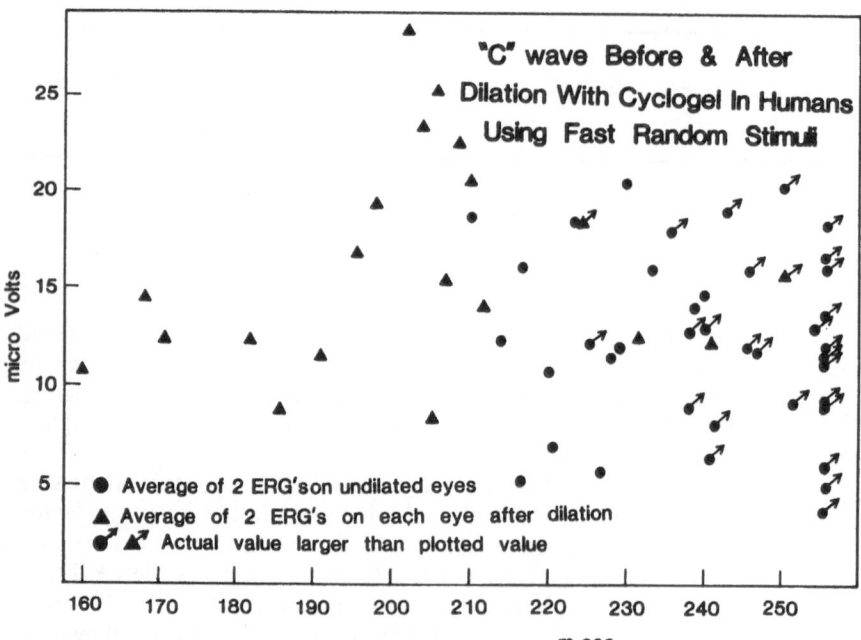

Fig. 3. Scattergram of 'C'-waves before and after dilatation.

330

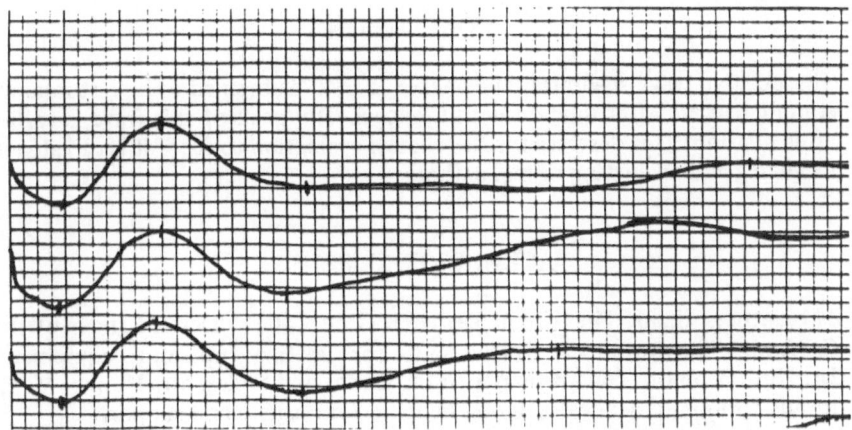

Fig. 4. These are three ERGs (tree runs from the same eye) obtained from a 44 year old patient diagnosed as having retinitis pigmentosa. No consistent positive wave is noted in the late portion of the ERG. Each vertical division represents 0.36 microvolts and each horizontal division represents 4 milliseconds.

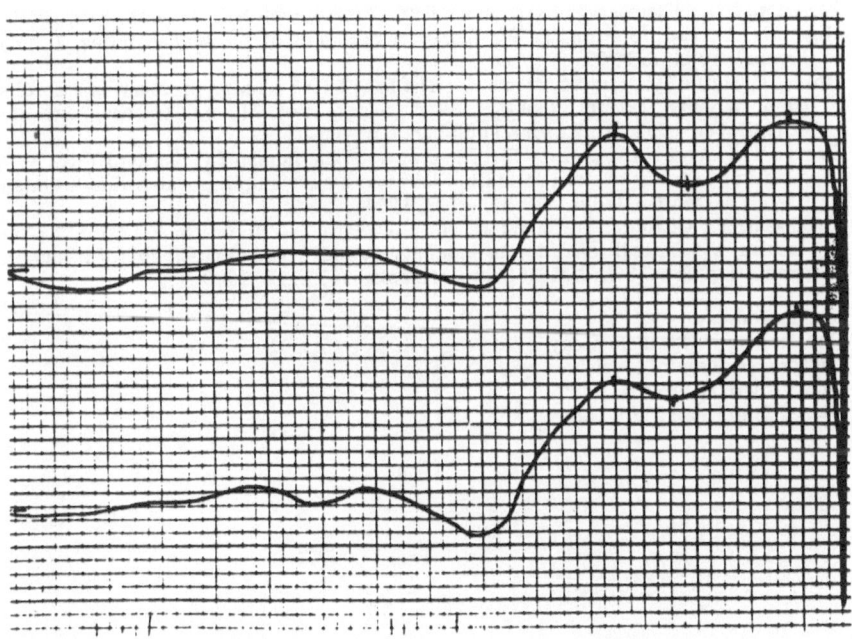

Fig. 5. This is the ERG (two runs from the same eye) of a teenaged patient diagnosed as having retinitis pigmentosa. Each vertical division represents 0.36 microvolts and each horizontal division represents 4 milliseconds.

CONCLUSION

The positive wave seen after the b-wave in ERG's obtained using fast random stimuli persists after dilation with Cyclogel. The peak of this wave is earlier after dilation. This deserves further clinical evaluation to see if it is of value in localizing and evaluating retinal pathology.

ACKNOWLEDGEMENTS

The authors thank The Vision Research Group of Dr. Derek Fender of the California Institute of Technology for setting up our equipment. Dr. Hiro Enomoto for his help with the graphs and tables, Mr. Thomas Merill for his photography and Dr. Irving Leopold for his help and support.

REFERENCES

Larkin, R. M., Klein, S., Ogden, T. E., and Fender, D. H.: Nonlinear kernels of the human ERG, Biological Cybernetics, 35: 145–160, 1979.

Marmor, M. F., and Hock, P. A.: A practical method for c-wave recording in man. Docum. Ophthal. Proc. Series, Vol 31, ed. by G. Niemeyer and C. H. Huber, 1982, Dr. W. Junk Publishers, The Hague.

Pearlman, J. T.: The c-wave of the human ERG, Arch of Ophthal., 68: 823–830, 1962.

Riggs, L. A., and Johnson, E. P.: Electrical responses of the human retina, J. Exp. Psychol. 39: 415, 1949.

Röver, J., Hüttel, M., and Schaubele, G.: The DC-ERG: Technical problems in recording from patients, Docum. Ophthal. Proc. Series, Vol 31, ed. G. Niemeyer and C. H. Huber, 1982, Dr. W. Junk Publishers, The Hague.

Skoog, K. O. and Nilsson, S. E. G.: The c-wave of the human DC registerd ERG. 1. A quantitative study of the relationship between c-wave amplitude and stimulus intensity, Acta Ophthal. (Kbh.) 52: 759–773, 1974.

Takahashi, Y., Ohtsuka, T., Sasamori, H., Takamatsu, T., Inomato, K., Mito, T., and Tazawa, Y.: DC-registered c-wave in human normal eyes and possibility of its clinical application, Proc. 16th ISCEV Symp. Moreoka, 113–118, 1979.

Mailing address:
Department of Ophthalmology
California College of Medicine
University of California, Irvine
Irvine, California 92717, U.S.A.

FAST RANDOM AND SLOW REGULAR STIMULUS ERG's IN RABBITS AFTER DILATATION WITH CYCLOGEL AND AFTER SODIUM IODATE INJECTION: A PRELIMINARY STUDY

D. V. SCHOON, M. P. HARRIS AND R. M. LARKIN

(Irvine, California, U.S.A.)

ABSTRACT

Microprocessor computers make the use of fast random stimuli, and the cross correlation of the stimulus and the response, a feasible method of obtaining electroretinograms. ERG's were done on thirty eyes of fifteen pigmented rabbits using fast random stimulation for 10 seconds and using slow regular (2 Hz) stimulation for 90 seconds. Eight of the rabbit eyes were then dilated using cyclogel and the dilated and undilated eyes were retested. The amplitude and implicit times of the ERG waves for the dilated and undilated eyes were reevaluated. Using this small sample, no significant difference between dilated and undilated eyes in the implicit time or amplitude of the major waves could be demonstrated. However, a positive wave following the b-wave was noted and this wave persisted after dilation.

Seven of the pigmented rabbits were given intravenous sodium iodate. In the rabbits receiving a heavier dose of sodium iodate (over 30 mg/Kg body weight), a slowing of the b-wave was observed along with a decrease in the amplitude of the b-wave. The positive wave following the b-wave showed a decrease in amplitude which was not statistically significant when fast random stimuli were used. Using slow regular stimuli, the wave became larger and slower after large doses of sodium iodate. Some of the improvements which might be helpful in future investigations are listed.

INTRODUCTION

We had noted a consistent positive potential following the b-wave in human subjects using fast random stimuli. In humans, this wave appeared in the ERG of subjects even after dilation. An animal study was undertaken to see if this positive potential was present and to see if it was modified after dilation or after intravenous sodium iodate. This study was done in parallel using slow regular and fast random stimuli so that the differences in the portion of the ERG between 100 and 256 msec after the stimulus could be observed. Noell (1953) had given intravenous sodium iodate to albino rabbits and found that this markedly changed the c-wave. Other investigators (Riggs and Johnson,

1949, Pearlman, 1962) had found that in humans what was called a c-wave in the ERG disappeared after dilation of the pupil.

METHOD

Fifteen pigmented (Rex) rabbits were used to obtain ERG studies of 30 eyes. The sex of the rabbits was not determined. The rabbits were all approximately 3 months of age.

A Henkes contact lens electrode was used over a high plus (+ 19 to + 26 diopters) soft contact (Tresoft) lens and this electrode was attached to a high Z probe in which isoswitches had been incorporated. It was necessary to manually hold the Henkes lens in place because suction could not be maintained with the soft contact lens under the Henkes lens. Spring clip gold electrodes were used to each ear. One ear served as ground and the other as a reference electrode. No anesthetic was used and no sedation was used.

The stimulus was obtained from a pulsed source (Chadwick-Helmuth Strobex Point Source Model 136). This has a relatively constant output of 0.15 joules per 20 microsecond flash with less than 2% variation of intensity between flashes (manufacturer's specifications).

The source was housed in a box lined with black felt and was placed approximately 60 cm from the rabbit's eye being evaluated. A circular aperture subtending just under 15° in diameter was located between the light source and the rabbit. A diffuser attenuated the flash by 0.45 log units. The rabbit was placed so that the light beam entered the pupil of the eye being tested as close as possible to the visual axis. (See Figure 1 for a schematic drawing of the apparatus used).

A Grass Model P511 H preamplifier was used with half amplitude filters set at 1 Hz (low) and 300 Hz (high). A 60 Hz line filter was used. An amplification of 50,000 was used. For the fast random stimuli, the flash was triggered in a rapid random binary fashion as described by Larkin et al., (1979). Time bins of 16 msec were used in which there was a flash triggered with a probability of 0.5. Two runs of 10 seconds were made on each eye. Each 10 second run included about 310 stimuli.

The computer weighted the potentials measured following a time bin with a stimulus with a factor of + 1. Following a time bin in which no stimulus was given a factor of − 1 was used as a weighting factor. Measurements of potential changes were made every millisecond and were weighted appropriately with the stimulus and summed to 256 msec after each stimulus time bin. The computer was hard wired to do only this task.

A Hewlet Packard Model 7015−B X−Y plotter was used to obtain a hard copy of the summed response.

For the slow regular stimuli, two 90-second sessions of 2 Hz stimulation were carried out on each eye. Thus each run was the sum of 180 responses. The timer of a Grass photostimulator was used (divided by 10) to supply the 2 Hz triggers to the power supply of the xenon flash. After the initial four ERG's on each eye (2 fast random and 2 slow regular), eight eyes were dilated using 1% cyclogel. The testing was then repeated on both the dilated and undilated eyes.

Block Diagram of Stimulus and Recording Apparatus for ERG

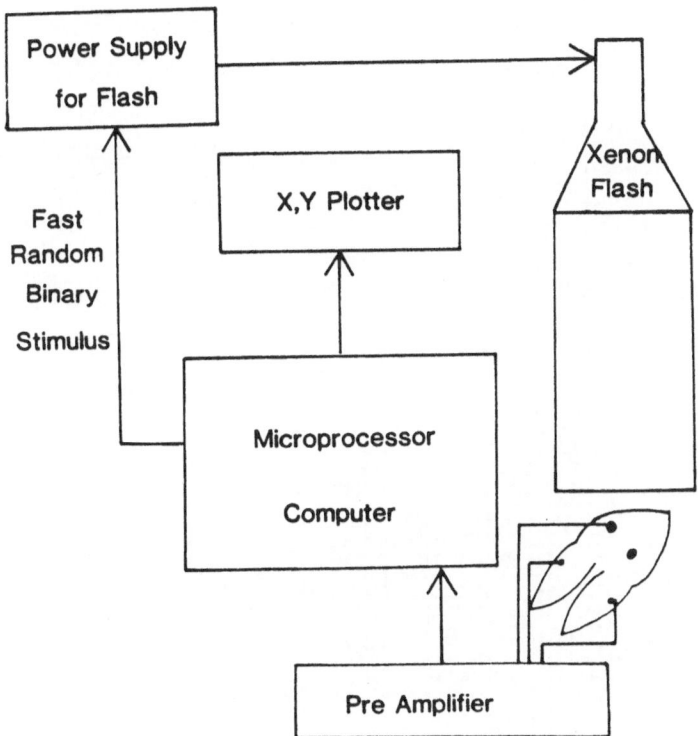

Fig. 1. Schematic of apparatus.

Sodium iodate 2% solution was injected into the marginal ear vein of seven rabbits (5 cc into each of five rabbits and 2 cc into each of two rabbits). The two rabbits receiving 2 cc had received a dosage under 20 mg/Kg body weight and the five rabbits receiving 5 cc received a dosage over 30 mg/Kg body weight.

RESULTS

Dilation study

The amplitude changes and implicit times changes were tabulated comparing before and after dilation for eight eyes. The fellow eye which was not dilated was also reevaluated and the changes from the first to the second evaluation

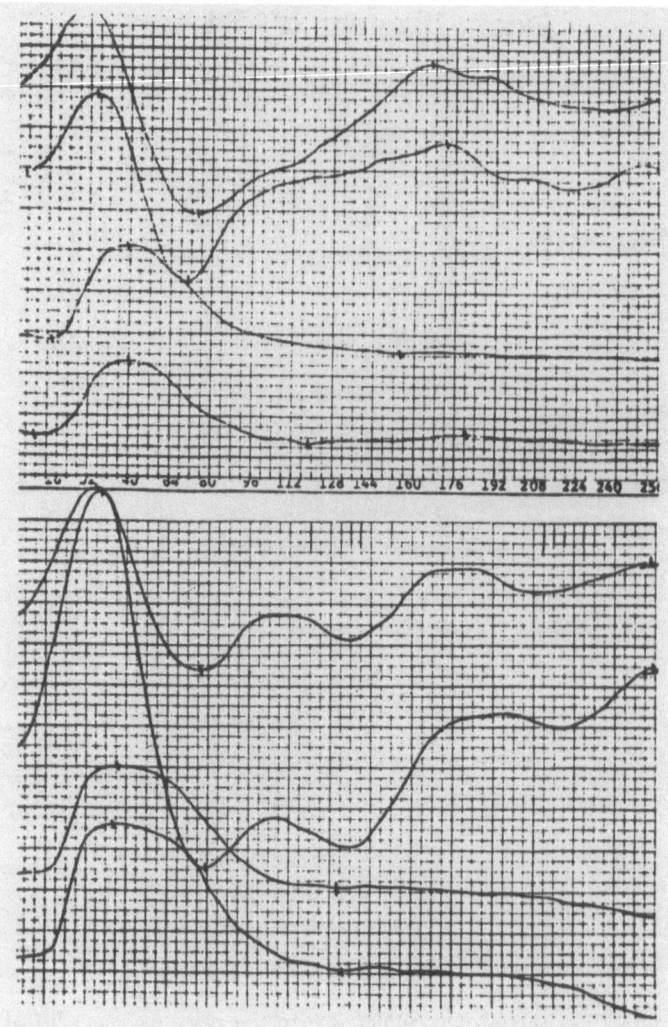

Fig. 2. The top half are the ERG's of a normal rabbit. The top two traces are repeat runs using fast random stimuli and the next two traces are responses to slow regular stimuli. The bottom half are the ERG's of the same eye after dilation. The same format is used as was used for the top half. For the runs using fast random stimuli each vertical division is 2.2 microvolts and for those using slow regular stimuli each vertical division is 14.7 microvolts. Each division on the horizontal (time) scale is 4 msec.

were noted. The positive wave seen following the b-wave persisted after dilation but no significant changes was noted in its amplitude or its implicit time when the ERG's before dilation were compared with those done after dilation. Figure 2 shows the ERG's of one eye prior to dilation and after dilation.

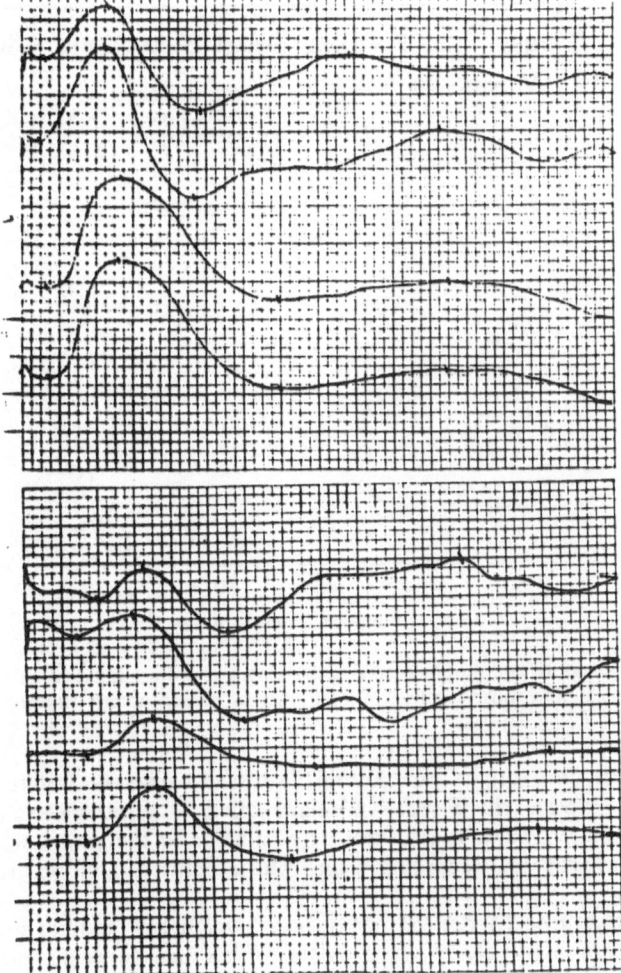

Fig. 3. The top half are the ERG's of a normal rabbit. The top two traces are repeat runs using fast random stimuli and the next two traces are responses to slow regular stimuli. The bottom half are the ERG's of the same eye after sodium iodate. The format on the bottom is the same as that used on the top. The scale is also the same as was used in Figure 2.

Sodium Iodate

Figure 3 shows the ERG of an eye after the rabbit received sodium iodate. Figure 4 shows the data obtained when the b-waves were measured before and after giving sodium iodate using fast random stimuli. Figure 5 shows the data obtained when the F waves were measured before and after sodium iodate. The means and standard deviations obtained using fast random stimuli and slow regular stimuli are listed in Tables 1 and 2. The units of amplitude are much smaller using fast random stimuli because we have in effect used a

337

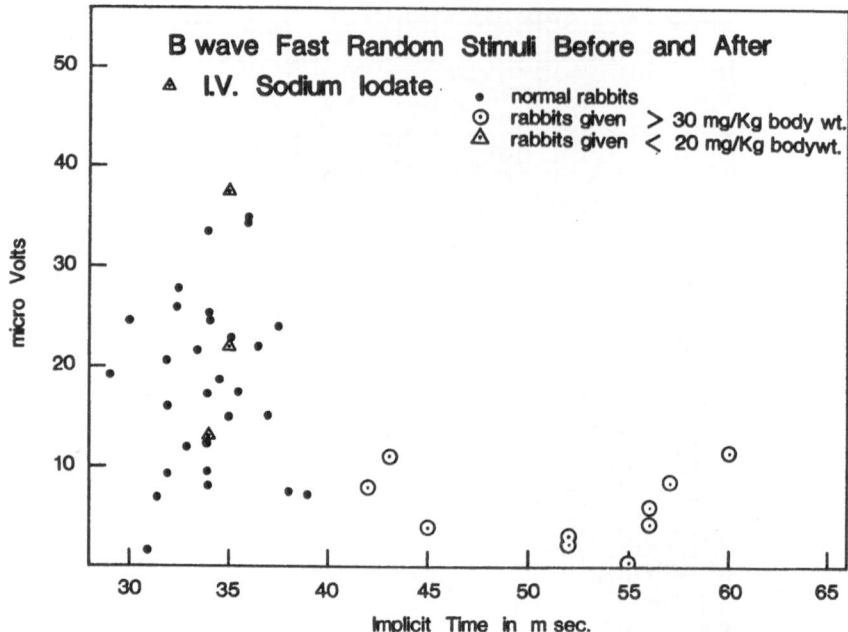

Fig. 4. The b-waves of the rabbits receiving low doses of sodium iodate are not different from the normals, and those receiving a large dose of sodium iodate showed prolonged implicit times.

small stimulus on a bright background. We have called the negative trough following the b-wave, the 'F-wave'. We have called the positive wave following the b-wave, the 'C'-wave. It may not be analogous to the slow c-wave which many laboratories are recording using DC amplifiers and relatively long stimuli.

After a low dose (under 20 mg/Kg body weight) of sodium iodate, the b-wave was not markedly changed. After a high dose (over 30 mg/Kg body weight), all of the waves show a slowing and a decrease in amplitude (although using fast random stimuli in only 10 seconds testing sessions, the significance of the change in the 'C' wave could not be verified).

Figure 6 shows the ERG of one rabbit given a large dose of sodium iodate and tested over a period of time.

CONCLUSIONS

With respect to the experimental plan, some of the conclusions we reached were the following:

(1) The sampling of 10 seconds of responses to fast random stimuli (approximately 310 responses) is not sufficient for the amplitudes of the major waves of the ERG to reach a highly reproducible level, although the implicit times of the waves appear to be reliable after that short testing. A

338

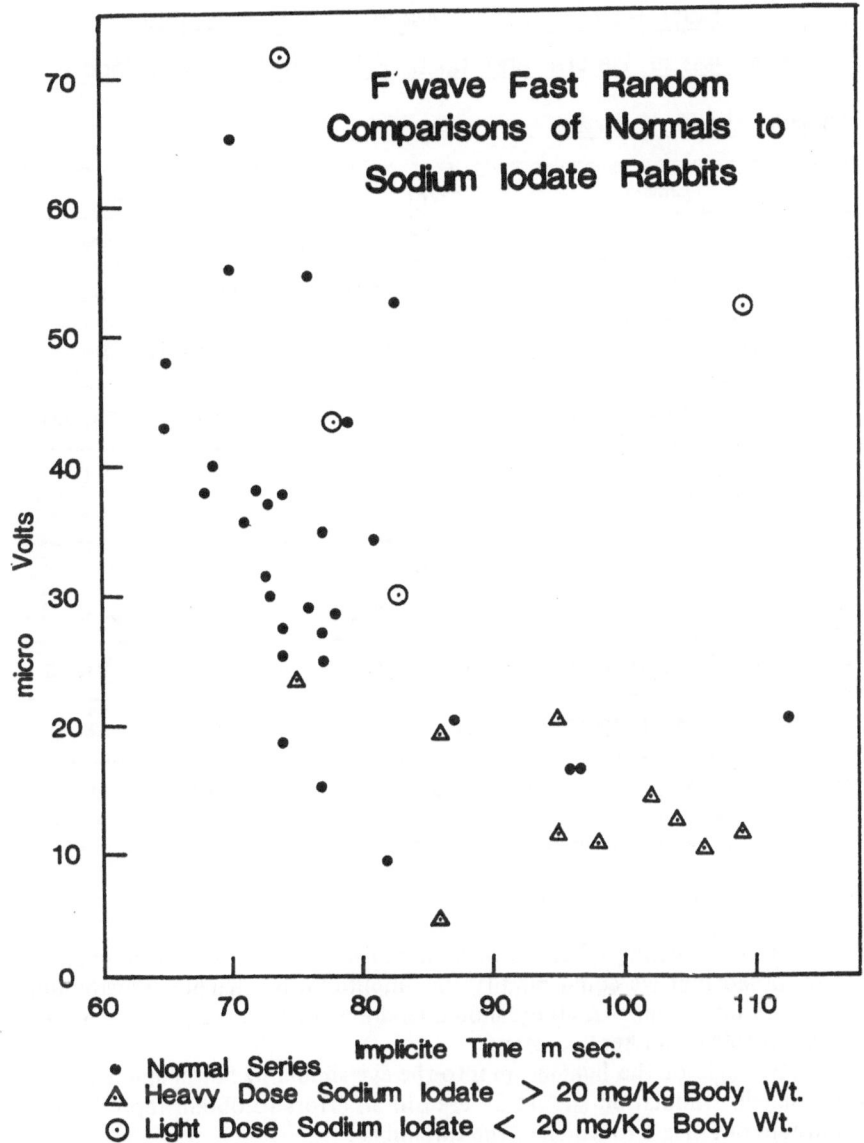

Fig. 5. The F waves of rabbits receiving large doses show prolongation of the implicit times.

test run of about 60 seconds is probably needed to reach a stable and reproducible level, although that must be determined by repeated testing of various durations.

(2) The amount of finger pressure on the contact lens electrode may cause the amplitudes of the waves to vary. Foulds and Johnson (1974) have

Slow Regular Stimuli Mean Values of Rabbits
ERG waves Before and up to 3 hr. after Sodium Iodate

Implicit Times in msec.

wave	N	Normals $\bar{X} \pm SD$	N	> 30 mg/Kg $\bar{X} \pm SD$	Significance	N	< 20 mg/Kg $\bar{X} \pm SD$	Significance
b-wave	30	41.7±2.9	10	53.6±5.0	P<.001	4	42.75±2.9	NS
F-wave	30	118.6±15.5	10	120.9±22.6	NS	4	125.9±3.4	NS
"C"-wave	30	195±25.90	10	218.4±18.7	P<.01	4	254.7±4.1	P<.001

Amplitudes in micro volts

wave	N	Normals $\bar{X} \pm SD$	N	> 30mg/Kg $\bar{X} \pm SD$	Significance	N	< 20 mg//Kg $\bar{X} \pm SD$	Significance
b-wave	30	131.7±41.47	10	59.4±42.1	P<.001	4	167.2±14.4	P<.05
F-wave	30	151.4±48.43	10	78.9±39.0	P<.001	4	171.7±60.3	NS
"C"-wave	30	16.5±12.0	10	36.7±18.3	P<.01	4	1.8±2.9	NS

NS = not significant at P<.05 level

Table 1.

described the lowering of the b-wave amplitude with ischaemia in rabbits, and we noted that we could modify the amplitudes by changing the amount of pressure on the lens. A study should be done in which the pressure on the lens is controlled and kept constant.

(3) The angle of the light beam into the eye should be better standardized or a ganzfeld stimulation should be used in an effort to obtain reproducible amplitudes or at least to decrease the variability.

(4) A larger series of test runs would be helpful in establishing the significance of changes in the ERG after dilation.

In spite of its shortcomings, this preliminary study does show the presence of a positive wave following the b-wave which persists after dilation. We could not demonstrate a significance in the changes which occurred after the injection of sodium iodate in the period up to 3 hours after the injection. Subsequent evaluation of ERG's done later will help to show what happens to the late positive wave over a period of time. One series of ERG's shows a flattening of the entire ERG and with no recovery after 7 months.

Fast Random Stimuli Mean Values ERG's in Normal Rabbits and Rabbits Given I.V. Sodium Iodate

Implicit Time in msec.

wave	N	$\bar{X}\pm SD$ (Normals)	N	$\bar{X}\pm SD$ (>30 mg/Kg)	Significance	N	$\bar{X}\pm SD$ (<20mg/Kg)	Significance
b-wave	30	34.3±3.1	10	51.8±6.0	P<.001	4	34.0±12.2	NS
F-wave	30	76.8±10.9	10	95.6±10.1	P<.001	4	86.1±13.6	NS
"C"-wave	30	215±37.5	10	217.9±27.9	NS	4	229.2±28.0	NS

Amplitudes in micro Volts

wave	N	$\bar{X}\pm SD$ (Normals)	N	$\bar{X}\pm SD$ (>30 mg/Kg)	Significance	N	$\bar{X}\pm SD$ (<20 mg/Kg)	Significance
b-wave	30	20.5±10.7	10	6.6±4.3	P<.001	4	33.1±14.9	P<.01
F-wave	30	36.9±17.6	10	15.4±5.9	P<.001	4	56.2±19.7	NS
"C"-wave	30	24.1±11.4	10	17.3±7.9	NS	4	34.9±13.2	NS

NS = not significant at P<.05 level

Table 2.

ACKNOWLEDGEMENT

The authors would like to acknowledge and express their thanks to the vision research group of Dr. Derek Fender at the California Institute of Technology for their help in setting up the apparatus used in these experiments, Dr. Irving Leopold for his help and support, Dr. Hiro Enomoto for his help in preparing the illustrations and Tom Merrill for his photography. We also wish to thank Debbie Hensen for her help with the actual experimentation.

REFERENCES

Foulds, W. S., Johnson, N. F.: Rabbit electroretinograms during recovery from induced ischaemia, Trans., Ophthalmol. Soc. U.K. 94: 383–393, 1974.
Larkin, R. M., Klein, S., Ogden, T. E., and Fender, D. H.: Nonlinear kernels of the human ERG, Biological Cybernetics 35: 145–160, 1979.

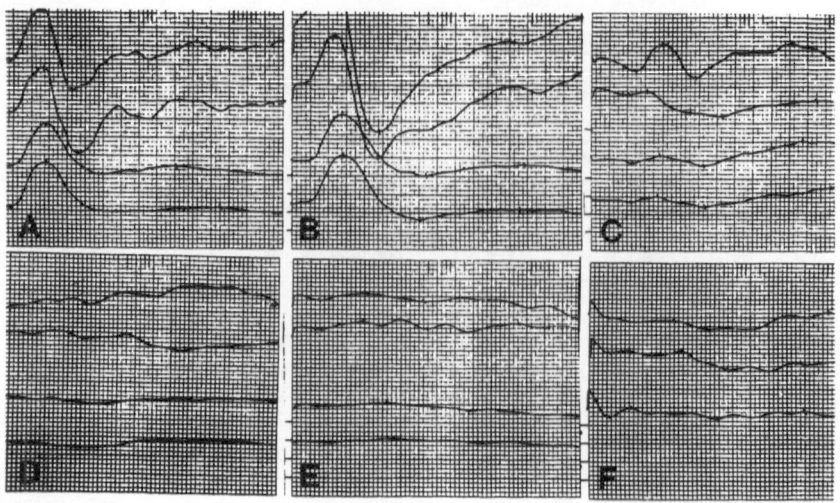

Fig. 6. (A) This shows the ERG of one eye prior to being given a large dose (over 40 mg/Kg body weight) of sodium iodate; (B) One hour after injection; (C) Three hours; (D) Five and one-half hours; (E) Seven months; (F) Three extra runs using fast random stimuli at seven months. For A–E, the format is the same as Figures 2 and 3.

Noell, W. K. (1953). Studies on the electrophysiology and the metabolism of the retina. U.S. Air Force. SAM Project 21–1201–0004, Randolph Field, Texas.

Pearlman, J. T.: The c-wave of the human ERG, Arch. of Ophthalmol. 68: 823–830, 1962.

Riggs, L. A. and Johnson, E. P.: Electrical responses of the human retina, J. Exp. Psychol. 39: 415, 1949.

Mailing address:
Department of Ophthalmology
California College of Medicine
University of California, Irvine
Irvine, California 92717, U.S.A.

342

A NEW DISPOSABLE ERG ELECTRODE UTILIZING A HYDROPHILIC SOFT CONTACT LENS WITH HIGH WATER CONTENT

K. YANASHIMA, S. OKISAKA, Y. INAGAKI AND H. KENJYO

Department of Ophthalmology, National Defense Medical College, Tokorozawa Department of Ophthalmology, Juntendo University, Tokyo Toray Co. Ltd., Ohotsu, Japan

A high water content soft contact lens (Toray) is used as an ERG electrode itself. The potentials are led off by carbonic fibers coated with a non-conductor without using any metal. The electrode can be worn with no local anesthesia and the visual acuity is not reduced. The cornea does not dry up. Blinking can be controlled. The length of the recording session does not appear to be limited by the use of this electrode. ERP, flash-ERG and pattern-ERG were recorded with this electrode which is thought to be the 'ERG electrode of the future.'

THE ERG IN RETINITIS PIGMENTOSA

A. SOLISH, J. HECKENLIVELY, AND D. MARTIN

Jules Stein Eye Institute, UCLA Center for Health Sciences, Los Angeles, California 90024, USA

The electroretinograms from 215 patients with Retinitis Pigmentosa (RP) were examined for recordability and presence of photopic flicker response. Ten diagnostic categories were established for the purpose of analysis, including rod-cone and cone-rod degenerations, choroideremia and Usher's syndrome. Rod-cone and cone-rod degeneration categories were differentiated by the pattern of the electroretinogram and by the final rod threshold values (patients with $\geqslant 2.0$ log units of elevation were placed in the rod-cone group).

Of 215 RP patients at least one component of the ERG was recordable in 89 patients (41.4%). There was a significant difference ($p < 0.001$) in recordability of ERG's between patients with rod-cone and those with cone-rod degeneration. In the cone-rod groups, more than 50% of patients had recordable ERG's, while every rod-cone group (including choroideremia), had less than 50% recordability.

Fourteen patients, representing 7 different diagnostic categories, had recordable photopic flicker responses despite a nonrecordable photopic, scotopic, or bright flash, dark-adapted ERG. In RP patients, the photopic flicker may be a more powerful stimulus to the retina than the diagnostic photopic or scotopic stimuli.

ALTERATIONS IN THE PHOTOPIC ERG AND OPTIC ATROPHY/DYSPLASIA IN CONGENITAL STATIONARY NIGHTBLINDNESS

J. HECKENLIVELY AND D. MARTIN

Jules Stein Eye Institute, UCLA Center for the Health Sciences, Los Angeles, California 90024, USA

Eight patients from six pedigrees have been identified with congenital stationary nightblindness in which there are similar changes, including congenital nightblindness, and myopia. The electroretinograms demonstrated photopic ERG's which are normal to subnormal in amplitudes and implicit times, and nonrecordable scotopic ERG's. The visual fields are normal for myopia.

The photopic ERG's were unique in that the oscillatory potentials are missing, leaving a characteristic 'squared-off' appearance to the a-wave. When the values are compared against an age-matched normal control group, the photopic b-wave amplitude was significantly smaller ($p \leqslant 0.004$), and the a-wave implicit time significantly longer ($p \leqslant 0.0001$). The bright flash, dark-adapted b-wave amplitude and implicit times were significantly smaller ($p \leqslant 0.0001$) and shorter ($p < 0.0001$). The a-wave amplitude and implicit time were significantly smaller ($p \leqslant 0.0002$) and longer ($p \leqslant 0.0001$).

All patients demonstrated optic atrophy and/or optic dysplasia, some of which looked 'tilted' but on examination with fluorescein angiography were found to have missing disc tissue even though papillary vessels were in their normal location.

SUPERNORMAL SCOTOPIC ERG IN MACULAR DYSTROPHY

K.R. ALEXANDER AND G.A. FISHMAN

University of Illinois Eye and Ear Infirmary, Chicago, Illinois 60612, USA

We have studied two patients with macular dystrophy who exhibit an unusual ERG response. When tested with bright light stimuli in the dark, both patients show a markedly increased ERG amplitude compared to normals. One patient appears similar to that reported earlier by Gouras et al. (ARVO, 1982), with an elevated rod ERG threshold and an increased slope of the amplitude-intensity function. The second patient with a supernormal scotopic ERG amplitude to bright-light stimuli showed a *normal* scotopic ERG response to less intense stimuli. Additional tests of visual function demonstrated other important differences between the two patients.

ERG AMPLITUDE AND LATENCY CHANGES DURING EARLY DIABETES MELLITUS IN RATS

W.M. KOZAK, L.G. DENEAULT AND J. ROGOWSKA

Biomedical Engineering Program, Carnegie-Mellon University, Pittsburgh, Pennsylvania 15213, USA

Electroretinograms (ERGs) were recorded in three insulin treatment groups of Wistar albino rats before and two to three weeks following the onset of Streptozotocin-induced diabetes mellitus, as well as in normal rats. 48 rats arbitrarily subdivided into four groups showed no significant inter-group differences between any ERG parameters at the start of the experiment, by two-tail t-test. Two week diabetic rats (no insulin) had significantly ($p < 0.03$ to 0.001) lower amplitudes of the a, b-waves and of the second wavelet and longer ($p < 0.02$ to 0.01) a-wave implicit time and of the first three averaged wavelets than the sex and age matched normal group. The same two week diabetic no insulin rats showed, to our surprise, higher b-amplitudes and wavelet amplitudes ($p < 0.002$ to 0.00002) and shorter ($p < 0.005$) a-wave implicit time than a matched group of rats injected once daily with $10 \, \text{u/Kg}$ insulin. Consequently, all amplitude parameters (a, b-waves, averaged 3 wavelets) were lower ($p < 0.01$ to 0.001) and the a-latency and wavelet latencies were longer ($p < 0.001$) in the once daily injection group than in the normal group. The latency to the b-intersection with the isopotential line and the parameters of the first wavelet were least different in the two groups. The a-wave and wavelet amplitudes and the a-, b-wave and wavelet latencies were the same in the normals and in rats receiving $3.3 \, \text{u/Kg}$ insulin thrice daily. The once daily insulin and the thrice daily insulin groups differed dramatically with respect to all amplitude parameters (thrice daily being higher, $p < 0.002$ to 0.0001) and all latency parameters (thrice daily being shorter, $p < 0.001$).

LUMINANCE EFFECTS ON LATENCY AND TOPOGRAPHY OF AVERAGE PATTERN-EVOKED POTENTIALS

E. ADACHI-USAMI AND D. LEHMANN

(Chiba, Japan and Zürich, Switzerland)

ABSTRACT

With decreasing target luminance (0 to 2.0 log unit density filters), the latency of the checkerboard reversal-evoked scalp potential component P1 increased non-linearly in a population of 17 healthy volunteers. It is suggested that the non-linear latency increase in the evoked potential reflects the gradual increase of rod activity at the lower luminance level.

INTRODUCTION

The latency of the pattern evoked cortical potential (EP) varies not only as a function of pathological conditions of the visual system (Halliday, 1973), but also as a function of age (Celesia and Daly, 1977, Shaw and Cant, 1980 and Sokol et al., 1981) and of stimulus condition.

In order to elucidate the latency changes in patients, a number of papers have investigated baseline data in normal subjects. It has been reported that defocussing (Duwaer and Spekreijse, 1978), contrast change (Spekreijse et al., 1979), spatial frequency (Parker and Salzen, 1977), target size (Spekreijse et al., 1979), retinal stimulus location (Lehmann and Skrandies, 1979), and mono- *vs* binocular viewing conditions (Adachi-Usami and Lehmann, 1982) influence EP latency. Some effects of target luminance on the latency of the pattern-evoked potentials were reported: Van der Tweel et al. (1979) investigated appearance-disappearance responses; Cant et al. (1978) and Halliday (1977) used checkerboard reversal stimuli, and reported 12 and 15 msec increases of latency per log neutral density filter unit. However, none gave data for a luminance dependency for the rate of the latency increase. We decided to re-examine the luminance effects on latency, including topography of the pattern reversal evoked potentials.

METHODS

Checkerboard reversal stimuli were presented via a feedback-controlled (no overshoot or ringing) mirror galvanometer projector system to 17 normal subjects (20–47 years old), using 50 cd/m² mean luminance, 94% contrast, 2/sec reversal rate, less than 0.5 msec reversing time, lower visual field semi-circular target field of 16 degrees in a diameter, 90 cm viewing distance, and check size of 56 min arc. Neutral density filters (Kodak Wratten Filters) with densities of 0.3, 1.0, 1.5 and 2.0 log units were placed in front of the eye to attenuate the pattern luminance. This means that the minimum luminance used in the present experiment was 0.5 cd/m². No pupil dilation or artificial pupil was used. We checked the pupil size in our experimental conditions by varying the luminance level for over 2 log units. No change of pupil size was measurable.

Scalp field potentials were sampled from four occipital midline electrodes between inion and 7.5 cm above inion, using an anterior reference at 30% nasion-inion. With a bandpass of 0.3–100 Hz, 93 responses were averaged in each run. Averaging was done either on-line with a CAT 1000, plotted, and measured by hand, or on-line or off-line (playback from analog tape) with a PDP 11/34 computer.

The latency of the evoked component P1 was determined in each run within a time window between 80 to 140 msec by searching for the time with the maximal, occipitally positive potential difference (Lehmann and Skrandies 1979, Lehmann et al, in press) between any two of the five electrodes. This measurement (without pre-selected reference) approximates global scalp field power, i.e. the unbiased determination of the maximal, global amount of relief and thereby of the maximal response strength in an electrical scalp field distribution map (Lehmann and Skrandies 1980), and avoids a pre-selection of an assumedly inactive reference electrode for evaluation (although a common reference is necessary for recording, another electrode than the anterior reference could have detected the most negative field value in a given run; actually this never happened in the present data). Using the component latency thus determined, the instantaneous voltage profile of the field distri-bution along the scalp midline can be plotted for unbiased topography of the component. In all measurements, technical zero (averaged short-circuited pre-amplifier input) of each channel was used as measurement zero baseline (Lehmann and Brown 1980, Lehmann et al. in press).

RESULTS

Actual VECPs recorded from the inion *vs* the anterior references to varied pattern luminance by inserting the neutral density filters of 0.3, 1.0, 1.5 and 2.0 log units in front of the eye are presented in Fig. 1. It is clearly seen that the latency of the major positive component around 100 msec (P1) increases as the pattern luminance decreases. Similar latency changes were found at the other three electrode positions, as shown in Figure 2 which demonstrates representative potentials evoked in 'no filter' and '2.0 log filter' conditions.

In Fig. 3, the mean P1 peak latency obtained from the data of the 17 normal subjects is plotted as a function of log luminance (indicated as log NDF inserted in front of the eye). Decreasing stimulus luminance from 0 to

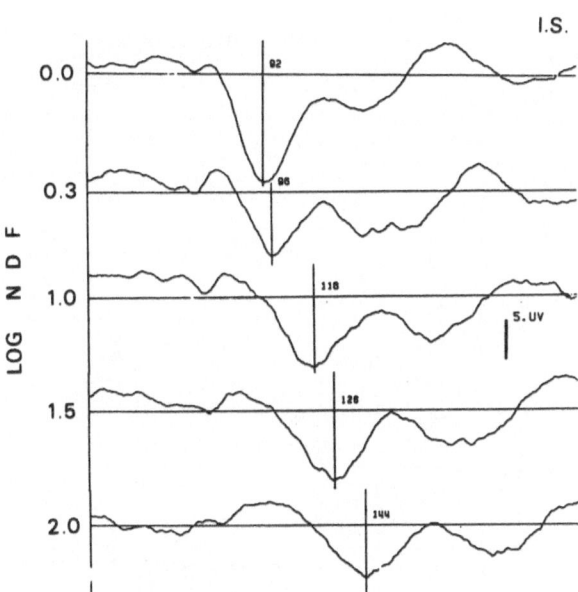

Fig. 1. Average pattern reversal evoked potentials of one subject, at five different levels of luminance (neutral density filters of 0.0, 0.3, 1.0, 1.5 and 2.0 log units in front of the eye). Electrodes at inion and 30% nasion-inion. Positivity at the inion is downward deflection. The maximum positive peak around the major positive component was determined and indicated with the vertical bar. Stimuli: Checkerboard pattern reversal 2 c/sec subtended 16 degrees semi-circular lower half field. 56′ check size, 94% contrast, the maximum mean luminance (without filter, indicated with NDF 0.0) 50 cd/m².

1.5 log units caused linear increases of the evoked potential latency of 18.1 msec per log unit luminance attenuation. However, further luminance attenuation to 2.0 log units increased the latency non-linearly by a rate of 19 msec per *0.5* log unit decrease of luminance. The mean latency values at 0, 0.3, 1.0 and 1.5 log units neutral density filter are almost perfectly fitted by a straight line. Linearly predicting the value for 1.5 log units from the other three values showed no significant deviation of the measured values from the predicted value. However, linearly predicting the value for 2.0 log units from the other four values resulted in a point (at 136 msec) from which the measured entries (mean 147 msec) deviated significantly (Wilcoxon single ended p near 0.005). Thus, the latency vs log luminance curve shows a kink at the luminance level of 1.5 log unit attenuation.

The topography of the mean evoked potential distributions over all subjects in the anterior-posterior direction along the midline is shown in Fig. 4 as voltage (amplitude) profiles at component latency. In order to compare directly the field profile data for the five luminance levels, the voltage (amplitude) profiles were scaled so that the maximal value equalled

355

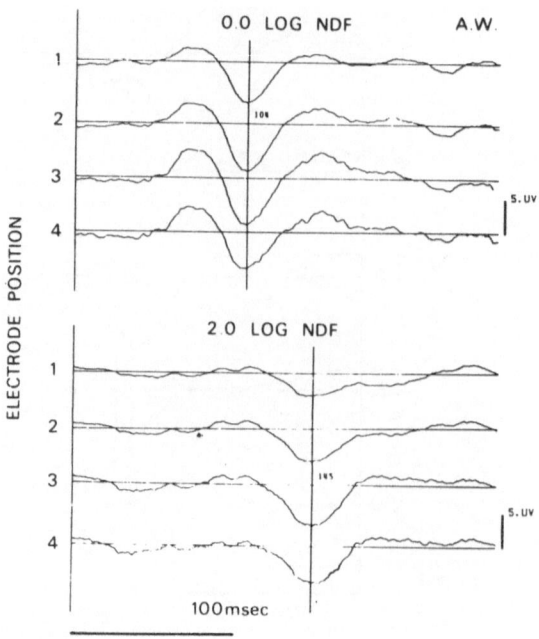

Fig. 2. Pattern reversal evoked potentials of one subject, recorded from 4 electrode positions along the midline (number 4: at the inion, 3: 2.5 cm above inion, 2: 5 cm above inion, and 1: as 7.5 cm above inion) for two different levels of the luminance. Without filter, the luminance was 50 cm/m², with 2.0 log ND Filter, 0.5 cd/m². Stimulus conditions were the same as described in the legend of Fig. 1.

100% for all cases. There was no significant difference between the data for the different luminance levels.

DISCUSSION

The increase of the latency per 1.0 log unit attenuation of the luminance was reported as 15 msec by Halliday (1977), 12 msec by Cant et al. (1978), 25 msec by Spekreijse et al. (1979) and 30 msec by Van der Tweel et al. (1979). None of the authors reported a change of the rate (i.e. non-linearity of the latency increase) as function of luminance. The reported results cannot be compared directly, since the luminance ranges and stimulus modes were different. Van der Tweel et al. (1979) and Spekreijse et al. (1979) employed high luminances (200 asb and 15,000 photopic trolands as maximum). However, in our data the rate of latency increase was smaller with higher than with lower luminances. Therefore, the latter authors' latency increase values of 25 msec and 30 msec per 1.0 log decrease of the luminance do not directly contradict our observations. The differences of the stimulus mode and the measured EP component wave (they used the main negative component of the appearance-disappearance response and we used the major positive

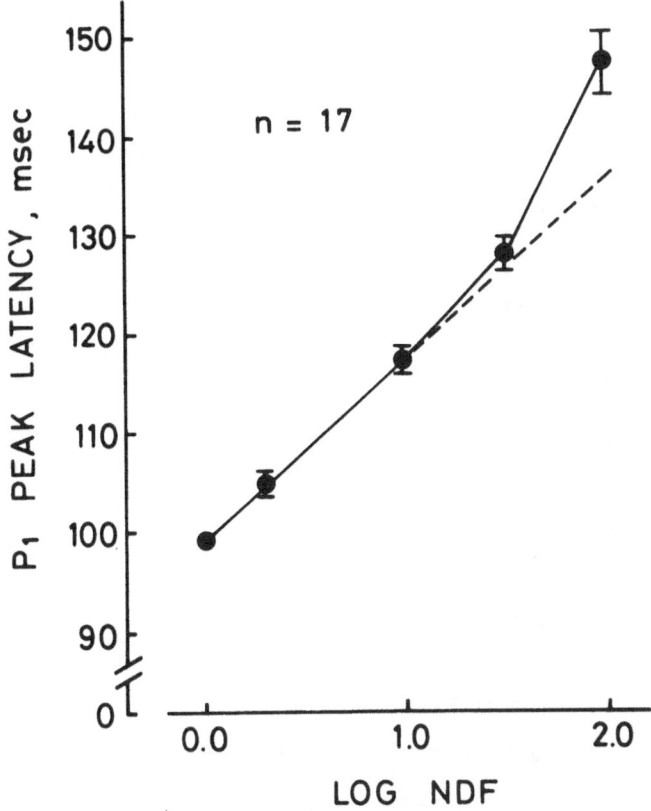

Fig. 3. Peak latency of the major positive component (P1) of the evoked potential as a function of luminance (given as neutral density filter). Mean data and standard error of 17 normal subjects. For stimulus conditions, see Fig. 1.

component of the pattern reversal EPs) likely contributed in addition to the divergence of results. Notwithstanding, it is noteworthy that van der Tweel (1979) found a constant value of increase of the latency for the luminous range over 6 log units; their lowest luminance of 6 log unit density filters was thus much lower than the luminance used in the present study, and the contrast which they used was 2.5 times threshold, obviously also much lower than ours. This might well be another reason for the disagreement with our results.

On the other hand, Halliday (1977) and Cant et al. (1978) employed nearly the same stimulus conditions as were used in the present study, but they did not report a luminance dependency for the rate of the latency increase. Halliday found 15 msec increase of latency per log unit decrease of luminance over the entire examined range of 5 log units; this implies that they used much lower luminances than we did. At lower luminance, we found a greater increase of latency than at high levels. Cant et al. (1978)

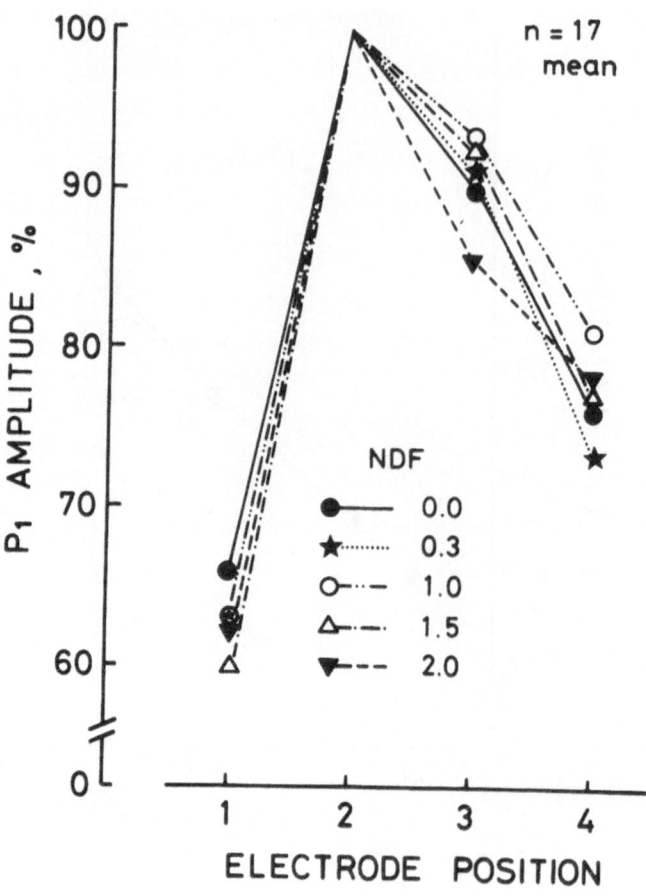

Fig. 4. Evoked potential field voltage (amplitude) profiles for P1, i.e. amplitudes plotted at P1 latency against electrode positions, along the midline (1 = most anterior, 4 = most posterior electrode). The profiles for the five different luminance levels were scaled to unity maximal values. Mean of 17 normal subjects.

did not test at luminance levels lower than 5 cd/m², corresponding to about 1.0 log units NDF in the present study. As to their results for the luminance range of 5 to 50 cd/m² (i.e. 0 to 1.0 log units NDF in our results), there was a good agreement with our data.

The greater increase of the latency observed by us at the lower luminance level suggests a crucial rod system contribution to the overhead potential. With lower luminances more rods will be activated. Thus, the greater increase of the latency might be caused by a substantial increase of rod activity coming into play at the luminance level of 0.5 cd/m², as incremental threshold studies with EP methods had suggested earlier (Adachi-Usami, 1974). This luminance level is, however, not yet in the absolute scotopic range, rather in a mesopic range.

In spite of this indication of an increased rod contribution to the cortical evoked potential waveform there was no significant shift of the maximum potential value to more anterior scalp locations, as one might have expected for a relative increase of more peripheral retinal upper hemiretina activation. Presumably, the luminances used at the mesopic level were not low enough to activate the rods selectively.

Van der Tweel et al. (1979) reported that there was no change in evoked potential wave shape when the stimulus luminance was attenuated over 6 log units. We used the evaluation procedure of Van der Tweel et al., shifting the potential wave shapes so as to align the peak point of the major positive component in the data of a subject (Fig. 5). Figure 5 shows that as luminance decreases, P1 is broadened, as indicated by the increasing time between preceding and following negative peak. This observation is similar to those reported by Spekreijse et al. (1973). We concur in the latter authors' explanation that most likely, the contrast change which was associated with the luminance change in Van der Tweel et al.'s (1979) experiments explains the difference in results.

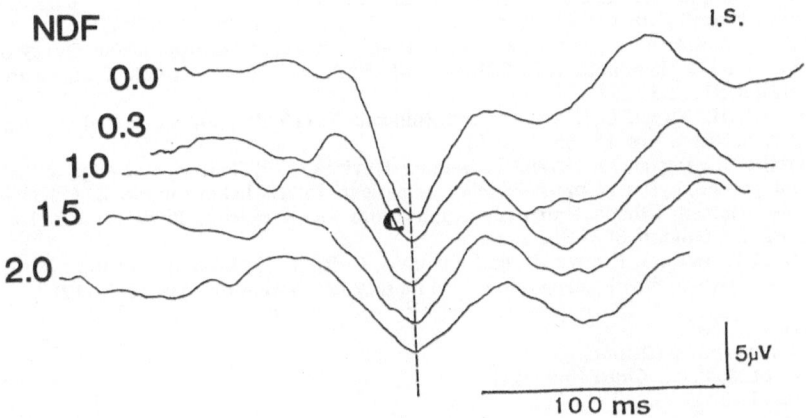

Fig. 5. Pattern reversal evoked potentials of one subject, recorded from the inion *vs* the anterior reference, at the five different luminance levels of the stimulus. The wave forms were shifted laterally to align the positive peaks. For stimulus conditions, see legend Fig. 1.

REFERENCES

Adachi-Usami, E. (1974) Incremental threshold as obtained by the visually evoked cortical potentials (VECP). Ophthal. Res. 6: 55–63.

Adachi-Usami, E. and Lehmann, D. (1982) Scalp field topography of monocular and binocular evoked potentials: upper and lower hemiretinal stimuli. Docum. Ophthal. Proc. Series, 31: 391–398.

Cant, B. R., Hume, Ann L. and Shaw, N. A. (1978) Effects of luminance on the pattern visual evoked potential in multiple sclerosis. Electroenceph. Clin. Neurophysiol. 45: 496–504.

Celesia, G. G. and Daly, R. F. (1977) Effects of aging on visual evoked responses. Arch. Neurol. (Chic.) 34: 403–407.

Duwaer, A. L. and Spekreijse, H. (1978) Latency of luminance and contrast evoked potentials in multiple sclerosis patients. Electroenceph. Clin. Neurophysiol. 45: 244–258.

Halliday, A. M., McDonald, W. I. and Mushin, J. (1973) Visual evoked response in the diagnosis of multiple sclerosis. Brit. med. J. 4: 661–664.

Halliday, A. M. (1977) Cortical EPs in man. Clinical observations. In: Spekreijse, H. and Tweel, L. H. van der (eds) Spatial Contrast, Report of a Workshop. North Holland, Amsterdam, pp. 84–89.

Lehmann, D. and Brown, W. S. (1980) How to measure evoked EEG potentials for topography. In: C. Barber (ed.) Evoked Potentials. MTP, Lancaster, pp. 143–148.

Lehmann, D. and Skrandies, W. (1979) Multichannel evoked potential fields show different properties of human upper and lower hemiretina systems. Exp. Brain Res. 35: 151–159.

Lehmann, D. and Skrandies, W. (1980) Reference-free identification of checkerboard-evoked multichannel potential fields. Electroenceph. Clin Neurophysiol. 48: 609–621.

Lehmann, D., Skrandies, W. and Adachi-Usami, E. (1982 in press) In: . . Rothenberger (ed.) Elsevier, Amsterdam.

Parker, D. M. and Salzen, E. A. (1977) Latency changes in the human visual evoked response to sinusoidal gratings. Vision Res. 17: 1201–1204.

Shaw, N. A. and Cant, B. R. (1980) Age-dependent changes in the latency of the pattern visual evoked potential. Electroenceph. Clin. Neurophysiol. 48: 237–241.

Sokol, S., Moskowitz, A. and Towle, V. L. (1981) Age-related changes in the latency of the visual evoked potential: Influence of check size. Electroenceph. Clin. Neurophysiol. 51: 559–562.

Spekreijse, H., Tweel, L. H. van der and Zuidema, T. (1973) Contrast evoked response in man. Vision Res. 13: 1577–1601.

Spekreijse, H., Duwaer, A. L. and Posthumus Meyjes (1979) Contrast evoked potentials and psychophysics in multiple sclerosis patient. In: D. Lehmann and E. Callaway (eds) Human Evoked Potentials Applications and Problems. Plenum Press, New York and London, 363–381.

Tweel, L. H. van der, Estévez, O. and Cavonius, C. R. (1979) Invariance of the contrast evoked potential with changes in retinal illuminance. Vision Res. 19: 1283–1287

Mailing address:
Department of Ophthalmology
School of Medicine, Chiba University
Inohana 1–8–1
280 Chiba, Japan

OCULOMOTOR BEHAVIOR IN HUMAN ALBINOS

P. APKARIAN, H. SPEKREIJSE AND H. COLLEWIJN

(Amsterdam and Rotterdam, The Netherlands)

ABSTRACT

In a recent visual evoked potential (VEP) investigation (Apkarian et al., 1982), asymmetry in the monocular VEP, reflecting abnormal retino-geniculo-cortical projections, was detected in all albinos with measurable responses and with zero false positives in non-albino controls. In contrast to monocular VEP asymmetry, oculomotor disturbances such as nystagmus, an established albino concomitant, are neither a specific nor an obligate albino pathognomonic. Because not all albinos demonstrate oculomotor disturbances whereas non-albinos may, the link between aberrant projections and organization of the oculomotor control centers in these patients is at question. To address this problem we have examined spontaneous eye movements, simultaneously recorded during VEP measurements, and stimulus induced optokinetic nystagmus (OKN) in albinos with nystagmus, an albino without nystagmus and a non-albino with nystagmus. As an objective confirmation of the clinical diagnosis, all subjects tested in this investigation were screened for VEP albino asymmetry. Simultaneously recorded EOGs indicated curious disjunctive eye movements; under certain conditions, the amplitude of the movement of one eye was significantly greater than that of the other eye. With OKN recordings, examined with both full-field and half-field conditions as a function of direction of target motion, inverted OKN was observed for an albino observer as well as for the non-albino control. One albino who did not show inverted OKN under any conditions, did show OKN directional asymmetry during partial-field stimulation. The variable OKN response patterns observed in our subject sample indicate that OKN disturbances, particularly inverted OKN and OKN directional asymmetry, necessitate further investigation to determine the relationship between aberrant retinal fiber projections and oculomotor control.

INTRODUCTION

Nystagmus and a high incidence of strabismus are well established clinical features of albinism (Bergsma, 1973). Concomitant with these oculomotor disturbances, striking visual pathway anomalies, most notably misrouted retinal fibers, are also manifest in albinism (Guillery et al., 1975). The presence of abnormal retinal to subcortical and cortical optic fiber projections is now well established anatomically and electrophysiologically in both human albinos (Creel et al., 1981; Coleman et al., 1979) and in several other species of albino mammals (Lund, 1965; Gross and Hickey, 1980; Guillery and Kaas, 1971; 1973).

Although we do not yet fully understand the etiology or the precise topography of the misrouting of retinal regions, particularly with respect to the oculomotor system, we do know that temporal retinal fibers which should remain ipsilateral erroneously decussate at the optic chiasm, subsequently producing reduced ipsilateral ganglion cell projections, throughout the visual pathways. Autoradiographic studies in tyrosinase-negative albino cats (Creel et al., 1982) have revealed aberrant ipsilateral input to the laminated dorsal and ventral lateral geniculate nucleus, medial interlaminar nucleus, retinal recipient zone of the pulvinar complex, pretectum and superior colliculus. Investigations in albino rats (Lund, 1965), Siamese cats (Weber et al., 1978) and albino guinea pigs (Giollo and Creel, 1973) have also revealed a paucity of ipsilateral projections to the pretectum and superior colliculus. These subcortical anomalies are preserved, at least in humans, at the cortical level (Guillery et al., 1975). Of clinical importance is that the resultant retinotopic cortical anomalies are reflected in the scalp recorded visual evoked potential (VEP) and can be used in the diagnosis of albinism. The basic electrophysiological albino feature is that the misrouted optic pathway projections produce visual evoked potential asymmetry across the occipital left and right hemispheres.

Under optimal test conditions, described in detail in a previous report (Apkarian et al., 1982) misrouted optic fiber projections could be detected in all albinos with measurable responses (N = 78) and with zero false positive in normal controls (N = 34), including heterozygote family members and non-albinos with comparable albino symptoms (e.g. nystagmus, reduced visual acuity). These results suggest that monocular VEP asymmetry can be considered a specific and obligate albino pathognomonic.

Whether oculomotor disturbances in albinism such as nystagmus are a consequence of the aberrant neural circuitry or rather a result of abnormal ocular factors, e.g. foveal hypoplasia, or high refractive error (Duke-Elder, 1963; Krill, 1977), has not yet been determined. Furthermore, as not all albinos manifest oculomotor disturbance like nystagmus whereas some non-albinos may, the link between aberrant projections and aberrant organization of the oculomotor control centers is at question. Although abnormal optokinetic nystagmus (OKN) has been reported for the albino rat (Precht and Cazin, 1979), rabbit (Collewijn et al., 1978) and human albino (Wildberger and Meyer, 1978), it is not known whether similar OKN anomalies can be detected or induced in albinos with asymptomatic oculomotor behavior.

In the oculomotor study of albino rabbits by Collewijn et al. (1978), a stable eye position and relatively normal OKN reactions were found when full-field stimulation was used. With partial-field stimulation eye position became dramatically unstable and the optokinetic eye movements were inverted i.e. the direction of pursuit was opposite to the direction of stimulus motion. Since this change in behavior did not occur in non-albino rabbits, this finding suggested that restricted retinal stimulation may help to reveal oculomotor anomalies which otherwise would remain undetected. With an oculomotor recording method developed by Collewijn (1977) and Van Die and Collewijn (1982) stimulation of selective retinal regions is possible (even in subjects with severe nystagmus) by means of a servo-control system which locks the stimulus field to eye position. With this experimental method we were afforded the opportunity to investigate various OKN properties with either full-field or partial-field stimulation in albinos with nystagmus, albinos without nystagmus and a non-albino control with congenital nystagmus. This paper presents our preliminary OKN findings. In addition we present examples of unusual EOG response profiles recorded while simultaneously recording VEPs.

METHODS AND MATERIALS

Subjects

The data presented in this paper are from six subjects ranging in age from 12 to 32 years. One subject was clinically identified as tyrosinase-positive oculo-cutaneous albino, one as tyrosinase-negative oculocutaneous albino and three as ocular albino. A non-albino control who suffered from congenital nystagmus, also participated. All subjects underwent a complete ophthalmic examination, phenotypic evaluation and pedigree analysis. Visual evoked potentials (VEPs) were recorded in all subjects to verify the present or absence of misrouting. Electro-oculography (EOG) recordings in response to VEP stimuli were obtained in three subjects (albinos ELS, BRD and ROO); opto-kinetic nystagmus (OKN) recordings were obtained in the remaining three (albinos STE and JHOU and non-albino, JON). A summary of the clinical history for each subject is presented in Table I.

			VEP FINDINGS	OPHTHALMOLOGICAL FINDINGS					
PATIENT	AGE/SEX	CLINICAL CLASSIFICATION	MONOCULAR ASYMMETRY	CORRECTED VISUAL ACUITY	FUNDUS PIGMENT	MACULAR REFLEX	IRIS TRANSLUCENCY	PHOTOPHOBIA	NYSTAGMUS
ELS	12/F	ty-pos albino	present	OD,.3, OS,.3	+	-	+	+	+
ROO	32/F	ty-neg albino	present	OD,.1, OS,.15	-	-	+	±	+
BRD	32/M	ocular albino	present	OD,.2, OS,.2	+	-	+	+	+
STE	27/M	ocular albino	present	OD,.1, OS,.12	+	-	+	±	+
JHOU	26/M	ocular albino	present	OD,.5, OS,.5	+	-	+	+	-
JON	28/M	non-albino	absent	OD,.4, OS,.5	+	+	-	-	+

ty-pos = tyrosinase positive oculocutaneous, ty-neg = tyrosinase negative oculocutaneous
present (+), absent (-)

Table 1. VEP results and clinical observations in our patients with albinism

STIMULUS AND RECORDING

VEP and EOG

For simultaneous VEP and EOG recordings, the stimulus consisted of white and black checkerboard patterns of approximately 100% contrast generated on a TV screen (Sony CVM-1810E, 50 Hz). The mode of stimulus presentation was pattern appearance (300 msec)/disappearance (500 msec) at a constant mean luminance of 64 cd/m^2. For more details see Spekreijse et al. (1973). Viewing distance was 100 cm, check size 55' of visual angle and field size 20° (horizontal) by 15° (vertical); a 10' red square centered within the stimulus field served as the fixation spot.

Both the VEPs and EOGs were recorded with tinned/copper cup electrodes of 8 mm diameter. For VEPs, 5 active electrodes were positioned with equal spacing of 3 cm in a horizontal row, one cm above the inion, across the left and right occiput. Reference for VEP electrodes was linked ears; the common ground electrode was located at the vertex. For EOGs two active electrodes were positioned near the outer canthi of the left and right eye; the reference electrode was positioned at the nasion. The EEG and EOGs were amplified (Medelec/Van Gogh) and filtered with a bandwidth of 0.5 to 70 Hz. Filtered EEG signals were averaged with a HP2100 computer; EOG signals were recorded with a penwriter.

Procedure: Binocular, left and right eye responses were recorded for each stimulus condition while the subjects were comfortably seated in an electrically-shielded room. Monocular recordings were obtained with total occlusion of the fellow-eye. EOG signals were simultaneously measured for both left and right eye regardless of stimulus condition.

OKN

Stimulus: For OKN recordings the stimulus consisted of a hemicylindrical screen with a radius of 0.80 m and a height of 1.25 m upon which a square-wave pattern (0.2 cycles/degree) was projected from an overhead rotating cylindrical grid. During this investigation the grid was rotated at a constant speed of 30 deg/sec either leftward or rightward. Partial-field occlusion was obtained by cylindrical masks placed at various angular positions around the grid. The occluded sector was locked to a particular retinal area by a servo mechanism which was driven by the eye position. With this procedure, the retinal area of stimulation is unaffected by eye movements. For more details see Van Die and Collewijn (1982).

Recording: Monocular horizontal eye position was measured by an electromagnetic technique described in full detail by Collewijn et al. (1977). The basic technique consists of phase detection of a signal induced in a scleral search coil by a rotating, homogeneous A.C. magnetic field. The induction coil is embedded in an annular silicone contact lens which adheres comfortably and firmly to the limbic area, concentric with the cornea (Collewijn

364

et al., 1975). Eye position and velocity were recorded on a penwriter and magnetic tape on-line digitized and analysed by a DEC PDP11/10 computer.

Procedure: For OKN measurements only one eye bore the recording annulus. Subjects were seated with the head supported by a chin rest in the center of the hemicylindrical screen and were instructed to attend to the moving stripes without attempting to deliberately pursue a single stripe.

RESULTS

Visual evoked potential screening

Results from the VEP screening are presented in Fig. 1. Albino asymmetry can be seen in Fig. 1A–E, by comparing the left eye responses (left columns) to those of the right eye (right columns). The peak of the potential distribution for the left eye is localized across the right hemisphere whereas the peak of the potential distribution for the right eye is localized across the left hemisphere. Albino asymmetry in the potential distribution can also be seen by a change in sign (see arrows) of the difference potential (bottom-most trace) from left to right eye stimulation. Whether oculocutaneous (Figs. 1A and B) or ocular (Figs. 1C and E), all albinos show asymmetry in the distribution of the responses across the scalp in contrast to the response profiles of the non-albino control (Fig. 1F). Note for this latter subject the stability of the location of the peak of the potential distribution in the monocular responses. Note also that there is no change in the sign of the difference potential (bottom-most traces, L–R). The comparable monocular hemispheric laterality seen in Fig. 1F is as expected due to the fact that under monocular whole field stimulation in non-albinos, both the left and right hemispheres receive nearly symmetric input from temporal and nasal retinal fiber projections.

EOG Observations

While monitoring eye movements during our visual evoked potential recording sessions, we serendipituously observed the curious oculomotor responses depicted in Fig. 2. In the examples presented, upper traces represent simultaneously recorded left (upper) and right eye (lower) EOGs during binocular viewing of an abruptly appearing/disappearing checkerboard pattern (check size was 55′). Middle traces represent left and right eye EOGs recorded during right eye stimulation (the fellow eye was totally occluded) and lower traces represent left and right eye EOGs with left eye stimulation. In the first response triad (binocular, monocular right eye open, monocular left eye open) for tyrosinase-positive oculocutaneous albino, ELS, the amplitude of the occluded left eye movement increased dramatically relative to the amplitude of the right eye. For this subject left and right eye movements remained comparable in type with either binocular or left eye stimulation.

365

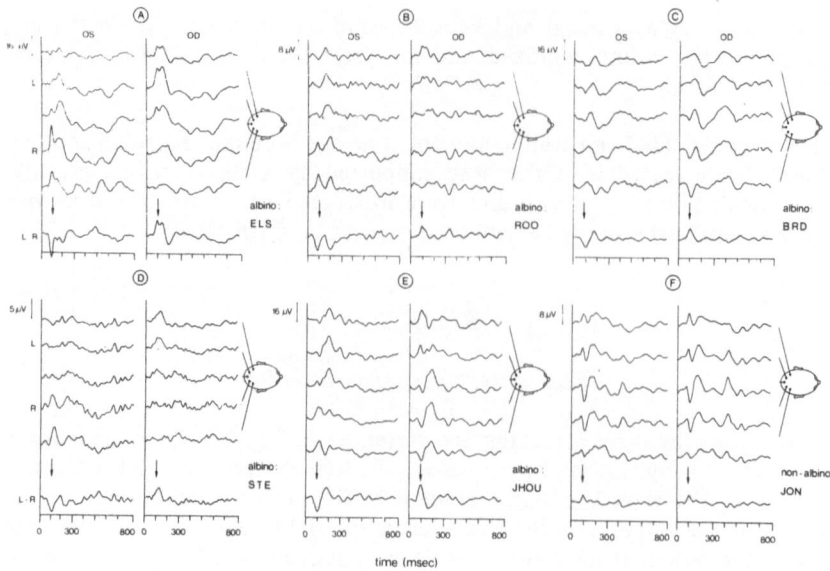

Fig. 1. Left eye (OS) and right eye (OD) responses to an appearing (300 msec)/disappearing (500 msec) checkerboard pattern for albinos (A–E) and a non-albino control (F). Each pattern element subtended 55'. The upper five traces for each condition represent monopolar responses derived from one of five electrodes; the bottom-most traces represent a bipolar derivation obtained by subtracting trace R (from a right hemisphere) from trace L (from a left hemisphere). For albinos (A–E), the location of the peak of the potential distribution within an early response component changes dramatically with left to right eye stimulation. Note also from the bipolar derivation the change in sign at 100 msec (see arrows). For the non-albino (F) the peak of the potential distribution across the scalp remains stable. Although hemispheric laterality is present, the difference potential does not change in sign from left to right eye stimulation.

The instability in eye movement frequency with binocular stimulation is inconsequential reflecting the high degree of oculomotor instability noted for albino subjects. The disjunctive amplitude effect seen here with left eye occlusion proved independent of stimulus condition. Similar effects were found with a reversal stimulus, smaller pattern sizes and even a homogeneous stationary field. Furthermore, within a given condition, the difference in amplitude could wax and wane, change from the occluded to non-occluded eye or disappear altogether. An example of an increased response amplitude for the non-occluded eye relative to the occluded eye is seen in the second response triad for tyrosinase-negative oculocutaneous albino, ROO. Following left eye occlusion the stimulated right eye shows a larger amplitude; following right eye occlusion, the left eye shows an amplitude increase. The disjunctive amplitude effect is also not restricted to a monocular situation. In the last response triad for ocular albino, BRD, an example of disjunctive left and right eye amplitude with binocular stimulation is presented. Note that the effect is no longer present during monocular stimulation of the right eye and only just noticeable during monocular stimulation of the left eye.

366

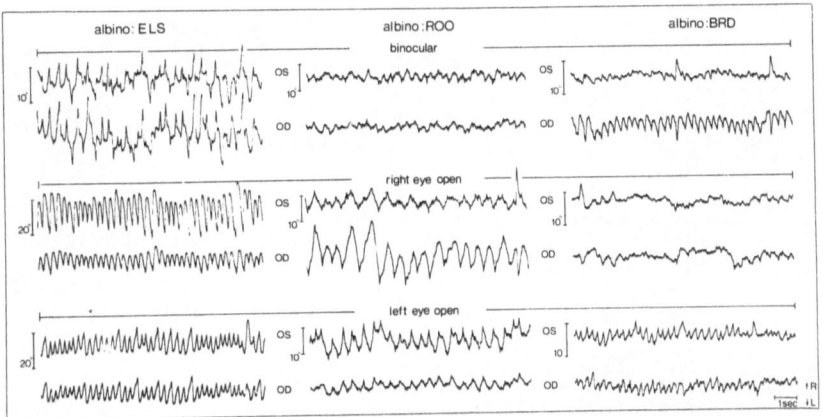

Fig. 2. Left (OS) and right (OD) eye movements in three albinos obtained while simultaneously recording VEPs. An increased amplitude of one eye relative to the fellow eye is present under monocular viewing conditions for either the occluded eye (first column, right eye open), or the open eye (second column, right or left eye open) and under binocular conditions (third column, both eyes open). Note that while the amplitude of the eye movements is disjunctive, phase and frequency appear to remain conjugate.

OKN Observations

Results from the investigation of optokinetic nystagmus in albino, STE, and non-albino, JON, are presented in Fig. 3. The recordings seen here were obtained from the left eye during binocular full-field stimulation. Direction of target motion is labeled above the traces of eye position (P) and eye velocity (V). The direction of the fast saccadic phase of the OKN is most clearly seen by inspection of the velocity traces. Fast phase in a left direction is represented by a large upward deflection. For an observer with normal OKN, the slow phase tracking movement follows the direction of the target motion and is interrupted periodically by a fast phase in the opposite direction. Both albino, STE and non-albino, JON, however, show inverted OKN responses. The direction of smooth pursuit tracking movement or slow phase is opposite to the target motion; the direction of the saccadic or fast phase is the same as that of the target motion. In contrast to these abnormal OKN responses we present, in Fig. 4 the OKN recordings of albino, JHOU, who shows normal tracking behavior in response to either binocular or monocular (left eye), full-field stimulation. For left and right target motion, OKN was in the normal direction.

Relatively normal OKN direction was also preserved in this subject with left eye half-field stimulation as seen in Fig. 5. Responses during temporal field (nasal retina) or nasal field (temporal retina) stimulation show a slow phase to the right, fast phase to the left with rightward target motion and a slow phase to the left and fast phase to the right with leftward target motion. Although half-field stimulation did not reveal an inverted OKN response. This stimulus condition did induce greater eye movement instability and

367

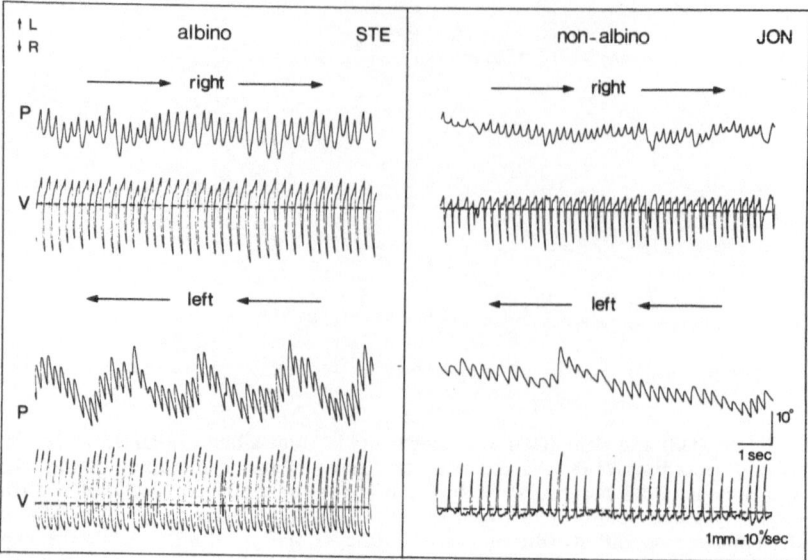

Fig. 3. Left eye recordings of OKN in albino, STE (left) and non-albino, JON (right) elicited by target motion to the right or left under binocular viewing conditions. Stimulus velocity was 30 deg/sec; recordings are from a curvilinear penrecorder. Upper traces in each group represent position (P), lower traces, velocity (V). Large deflections in the velocity traces above the zero line (dashed line) represent fast phase to the left, large deflections below the zero line represent fast phase to the right. Note that inverted OKN was elicited in both subjects with either leftward or rightward motion of the stimulus pattern.

directional asymmetry (i.e. the OKN is driven better in one horizontal direction in the visual field than in the other). Responses from centrifugal stimulation (target motion away from the macular region) are more stable and show relatively normal pursuit compared to responses from centripedal stimulation (target motion towards the macular region). Asymmetric OKN from partial-field stimulation as seen here was not present in subject, JHOU, with monocular full-field stimulation (Fig. 4).

DISCUSSION AND CONCLUSIONS

A recent investigation of 78 albinos (Apkarian et al., 1982) indicated that with optimal stimulus and recording conditions, misrouted optic fibers as reflected in the monocular potential distributions could be detected in all of the albinos tested. The results indicated that VEP asymmetry is a decisive clinical measure for the differential diagnosis of albinism. Using this diagnostic VEP protocol, we performed an objective screening for the patients who participated in this investigation of oculomotor disturbances. While all five albinos with or without spontaneous nystagmus showed the expected pattern of monocular VEP asymmetry the response profiles from

368

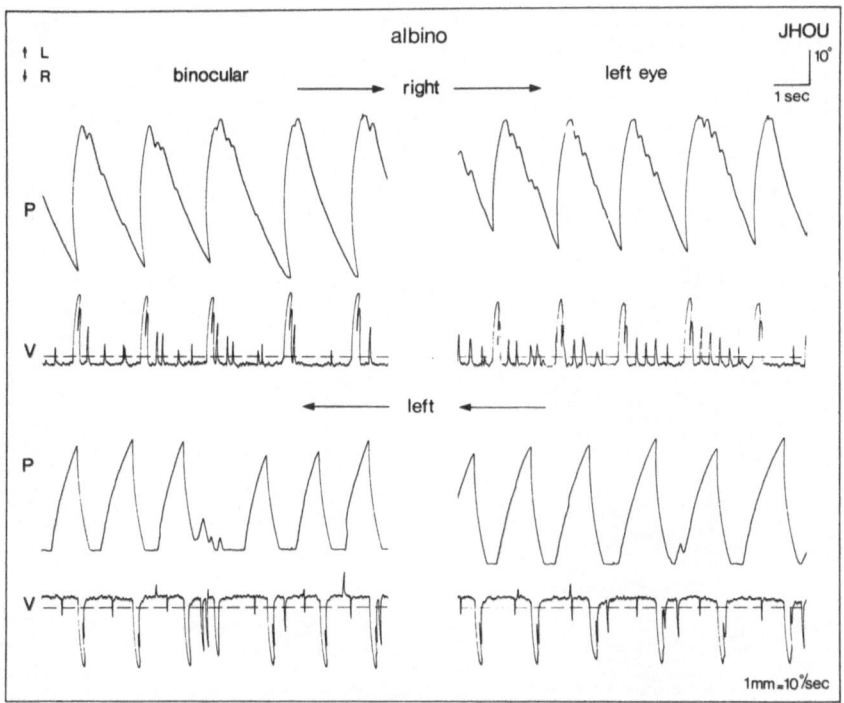

Fig. 4. Left eye recordings of OKN in albino JHOU elicited by full-field target motion to the right or left under binocular (left column) and left eye (right column) viewing conditions. For other details see Fig. 3. Note the relatively normal OKN response; regardless of pattern direction or viewing condition, the slow phase is in the direction of target motion and the fast phase is in the opposite direction.

the non-albino with nystagmus were normal. Having thus verified the presence or absence or retino-geniculo-cortical misrouting we were confident in our albino and non-albino diagnoses.

During the course of the VEP albino screening, left and right eye movements were simultaneously monitored. The spontaneous eye position instability and disjunctive eye movements which we observed prompted a more systematic investigation of optokinetic nystagmus (OKN), a subsystem of oculomotor stabilization. As expected from OKN investigations in the albino rabbit (Collewijn et al., 1978), one of the albinos from the present study demonstrated inverted OKN. Inverted OKN, however, proved to be a non-specific pathognomonic for albinism since it was also obtained in the non-albino. Furthermore, the albino with no nystagmus demonstrated relatively normal OKN with binocular or monocular full-field or monocular half-field stimulation. Although it is tempting to suggest that albinos with nystagmus have inverted OKN while those without do not, our continuing investigations in a larger sample of albinos indicate that inverted OKN is not always manifest, at least under the condition tested, even when spontaneous nystagmus is.

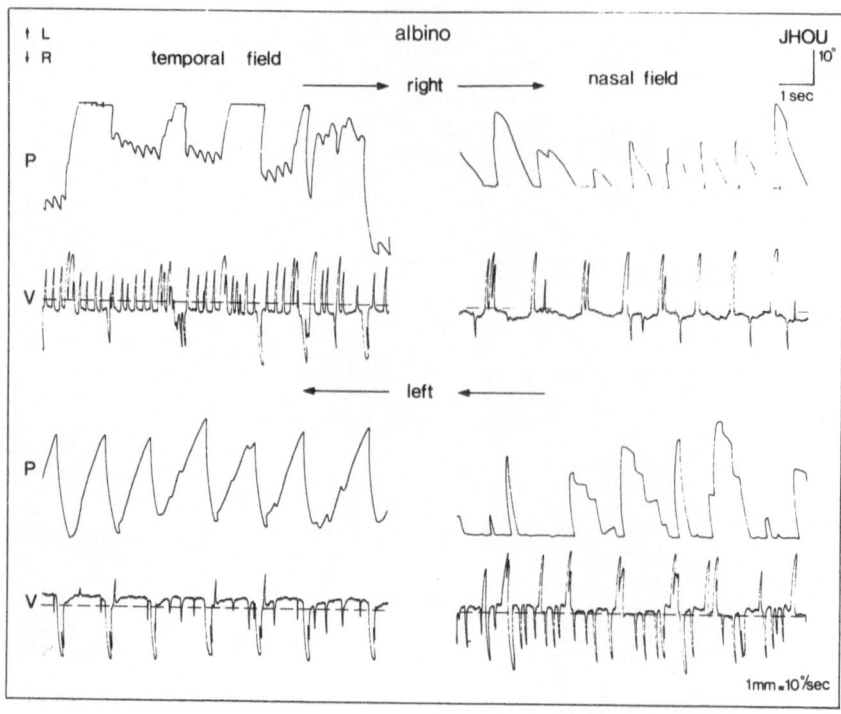

Fig. 5. Left eye recordings of OKN in albino JHOU elicited by half-field stimulation (temporal field, left column; nasal field, right column) under left eye viewing conditions. For other details see Fig. 3. Note that although the OKN is not inverted, half-field stimulation induced greater eye movement instability and OKN directional asymmetry.

In the albino who did not show inverted OKN we were able to induce OKN directional asymmetry and irregular saccades by restricting the visual field. The OKN in this subject was better driven in one horizontal direction in the visual field than in the other. Although we do not yet understand the relationship between misrouted retinal fibers and OKN directional asymmetry, the occurrence of directional asymmetry in subject samples and animal models with reduced visual acuity and immature or impaired binocular function may be of related importance. Asymmetric monocularly elicited OKN has been reported for strabismic or anisometropic amblyopes (Schor and Levi, 1980), human rod monochromats (Baloh et al., 1980), human and monkey infants (Wakusawa and Sato, 1974; Atkinson, 1979), cats reared with monocular deprivation (Van Hof-van Duin, 1976; Hoffman, 1979) or visual field ablation (Wood et al., 1973) and a large sample of afoveate mammals, birds and reptiles including rabbit (Collewijn, 1969), guinea pig (Smith and Bridgeman, 1943) and pigeon (Mowrer, 1936).

In the study of optokinetic nystagmus in human and monkey infants, Atkinson (1979) suggested that the development of functional cortical binocularity as tested by stereoscopic performance may be correlated with

370

the development of symmetric OKN. In this report, albino, JHOU, who showed asymmetric OKN under partial-field stimulation, also demonstrated stereoscopic vision when tested with Julesz random dot patterns (Julesz, 1964). Thus, in this case, abnormal binocularity is not a concomitant of OKN asymmetry.

The variable OKN response patterns observed in our subject sample thus far, indicate that OKN disturbances, particularly inverted OKN and OKN directional asymmetry, are not as yet reliable diagnostic indices of human albinism. Further research in this area is required to determine the presence and consequences of aberrant projections and organization of the oculomotor control centers of albinos as well as of non-albinos with comparable oculomotor symptoms.

ACKNOWLEDGEMENT

The authors wish to thank Peter Brassinga and Ernst Peter Tamminga for their technical assistance, Els Borghols and Trees Scholt-Klerks for secretarial assistance. Special thanks are due to Wim van Veenendaal and T.J.T.P. van den Berg for their critical reading of the manuscript and to B. Bastiaenen for her invaluable support during the manuscript preparation.

REFERENCES

Apkarian, P., Reits, D., Spekreijse, H. and Dorp, D. van. A decisive electrophysiological test for human albinism. Electroenceph. clin. Neurophysiol. (submitted) 1982.

Atkinson, J. Development of optokinetic nystagmus in the human infant and infant monkey: an analogue to development in kittens. In: Freeman, R. H. (ed.) Developmental Neurobiology of Vision, 277–287, Plenum Press, New York, 1979.

Baloh, R. W., Yee, R. D. and Honrubia, V. Optokinetic asymmetry in patients with maldeveloped foveas. Brain Res. 186: 210–216, 1980.

Bergsma, D. Birth Defects, Atlas and Compendium. The National Foundation. White Plains, New York, 1973.

Coleman, J., Sydnor, C. F., Wolbarsht, M. L. and Bessler, M. Abnormal visual pathways in human albinos studied with visually evoked potentials. Exp. Neurol. 65: 667–679, 1979.

Collewijn, H. Optokinetic eye movements in the rabbit: input-output relations. Vision Res. 9: 111–132, 1969.

Collewijn, H. Eye- and head movements in freely moving rabbits. J. Physiol. 266: 471–498, 1977.

Collewijn, H., Winterson, B. J. and Dubois, M. F. W. Optokinetic eye movements in albino rabbits: inversion in anterior visual field. Science 199: 1351–1353, 1978.

Collewijn, H. Mark, F. van der, Jansen, T. C. Precise recording of human eye movements. Vision Res. 15: 447–450, 1975.

Creel, D., Hendrickson, A. E. and Leventhal, A. G. Retinal projection in tyrosinase-negative albino cats. J. Neurosci. 2: 907–911, 1982.

Creel, D., Spekreijse, H. and Reits, D. Evoked potentials in albinos: efficacy of pattern stimuli in detecting misrouted optic fibers. Electroenceph. clin. Neurophysiol. 52: 595–603, 1981.

Duke-Elder, S. System of opthalmology, vol. 3 Normal and abnormal development, part 2 Congenital deformities. Mosby, St. Louis, Mo. 1963, 803–813.

371

Giolli, R. A. and Creel, D. J. The primary optic projections in pigmented albino guinea pigs: an experimental degeneration study. Brain Res. 55: 25–39, 1973.

Gross, K. J. and Hickey, T. L. Abnormal laminar patterns in the lateral geniculate nucleus of an albino monkey. Brain Res. 190: 231–237, 1980.

Guillery, R. W. and Kaas, J. H. A study of normal and congenitally abnormal retino-geniculate projections in cats. J. Comp. Neurol. 143: 73–100, 1971.

Guillery, R. W. and Kaas, J. H. Genetic abnormality of visual pathways in a 'white' tiger. Science 180: 1287–1289, 1973.

Guillery, R. W., Okoro, A. N. and Witkop, C. J. Jr. Abnormal visual pathways in the brain of a human albino. Brain Res. 96: 373–377, 1975.

Hoffman, K. P. Optokinetic nystagmus and single-cell responses in the nucleus tractus opticus after early monocular deprivation in the cat. In: Freeman, R. H. (ed.) Developmental Neurobiology of Vision, 63–72, Plenum Press, New York, 1979.

Julesz, B. Binocular depth perception without familiarity cues. Science 145: 356–362, 1964.

Krill, A. E. Hereditary Retinal and Coroidal Diseases. Vol. II Clinical Characteristics, Harper and Row Publ. Hagerstown, Maryland, 1977, 645–664.

Lund, R. D. Uncrossed visual pathways in hooded and albino rats. Science 149: 1506–1509, 1965.

Mowrer, O. H. A comparison of the reaction mechanisms mediating optokinetic nystagmus in human beings and in pigeons. Psychol. Monogr. 47: 294–305, 1936.

Precht, W., Cazin, L. Functional deficits in the optokinetic system of albino rats. Exp. Brain Res. 37: 183–186, 1979.

Schor, C. M. and Levi, D. M. Disturbances of small-field horizontal and vertical opto-kinetic nystagmus in amblyopia. Invest. Ophthalmol. Vis. Sci. 19: 668–683, 1980.

Smith, K. U. and Bridgeman, M. The neural mechanisms of movement vision and optic nystagmus. J. Exp. Psychol. 33: 165–187, 1943.

Spekreijse, H., Tweel, H. van der and Zuidema, Th. Contrast evoked responses in man. Vision Res. 13: 1577–1601, 1973.

Van Die, G. and Collewijn, H. Optokinetic nystagmus in man. Role of central and peripheral retina and occurance of asymmetries. Human Neurobiol. 1: 111–119, 1982.

Van Hof-van Duin, J. Early and permanent effects of monocular deprivation on pattern discrimination and visumotor behavior in cats. Brain Res. 111: 261–276, 1976.

Wakusawa, S. and Sato, Y. Development of optokinetic response in the human infant. Jap. J. Ophthalmol. 18: 299–310, 1974.

Weber, J. T., Kaas, J. H. and Harting, J. K. Retinocollicular pathways in Siamese cats: an autoradiographic analysis. Brain Res. 148: 189–196, 1978.

Wildberger, H. and Meyer, M. Zur augenmotorischen Störung des Albino. Klin. Monatsbl. Augenheilk. 172: 487–490, 1978.

Wood, C. C., Spear, P. D. and Braun, J. J. Direction-specific deficits in horizontal opto-kinetic nystagmus following removal of visual cortex in the cat. Brain Res. 60: 231–237, 1973.

PATTERN VECP TOPOGRAPHY TO RIGHT AND LEFT HALF FIELD

H. YAMAZAKI, E. ADACHI-USAMI AND N. KURODA

(Chiba, Japan)

ABSTRACT

The topographical distribution of pattern VECPs to stimulation of the right and left half visual field were studied in normal subjects and cases having homonymous hemianopia caused by intracranial diseases. Simultaneous 16 channel recording system and a topography program manufactured by Nihon-Kohden were used to produce topograms. Amplitude differences at around 100 msec were displayed topographically on a color television monitor. Thirteen out of sixteen normals showed responses that started at the ipsilateral hemisphere relative to the side of the visual field that was stimulated and spread towards the contralateral hemisphere. In patients with homonymous hemianopia, the topograph showed a retention of activity at the impaired brain hemisphere when the impaired visual field was stimulated.

INTRODUCTION

It is well known that human VECPs are clearly recorded with an electrode placed on the occipital scalp. However, only a few reports are available on their scalp distribution. This may be because of the technical difficulties of averaging many channels simultaneously. Recently, several recording systems have been developed for this. In this report, we studied the topography of pattern VECPs to the right and left half field stimulation in normal subjects and patients with homonymous hemianopia caused by intracranial diseases using a simultaneous 16 channel recording system made by Nihon-Kohden.

METHODS

Checkerboard pattern stimuli subtending a total visual angle of $19° \times 26°$ were presented on a TV monitor. Individual checks subtended $112'$. The pattern reversed at a rate of $1.6\,Hz$, with square wave modulation. The contrast of the checkerboard was kept at 98%, the mean luminance was

46 cd/m^2. Subjects and patients looked monocularly at a fixation point on the center of either the right or left border of the visual field. The viewing distance was 75 cm. VECPs were recorded from 16 silver cup electrodes placed on a scalp with a reference electrode placed at Fz as shown in Fig. 1. The inter-electrode distance was set at 3 cm.

The responses were amplified with an EEG amplifier (EEG 6518, Nihon-Kohden) with a band pass of 0.3–120 Hz. 100 responses were averaged and recorded on magnetic tape. Later, the data were reproduced and written with an X-Y plotter, and VECP topograms were made by using programs of Nihon-Kohden. Topographs were written by a serial printer (SD-120, N.K.) and displayed on a color TV monitor.

In this study, each case showed a clear surface positive wave (P1) at around 100 msec after reversal of stimuli and surface negative waves (N1, N2) at around 70 msec and 130 msec. The amplitude topograms were thus obtained at fixed time windows between N1 and N2. The amplitude at the

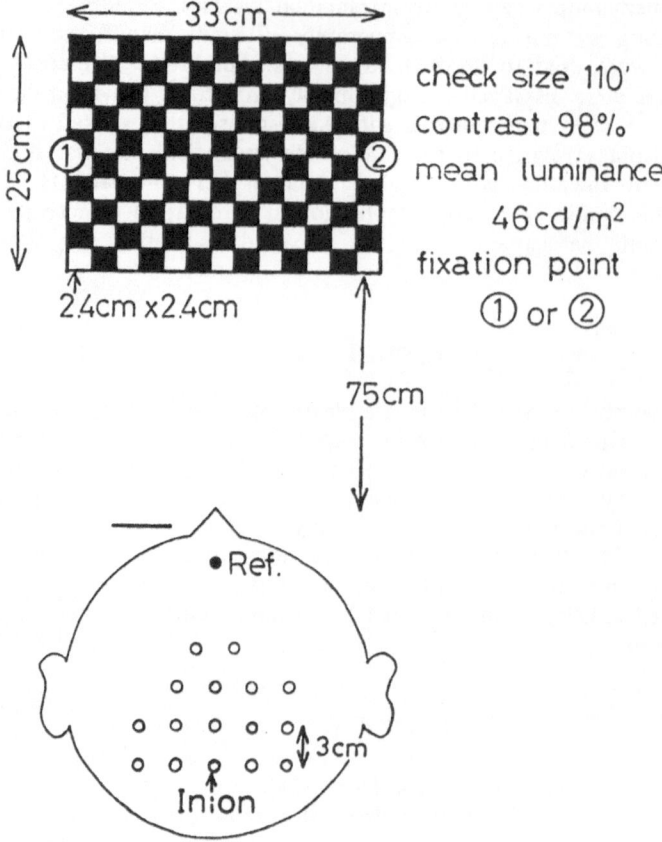

Fig. 1. Schematic arrangement for the recording and topographic display of pattern VECPs.

374

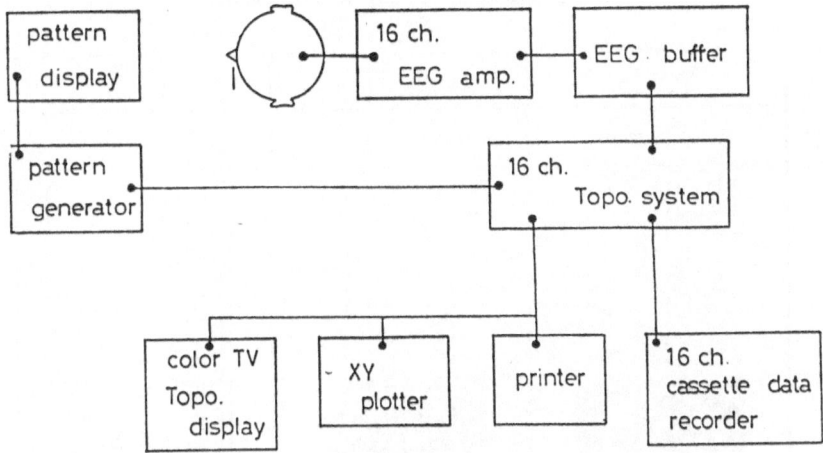

```
pattern          16 ch.          EEG  buffer
display          EEG  amp.

pattern                    16 ch.
generator                  Topo. system

color TV      XY        printer      16 ch.
Topo.         plotter                cassette  data
display                              recorder
```

Fig. 2. 16 electrode positions and pattern stimuli employed. Numbers 1 and 2 on the pattern edge indicate the fixation point for right and left half field stimulation.

trigger point of the stimulus was defined as $0\mu V$. The largest difference of the amplitudes between any two responses was divided in 10 parts and an equi-potential map was displayed with 10 different densities at each 2 msec. The darkest portion indicates the maxima of the positive wave or the minima of the negative wave.

Eight normal subjects were examined. Their visual acuities were better than 1.0 with correction. Three patients with hemianopia caused from intra-cranial diseases were examined. Table 1. Two of them had a cerebral vascular accident and their visual fields showed left hemianopia with macular sparing. A third case had an occipital meningioma with right hemianopic depression. The visual acuities of the patients were all above 0.7.

RESULTS

1. VECP topography in normal subjects

Fig. 3 shows VECPs from subject H.E. A clear positive wave with a latency of around 100 msec, i.e. P1, is observed at each channel. P1 was present in all 7 subjects.

(i) P1 latency: Table 2 shows the mean P1 latencies obtained from electrodes on ipsi- and contralateral hemispheres to the stimulated half field. P1 latencies from the ipsilateral hemisphere are significantly shorter than those from the contralateral hemisphere. ($p < 0.005$: Wilcoxon test).

(ii) Topography: the actual topogram of subject H.E. is shown in the upper half of Fig. 5. In this case, the maxima (indicated with the darkest portion) moved from the ipsilateral to the contralateral hemisphere with respect to the stimulated half field, i.e. the maxima moved from the right to the left hemisphere when the right half field was stimulated and vice versa for left

375

Table 1. 3 cases of homonymous hemianopia

case	Y. S.	K. T.	G. S.
age sex	60y, male	55y, female	64y, male
V A	VD = 0.8 (1.0) VS = 0.9 (1.2)	VD = 0.7 (n.c.) VS = 1.0 (n.c.)	VD = 0.7 (n.c.) VS = 0.9 (n.c.)
V F			
C T			
diag	Rt PCA infarction	Rt PCA infarction	Lt occipital meningioma

half field stimulation. These movements from the ipsilateral to the contra-lateral hemisphere were observed in 13 out of 16 normal subjects.

2. VECP topography in the patients with hemianopia

Although 10 patients were examined, 7 of them didn't show the clear VECPs. This might be because of their difficulty in maintaining fixation. Topographical studies were performed in 3 patients who showed the distinct VECPs. Fig. 4 shows the actual VECPs of the patient Y. S. VECPs were obtained from all electrodes and a surface positive wave at around 100 msec was observed even on the scalp of the affected hemisphere.

(i) P1 latency: Table 3 shows the mean P1 latencies obtained from each hemisphere. The mean P1 latencies from the affected hemisphere seemed to be longer than those from the normal hemisphere.

(ii) VECP topography: The VECP topography of Y. S. is shown in the lower half of Fig. 5. In this case, the maxima travelled back and forth from the contralateral to the ipsilateral and then returned to the contralateral hemisphere when the non-affected right half field was stimulated. On the other hand, stimulation of the affected half field did not produce a shift of the maxima of the affected hemisphere.

The other cases also showed a similar asymmetric movement. This was not observed in normal cases. When their non-affected half field was stimulated, two of the cases showed pendular movement and one showed the maxima to stand still in the affected hemisphere as just described. When the affected half fields were stimulated, the maxima moved from the ipsi- to the

376

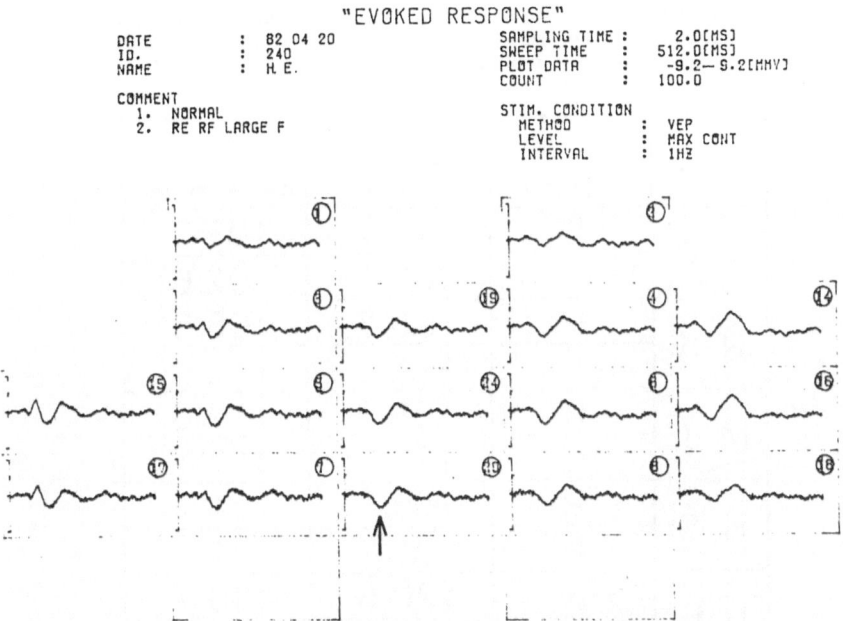

"EVOKED RESPONSE"

DATE   : 82 04 20   SAMPLING TIME :   2.0[MS]
ID.   : 240   SWEEP TIME   : 512.0[MS]
NAME   : H.E.   PLOT DATA   :   -9.2— 9.2[MMV]
                                 COUNT   : 100.0
COMMENT
   1. NORMAL   STIM. CONDITION
   2. RE RF LARGE F   METHOD   : VEP
                                    LEVEL   : MAX CONT
                                    INTERVAL   : 1HZ

Fig. 3. Actual VECPs obtained from 16 scalp electrode positions of normal subject, H.E. arrow indicates the major positive wave (P1) at about 100 msec–120 msec.

contralateral hemispheres in two cases, and one case showed no movement on the affected hemisphere.

DISCUSSION

Spatial distribution studies of the VECP on the scalp to right and left half field stimulation make it possible to investigate the function of the cerebral hemisphere with respect to the location of patterned stimuli. Cobb and Morton (1970) reported a greater amplitude of the VECP on the contralateral hemisphere to the stimulated half field. Lesevre and Joseph (1979) confirmed their results. On the other hand, Blumhardt et al. (1976, 1977, 1978) showed, with a larger visual field and coarser patterns, that the amplitude of the P100 component of the pattern reversal VECPs was greater on the ipsilateral hemisphere with respect to the stimulated half field. Lehmann and Skrandies (1979), using their 48 channel simultaneous recording system, also reported that the maxima of the VECP were distributed topographically in a manner similar to that observed by Blumhardt et al. Pattern stimuli have also been applied to the patients with hemianopia by several authors. Wildberger et al. (1976) and van Lith et al. (1980) reported that VECP amplitudes were reduced in the affected hemisphere. Blumhardt et al. (1977) however showed larger VECP on the ipsilateral hemisphere regardless of the affected side.

The present study showed that P1 latencies in normal subjects were

377

Table 2. The mean peak latencies obtained at ipsi- or contralateral hemisphere to the visual field stimulated in 8 normal subjects. The latencies at ipsilateral hemisphere are significantly (p < 0.005) shorter than contralateral ones.

name	stimulated half field	peak latency, msec	
		ipsi-hemisph.	contra-hemisph.
J. C.	R	97.7	103.0
	L	103.3	102.6
N. K.	R	95.7	105.0
	L	111.7	112.0
M. I.	R	106.6	117.0
	L	112.7	117.1
H. S.	R	109.7	121.7
	L	91.7	91.4
H. E.	R	120.6	130.7
	L	102.0	110.3
N. F.	R	122.0	123.0
	L	112.7	120.0
K. S.	R	94.3	94.0
	L	90.7	93.4
N. S.	R	103.7	114.3
	L	118.7	124.9

Wilcoxon test: ipsi<contra significant (<0.005)

shorter in ipsilateral than contralateral hemisphere. Furthermore, sequential topography between 70 msec and 130 msec showed the movements of the maxima from the ipsi- to the contralateral hemisphere. This might confirm a shorter latency on the ipsilateral hemisphere.

As for clinical findings, three patients with hemianopia showed a delay of the P1 latency in the affected hemisphere and their sequential topography was abnormal. Obviously, our data are not extensive enough for broad generalizations, but they do point to an abnormality of the visual fields that is related to the affected side. Further, it is interesting in regard to the source of VECPs, that clear responses were recorded on both hemispheres including the affected side. Considering the fact that all of the patients examined in the present study had macular sparing, one might have anticipated results similar to those of normal subjects. However, their topography showed clear differences from normals.

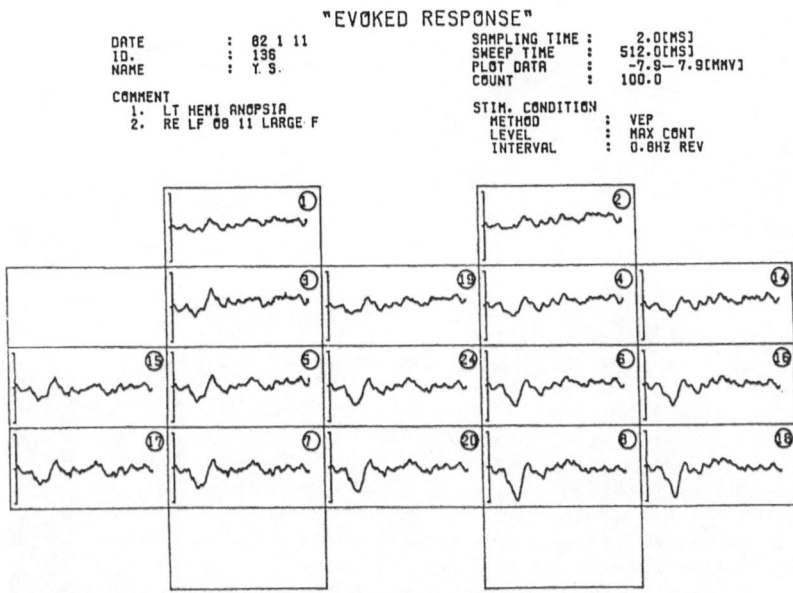

"EVOKED RESPONSE"

DATE   : 82 1 11   SAMPLING TIME :   2.0[MS]
ID.   : 136   SWEEP TIME   : 512.0[MS]
NAME   : Y. S.   PLOT DATA   :   -7.9— 7.9[MMV]
                                  COUNT   : 100.0
COMMENT
  1. LT HEMI ANOPSIA   STIM. CONDITION
  2. RE LF 08 11 LARGE F   METHOD   : VEP
                                   LEVEL   : MAX CONT
                                   INTERVAL   : 0.8HZ REV

Fig. 4. Actual VECPs of a case of left homonymous hemianopia, Y.S.

Table 3. The mean P1 peak latencies obtained at right and left hemisphere for each half field stimulation in 3 cases of homonymous hemianopia demonstrated in Table 1

name	age sex	visual field	stimulated eye	stimulated half field	peak latency, msec	
					R-hemisph.	L-hemisph.
Y. S.	60 M	Lt hemi- anopsia	R	R	79.4	78.0
				L	101.1	87.0
			L	R	102.0	109.0
				L	104.6	104.2
K. T.	55 F	Lt hemi- anopsia	R	R	100.0	92.0
				L	118.6	115.0
			L	R	106.6	82.3
				L	123.4	118.6
G. S.	64 M	Rt hemi- anopsia	R	R	128.3	137.0
				L	134.9	132.7
			L	R	130.3	131.0
				L	121.6	122.1

379

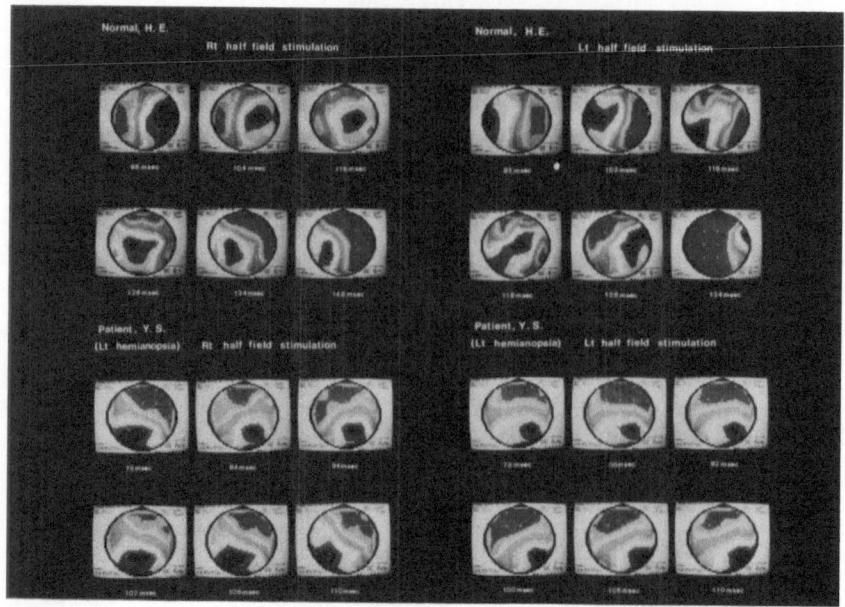

Fig. 5. Sequences of the amplitude topographs for right and left half visual field stimulation of normal subject and those of a patient with left homonymous hemianopia in the lower half.

In making measures of this sort, one must decide where the 'baseline' of the recordings is. Many authors have suggested different methods. Lehmann and Brown (1980) offered a 'technical zero' method and Shagass et al. (1976) used the mean amplitude at some fixed duration after pattern alternation as a OμV. We used the amplitude at the triggering point of the stimulus as a OμV. Baseline problems are minimized in the present case since the primary concern is with differences between potentials. Certain basic problems concerning clinical topography of VECPs still remain. However, we believe that our data point to a way of obtaining information for diagnosing hemianopic patients with pattern VECP topography.

REFERENCES

Cobb, W. A. & Morton, H. B. Evoked potentials from the human scalp to visual half-field stimulation. J. Physiol., 208: 39–40, 1970.
Barrett, G., Blumhardt, L., Halliday, A. M., Halliday, E. and Kriss, A. A paradox in the lateralization of the visual evoked response. Nature, 261: 253–255, 1976.
Blumhardt, L. D., Barrett, G. and Halliday, A. M. The asymmetrical visual evoked potential to pattern reversal in one half field and its significance for the analysis of visual field defects. Brit. J. Ophthalmol. 61: 454–461, 1977.
Blumhardt, L. D., Barrett, G., Halliday, A. M. and Kriss, A. The effect of experimental 'Scotoma' on the ipsilateral and contralateral responses to pattern reversal in one half field. Electroenceph. clin. Neurophysiol. 45: 376–392, 1978.

Lehmann, D. and Skrandies, W. Multichannel mapping of spatial distributions of scalp potential fields evoked by checkerboard reversal to different retinal areas. In: Human Evoked Potentials, Applications and Problems (Ed. Lehmann, D. and Callaway, E.) 201–214, Plenum Press, New York and London, 1979.

Lehmann, D. and Brown, W. S. How to measure evoked EEG potentials for topography. Evoked Potentials (Ed. Barber, C.) pp. 143–146, MTP Press Ltd. England, 1980.

Lesevre, N. and Joseph, J. P. Modifications of the pattern-evoked potential (PEP) in relation to the stimulated part of the visual field (clues for the most probable origin of each component). Electroenceph. clin. Neurophysiol., 47: 183–203, 1979.

Shagass, C., Amedeo, M. and Roemer, R. A. Spatial distribution of potentials evoked by half-field pattern reversal and pattern onset stimuli. Electroenceph. clin. Neurophysiol., 41: 609–622, 1976.

Van Lith, G. H. M., Henkes, H. E. and Vijfvinkel-Bruinenga, S. M. Asymmetric pattern evoked responses and stimulus parameters. Docum. Ophthal. Proc. Series., 23: 249–253, 1980.

Wildberger, H. G. H., van Lith, G. H. M., Wijngaarde, R. and Mak, G. T. M. Visually evoked cortical potentials in the evaluation of homonymous and bitemporal visual field defects. Brit. J. Ophthal., 60: 273–278, 1976.

Mailing address:
Department of Ophthalmology
School of Medicine, Chiba University
280 Chiba, Japan

VECTOR ANALYSIS OF PATTERN VEP OF PATIENTS WITH HEMIANOPIA

Y. OGUCHI AND M. TOYODA

(Tokyo, Japan)

ABSTRACT

A method of vector analysis of pattern VEP was already reported at the ISCEV symposium in 1980. The initial major vector component elicited by full field stimulation of normal subjects extends longitudinally and stretches from anterior to posterior. The initial major vector component produced by half field stimulation and ipsilaterally and anterior-posteriorly tilted vector. The vector analysis was carried for pattern VEP obtained from 20 patients with hemianopsia. Eleven among 12 homonymous hemianopic patients showed the expected vector components. However, in the left eye of one patient the tilted vector component was absent. Six among 8 bitemporal hemianopic patients showed the expected vector components. However, in two eyes of two patients, vector analysis of VEP was meaningless because the VEPs were hardly recordable due to very low visual acuity and/or very constricted visual fields.

INTRODUCTION

A method for vector analysis of pattern VEP was already presented in previous reports (Oguchi and Toyoda 1981; Oguchi 1981). The initial major vector component elicited by full field stimulation of normal subjects extends longitudinally and stretches from anterior to posterior. The initial major vector component triggered by half field stimulation exhibits ipsilaterally and anterior-posteriorly tilted vectors. From this result, a clinical application of vector VEP for detecting visual field defects such as hemianopia will be expected. In this paper twenty hemianopic and suspected hemianopic patients were studied.

METHOD

Twenty patients (3 females and 9 males from 2 years and 6 months to 79 years old) who showed homonymous hemianopia and suspected homonymous hemianopia participated in this study. Eight patients (2 females and 6 males from 3 years and 2 months to 63 years old) who showed bitemporal hemi-anopia were also studied. The method of vector analysis of pattern reversal VEP was already described (Oguchi and Toyoda 1981). In this experiment the 40 minute squares were used instead of 92 minute squares. The patients were asked to look at the center of the TV screen. In order to check for abnormalities of the vector VEP elicited by full field stimulation, the vector VEPs from 15 normal subjects were recorded. When the maximum ampli-tude on the Y-component in each patient is set at 100%, each amplitude at 17 points for a latency of 72 to 97.9 msec. can be represented as percentage amplitude. The same can be done for the X-component. From these values of each percentage amplitude, the averaged percent values of the amplitude on the X and Y axes and the standard deviations were calculated and plotted at 17 points for normal subjects after full field stimulation. Fig. 1 shows the averaged vector VEP and standard deviations obtained from right eyes and

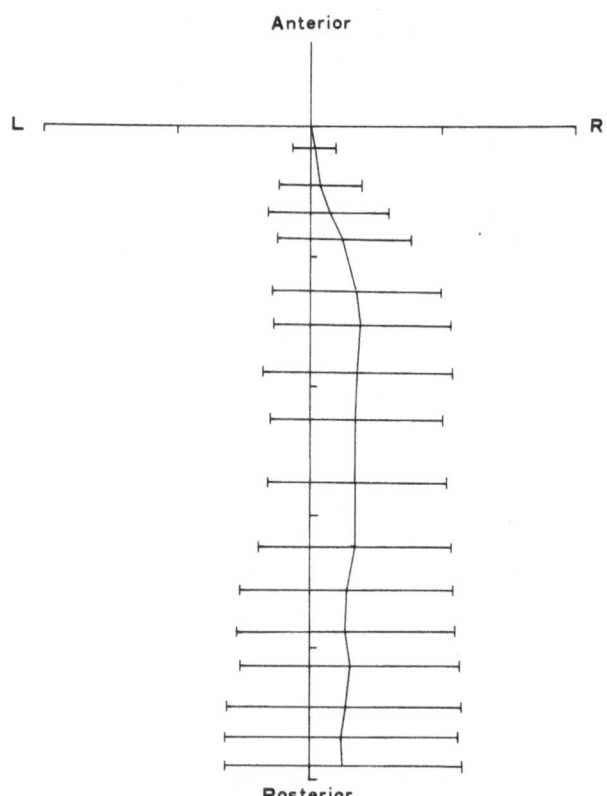

Averaged Vector VEP
(Full screen in the R-eye)

Fig. 1. Major vector component of the averaged vector VEP and standard deviation ob-tained from 15 normal subjects after full field stimulation of the right eye.

384

Averaged Vector VEP
(Full Screen in the L-eye)

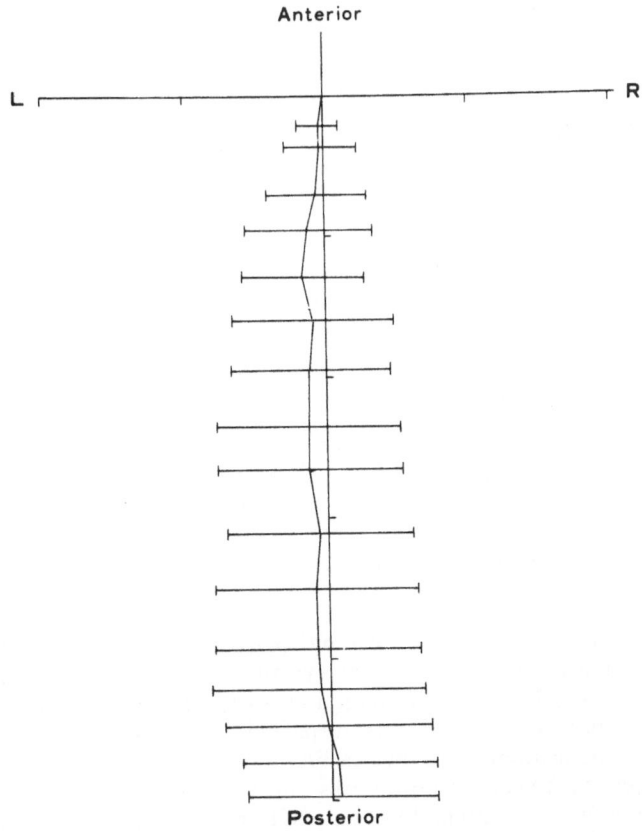

Fig. 2. Major vector component of the averaged vector VEP and standard deviation obtained from 15 normal subjects after full field stimulation for the left eye.

Fig. 2 from left eyes. In this study these standard values of the vector VEP were used for judging abnormalities of the vector VEP in patients.

RESULTS

In 11 among 12 patients homonymous hemianopia was confirmed by perimetry and in one case of homonymous hemianopia it was suspected from physical symptoms. Among these patients, there are 8 cases of cerebral vascular disease, 2 head injuries, 1 after partial occipital lobectomy for an astrocytoma and 1 of unknown origin. Eleven among 12 cases showed the expected vector VEP. The major vector component tilted nasally or temporally from the normal vector component after full field stimulation. Fig. 3

385

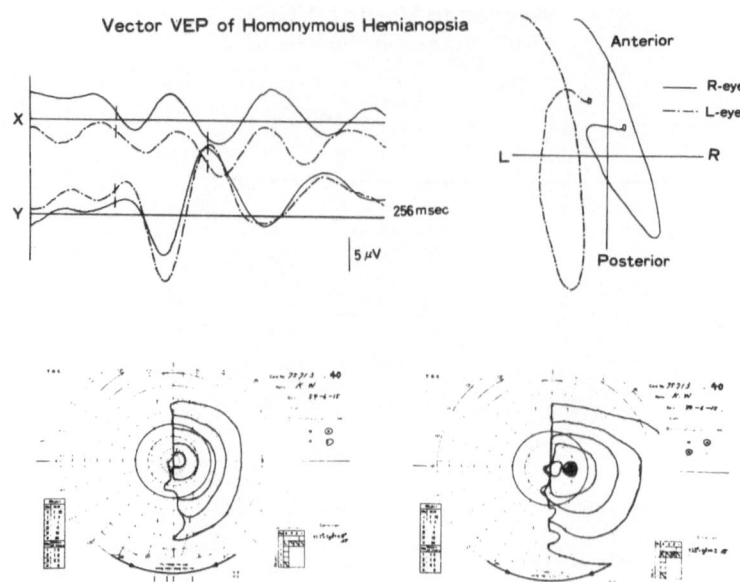

Fig. 3. Vector VEP and visual field of a 42 year old male patient after partial occipital lobectomy for an astrocytoma.

shows the vector VEP of a 42 year old patient after left partial occipital lobectomy for astrocytoma. In either eye the major vector component was shifted toward the left posterior direction. From this result an abnormality of the right half visual field was suspected. Perimetry revealed the left homonymous hemianopia as shown in Fig. 3. Fig. 4 demonstrates the vector VEP of an infant 2 years and 6 months old. She had a right hemiparesis on the arm and aphasia. Examination of the CT scan revealed no abnormalities. The vector VEP after full field stimulation to both eyes shows a left posteriorly tilted vector component which suggested an abnormality of the right half visual field. This finding coincided with her physical symptoms. Fig. 5 demonstrates the vector VEP of a 40 year old female patient who had a left homonymous hemianopia. The major vector component of the right eye tilted right posteriorly. But in the left eye it aimed first in a longitudinal direction and then tilted right posteriorly. For the left eye, the vector component was estimated to be within normal limits. The CT scan suggested a small infarct of posterior cerebral artery.

In another 8 patients, there are 5 cases of pituitary adenoma and 3 cases of craniopharyngioma. In 6 among 8 patients bitemporal hemianopia was ascertained and in 2 infant patients bitemporal hemianopia was suspected from their physical symptoms. Fig. 6 demonstrates the vector VEP of a 3 years and 2 months old boy with suspected craniopharyngioma. The visual acuity and visual field could not be examined due to limited cooperation. The vector component after full field stimulation for the right eye is tilted toward the left posterior direction, and that for the left eye toward

386

Vector VEP of a Patient
with r-Hemiparesis and Aphasia

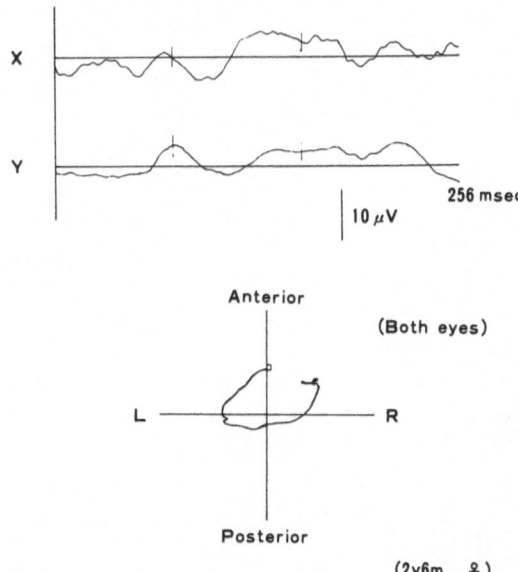

Fig. 4. Vector VEP of a 2 years and 6 months old infant with physical signs of right hemiparesis of the arm and aphasia.

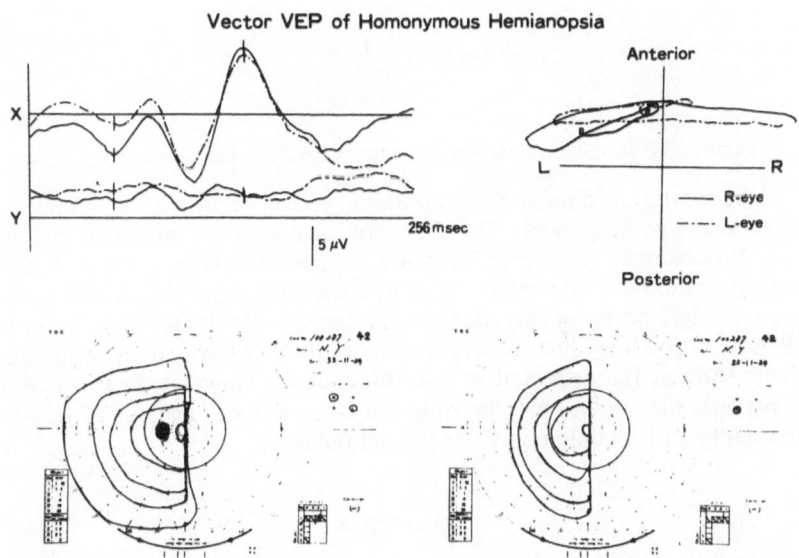

Fig. 5. Vector VEP and visual field of a 40 year old female patient with a small infarct of the posterior cerebral artery.

387

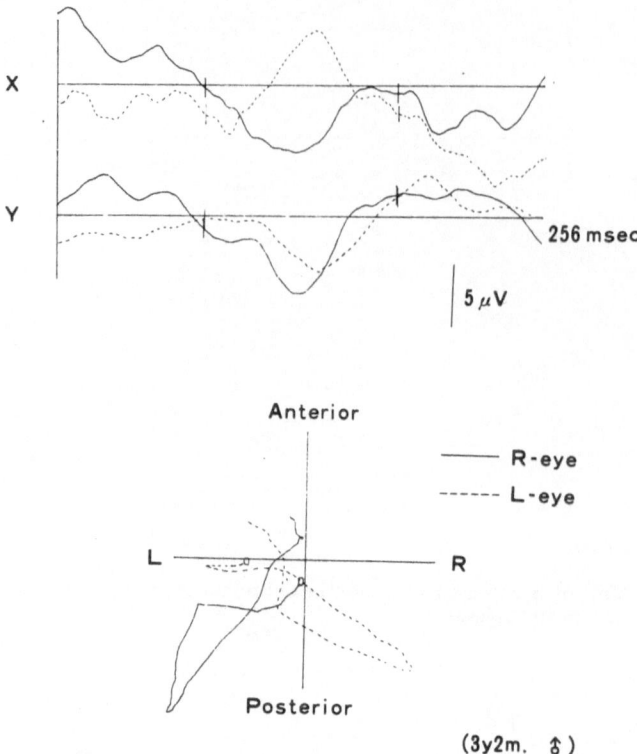

Vector VEP of a Patient with
Suspecting Craniopharyngioma

X

Y

256 msec

5 μV

Anterior

—— R-eye
------ L-eye

L

R

Posterior

(3y2m. ♂)

Fig. 6. Vector VEP of a 3 years and 2 months boy with a craniopharyngioma.

the right posterior direction. From these vector components, bitemporal hemianopia was suspected. The CT scan suggested a craniopharyngioma. Fig. 7 demonstrates the vector VEP of a 54 year old patient affected with a pituitary adenoma. Only in the right eye was the major vector component toward the left posterior direction. In the left eye the vector analysis of the VEP was impossible due to very low potentials. Fourteen eyes among 8 patients showed the expected vector components. However, in two eyes of two patients the vector analysis could not be carried out because of very low visual acuity and severely constricted visual fields.

DISCUSSION

Previously the authors reported that the initial major vector component elicited by full field stimulation is longitudinal in orientation and large,

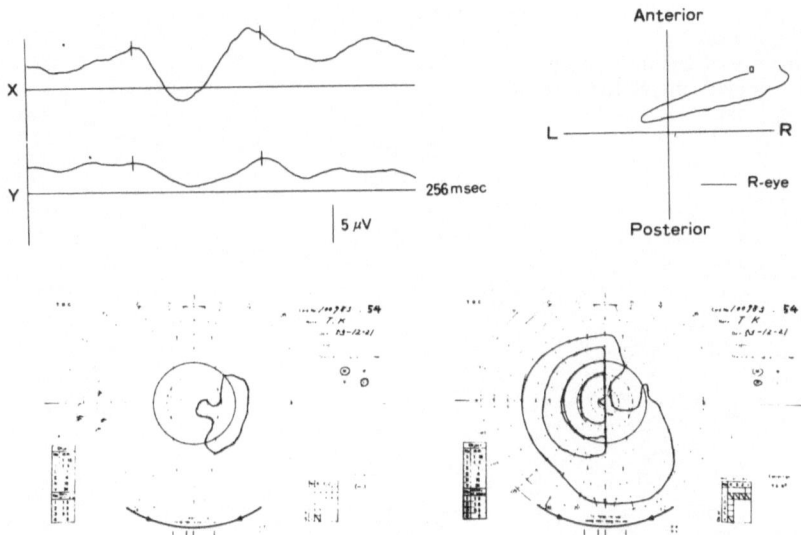

Fig. 7. Vector VEP and visual field of a 54 year old male patient with a pituitary adenoma.

stretching from anterior to posterior (Oguchi and Toyoda 1981; Oguchi 1981). However, in normal subjects there are some variations of the vector component. Therefore in this paper the averaged vector VEP and standard deviation were calculated. In the group with homonymous hemianopia there is only one case which does not show the expected vector component. Why only one exception exists cannot be explained. But this patient had a small infarction in the posterior cerebral artery region. On perimetry macula sparing was found. It seems that the vector component is mostly influenced by stimulating the central 10 to 18 degrees after pattern stimulation (Behrmann 1972, Katsumi et al., 1980). From this point of view, hemianopic scotoma might be detected more easily than hemianopia with macula sparing. Another difficulty to evaluate the vector VEP is that the vector analysis of the VEP is impossible when the visual acuity is low and the residual visual field severely constricted. In the present study a reliable vector VEP was obtained when the visual acuity was at least 0.09.

REFERENCES

Behrman, J., Nissim, S. and Arden, G. B. A clinical method for obtaining pattern visual evoked responses. (1972), pp. 199–206, in: G. B. Arden (ed.) Advances in Experimental Medicine and Biology. Vol. 24. Plenum Press, New York.

Katsumi, O., Matsuhashi, M. and Oguchi, Y. Effect of stimulus parameters on the pattern reversal VECP. Acta soc. ophthal. Japonica, 84: 1723–1730, 1980.

Oguchi, Y. Vector analysis of pattern VEP. Ophthal. Res. 13: 151–159, 1981.
Oguchi, Y. and Toyoda, M. Vector analysis of pattern VEP. Doc. Ophthal. Proc. Series, Vol. 27, 239–245, 1981.

Mailing address:
Department of Ophthalmology
School of Medicine, Keio University
Tokyo, Japan

EARLY/LATE COMPONENT RATIO IN PATTERN-REVERSAL VEP: NORMATIVE DATA AND CLINICAL APPLICATIONS

C. T. WHITE, C. L. WHITE AND R. W. HINTZE

(San Diego, California, U.S.A.)

ABSTRACT

It has been well-established that there is a quite reliable implicit time to a positive component (ca 100 msec) in respect to pattern reversal. This has been used as a neurological test of the integrity of the visual system. Our own findings indicate, however, that sub-cortical activity contributes strongly to that component.

Recent data suggest that activity around 200 msec is a more useful measure of the cortical response to pattern alternation. We have carried out a normative study of the relative amplitudes of the two components. Among normal adults activity around 200 msec is directly related to spatial frequency, increasing markedly in amplitude with higher spatial frequencies. This is in sharp contrast to the earlier component, which does not exhibit such sensitive size differentiation. This corresponds with our earlier transient pattern work, in which the late positive component (ca 200 msec) was always more sensitive to both high spatial frequency and binocular summation.

Recently we have used the ratio between the late and early component amplitudes as a quantitative indicator of the efficiency of higher-level processing of pattern formation. We will present our normative data and also illustrate the effects of various visual problems on this measure.

METHODS AND RESULTS

All the VEPs for this study were obtained using the Nicolet 1170 and pattern-reversal stimuli were generated by the Nicolet 1006. Preliminary studies showed that satisfactory responses could be obtained with a medium contrast situation, so the brightness setting of #3 (Nicolet 1006) was used for all subjects. The rate of 2.06 reversals/second was used at all times.

For the present study the results from ten normal subjects were used. All had 20/20 corrected acuity. These subjects were the authors and other volunteers. The patient data were obtained from records of patients who had been sent to the Electrophysiology Laboratory of the Mercy Hospital Eye Center for evaluation. The records of 12 such patients were selected at random. The only requirement was that a complete set of responses had been obtained in each case. Because of the small number of individuals involved, the results should be considered at tentative. However, the overall findings suggest that the approach is a valid one.

The normal subjects were studied at both 1 m and 2 m viewing distance. Responses were obtained for both single eyes and for binocular stimulation. The patient's responses were obtained only for single eyes at the 1 m distance. Figure 1 shows the responses of three of our normal group at the 2 m distance. Our special interest is the relationship of the two major positive components in the responses. It can be seen that across the variations in visual angle the P-100 process remains fairly stable in latency and amplitude by comparison with the second positive complex. This was generally true for all of our normal group. The exception is subject RWH, whose P-100 is seen to be quite irregular in amplitude. A further study with this subject showed that his upper and lower visual field responses were markedly out of phase around 100 msec thus creating the irregular central visual field results. For each of the subjects shown the second positive complex tended to occur later as the spatial frequency of the stimulus was increased. A closer inspection of the waveforms indicates that this second major positive complex is not a single

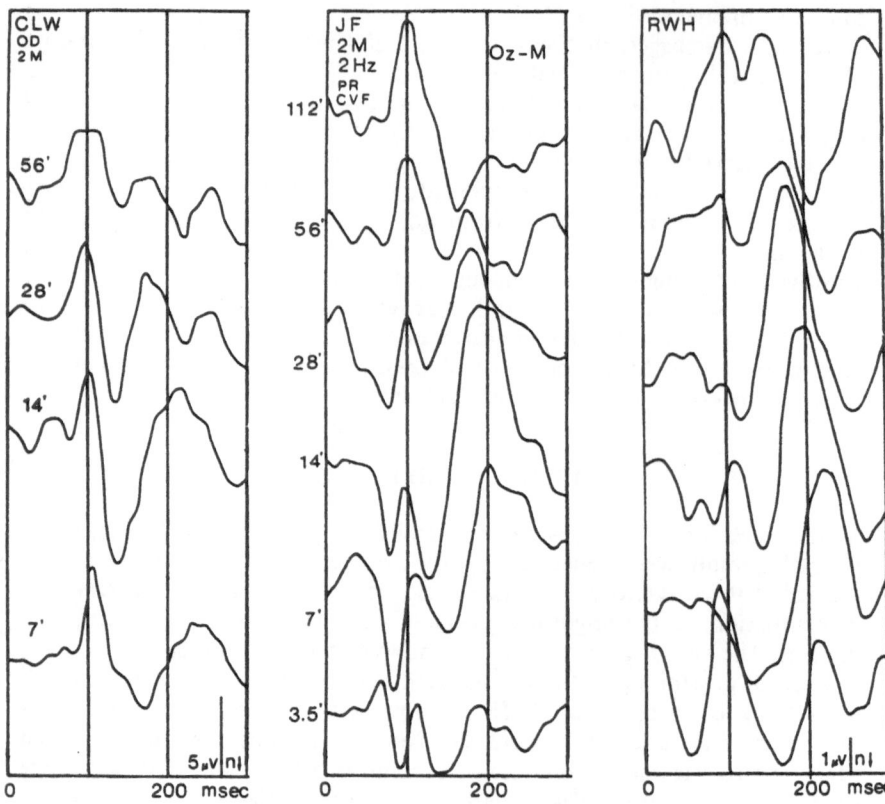

Fig. 1. Pattern-reversal responses of three normal individuals to changes in spatial frequency. (Note P100/P200 comparisons).

392

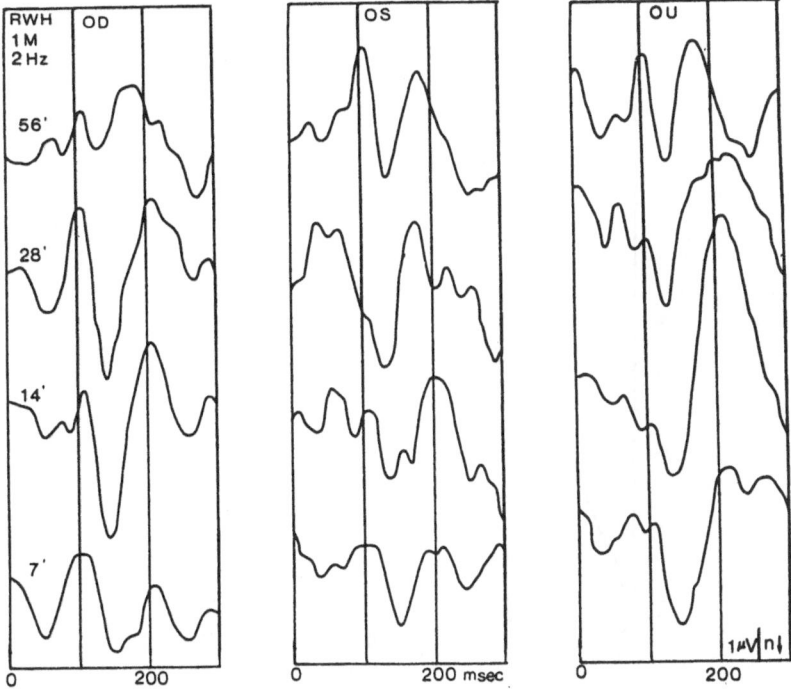

Fig. 2. Monocular and binocular response to pattern-reversal varying spatial-frequency. (Note multiple components in P200 wave complex).

entity, but instead consists of a number of components. This fact can be more clearly seen in Fig. 2, which presents the responses for RWH at 1 m. Here, especially in the OS responses, the multiple components are apparent for the 28′ and 14′ conditions. Three of these sub-components were chosen for further study: at 175, 200 and 224 msec. When we measure the amplitudes at these three latencies for RWH's 2 m responses we produce the curves shown in Fig. 3, which indicate the presence of three components rather sharply tuned to spatial frequency. We have carried out this same procedure for a number of our normals, with the same general result. In each case we obtained a series of sharply tuned components, with those tuned to the higher spatial frequencies occurring later in time. This would seem to explain the apparent shift in latency of the second positive complex as the spatial frequency of the stimulus pattern is increased.

Fig. 4 is a diagram of the normal group's mean amplitudes for components P-100 and P-200 (the latter was measured always exactly at 200 msec) over a range of visual angles with subjects at 2 m. It can be seen that the P-200 response for both the binocular and single eye conditions shows a sharp peak at 14′ visual angle, whereas the P-100 response, both binocular and monocular do not exhibit such peaking. The differences between P-100 and P-200 at 14′ are significant for both binocular and single eye data, with the greatest

393

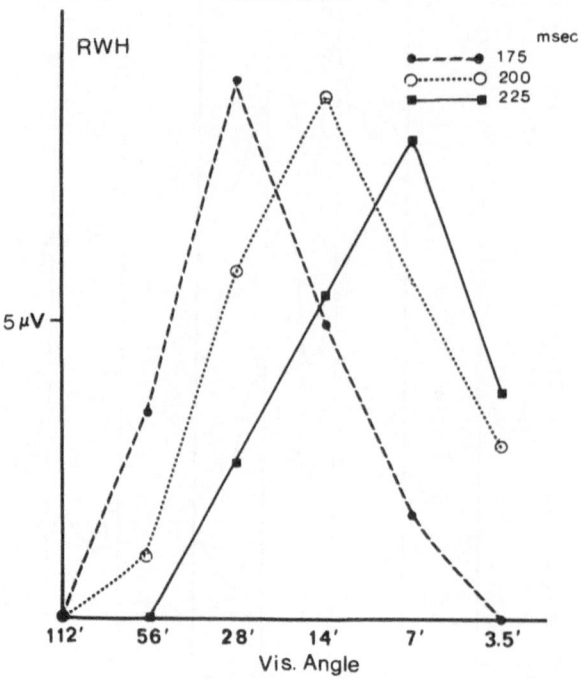

Fig. 3. Example of spatial frequency sensitivity function, 'tuning' of three temporal components of the pattern-reversal VEP for one subject.

significance for binocular results, when tested by Student's t-test for paired data. Significance for the binocular situation was p < 0.01.

Fig. 4 also includes a diagram of the ratio between the P-100 and the P-200 measures. This ratio is suggested as a possibly useful technique to employ since it would help to minimize the large variation in absolute amplitudes found in any group of individuals.

Fig. 5 contains the same information as does Fig. 4, but for the 1 m viewing condition for our normal group.

Fig. 6 presents a comparison of the mean amplitude from the twenty eyes in our normal group with the 24 eyes from the patient group for a range of visual patterns viewed at 1 m. The first thing to notice is that the P-100 is consistently larger for the patient group than for the normals. P-200, however, is another story: somewhat larger for the lowest spatial frequency stimulus used but steadily losing ground as the pattern elements become smaller. For the smallest pattern elements routinely used in our testing procedure, 14' visual angle, the normal amplitudes are significantly larger than those from p < 0.01 patient group. Because of the skewed distribution of patient data χ^2 tests of group differences were made for frequency of low or high response amplitude and for the P-200/P-100 ratios.

Fig. 7 shows the distribution of P-200 amplitudes of the two groups.

394

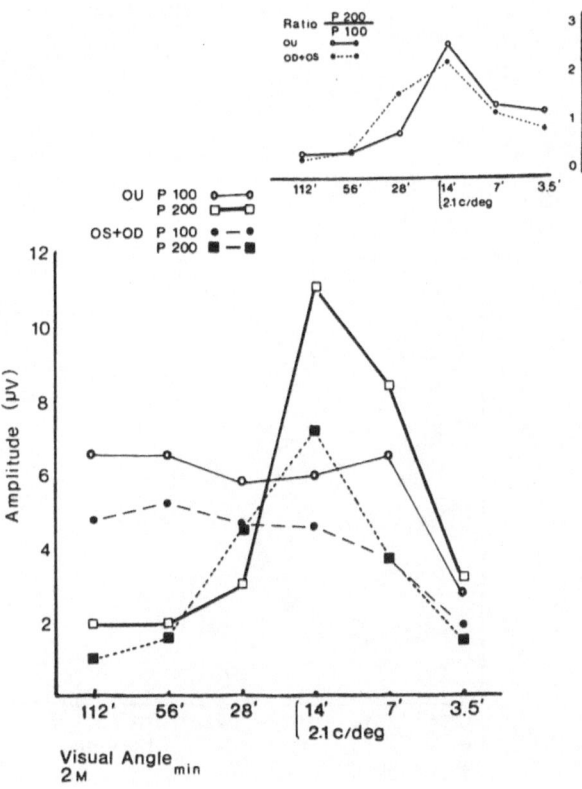

Fig. 4. Data for ten normal subjects, binocular and monocular, P100 and P200 amplitudes as a function of spatial frequency at 2 m, with ratios of P200/P100.

The use of the ratio, shown on Fig. 6, between P-200 and P-100 is seen to be of possible value. In this case its magnitude for the normal eyes is significantly greater than is the ratio for the patient group when the optimum spatial frequency stimulus pattern was used, with $p < 0.001$.

Fig. 8 presents records for four of the patient group who were referred because of unexplained losses in visual acuity. All were presented with the optimum stimulus for the normal group. It can be seen that there is little, if any, activity at 200 msec, whereas most of the group have sizeable P-100 components. The records on the right side of the Fig. 8 are for one of the group. In this case we summated responses for a wide range of stimulus patterns to see if any consistent components would become obvious. Only with the smaller patterns do we begin to see a minimum build-up at 200 msec. This particular patient has been examined extensively by visual specialists, and his best acuity is consistently no better the 20/200 corrected.

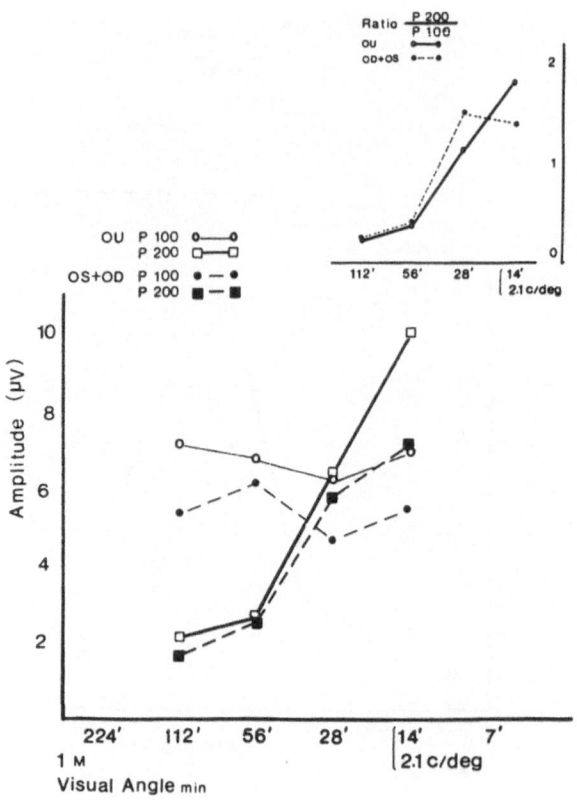

Fig. 5. Data for ten normal subjects, binocular and monocular, P100 and P200 amplitudes as a function of spatial frequency at 1 m, with ratios of P200/P100.

DISCUSSION

On the basis of the results reported here we have decided that the approach of using the P-200/P-100 ratio to quantify an individual's pattern response neurophysiologically is feasible. Although we did find a very significant difference in this measure between our normal and patient groups when the optimum check size was presented (14' of arc, or about 2.1 cycles/degrees), the difference would have been even more dramatic if we had limited our patient group to only those with well-established decrements in visual acuity. When we checked the records of those few who had high amplitude P-200s we found that this group included those who only had shown some inconsistency in their Snellen readings, and two were suspected malingerers.

Our decision to measure the secondary wave at precisely 200 msec based on the responses of the first few of our normals to be tested in detail, turned out to be correct, since was found that the large components occurring prior to that (if any) appear to be related to processes sensitive to only the lower spatial frequencies.

396

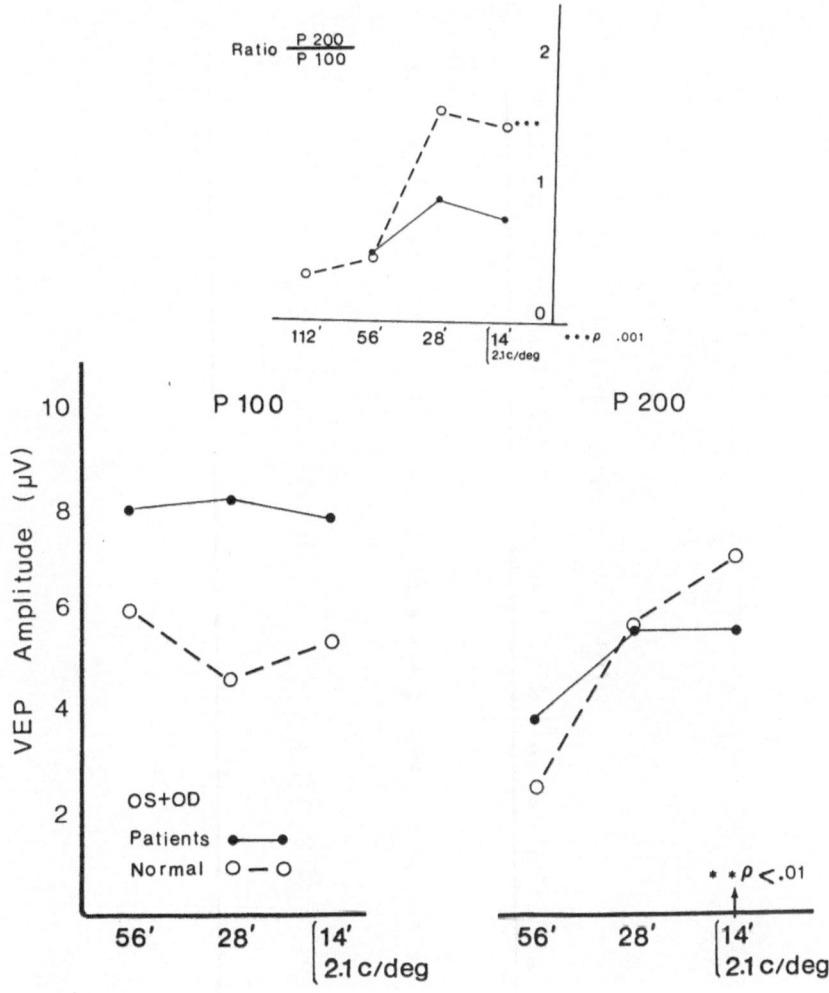

Fig. 6. Comparison of normal and patient groups, P100 and P200 amplitudes and P200/P100 ratios at 1 m.

It is believed that perhaps the most important result of this work was the finding that the secondary positive wave complex was not a unitary entity, but instead consisted of a number of sub-components with different sensitivities to spatial frequencies, and that those sensitive to the higher spatial frequencies occurred later in time, with the optimum sensitivity characteristic components being at 200 msec or slightly later.

A very detailed study of a number of our normal individuals showed that

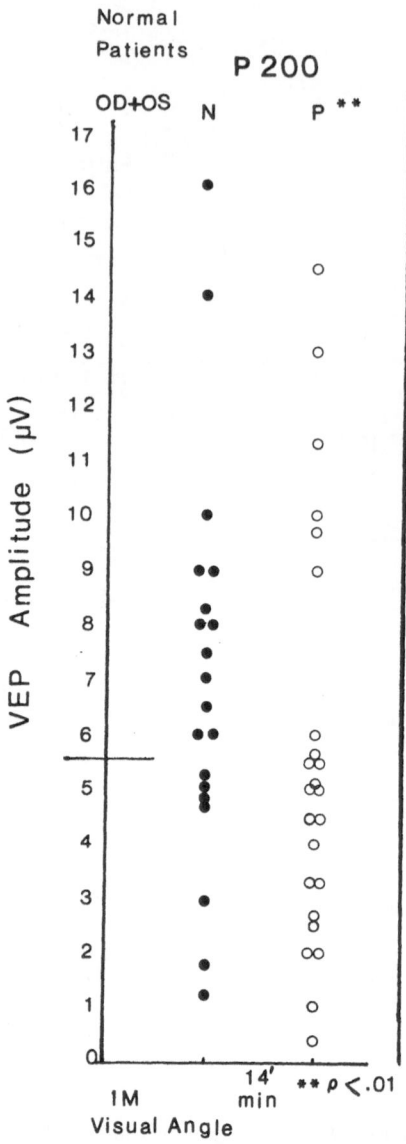

Fig. 7. Frequency distribution of P200 amplitude of normal vs patient eyes in response to optimal check size (14′ min/arc) at 1 m.

the responses of specific components around 200 msec were very sensitive to changes in the visual stimulus. For example one of the authors, RWH, required a slight correction for the left eye in order to bring both eyes up to 20/20. When the optimum stimulus pattern was presented to him binocularly with and without his glasses an interaction was to be seen among the

398

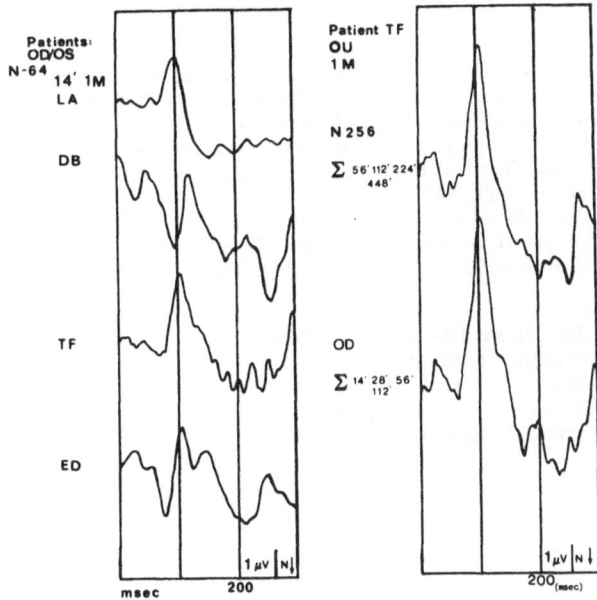

Fig. 8. Examples of pattern-reversal VEPs for 4 patients with unexplained visual acuity loss.

major subcomponents at 175, 200 and 225 msec. Without the glasses all three components were prominent, but the 175 was larger than the others. With the glasses, however, the 175 component fell in amplitude and the other two rose markedly, with the 200 msec component now being the largest. This was consistent enough for us to use it as a demonstration for interested visitors to the laboratory.

These findings seem to fit in very well with the previously reported fact that the secondary positive wave evoked by pattern reversal in an amblyopic eye tends to peak earlier than that of its unaffected mate (Sokol, 1982). It is clear that processes sensitive to the higher spatial frequencies (and occurring later in time) are selectively deactivated under such a condition.

Our other findings presented at this conference relating the P-100 to processing on a sub-cortical level, presumably the LGN, and the P-200 complex to cortical processing must also be considered here. They seem to add even more evidence for the role of selective cortical deficits in the development of amblyopia (De Valois, 1977; White, et al. 1982b).

Although the present findings are quite striking, and hopefully will prove to be of some value to those working in this field, many more very basic problems must be addressed in the future. What, for instance, is the nature of the slow potential upon which the spatially tuned components are superimposed, but which is seemingly not present in certain individuals who otherwise seem to have normal acuity and good vision in general? Also, the current findings seem to call for a close look at the ubiquitous P-100 (and its subcomponents) and how it relates to visual perception.

REFERENCES

De Valois, R. L., Albrecht, D. G. and Thorell, L. G. Spatial tuning of LGN and cortical cells in monkey visual system. In: H. Spekreijse and L. H. van der Tweel (Eds.) Spatial Contrast. Amsterdam, North Holland, 60–63 (1977).

Sokol, S. Pattern evoked potentials in visually normal and abnormal infants and young children. Docum. Ophthal. Proc. Series, Vol 31, Eds. G. Niemeyer and C. Huber. The Hague: Dr. W. Junk, 449–460 (1982).

White, C. T., White, C. L. and Hintze, R. W. Sub-cortical components of the VEP in adults and infants. In Docum. Opthal. Proc. Series, Vol 31, Eds. G. Nieymeyer and C. Huber. The Hague: Dr. W. Junk, 483–489 (1982).

Mailing address:
University of California Medical Center, San Diego
Department of Pediatrics, H-638-A
University Hospital
225 Dickinson Street
San Diego, California 92103, U.S.A.

CORTICAL VS SUB-CORTICAL COMPONENTS OF THE PATTERN VEP

C. T. WHITE, C. L. WHITE AND R. W. HINTZE

(San Diego, California, U.S.A.)

ABSTRACT

In a number of previous papers our group has shown that wavelength-related VEPs can be recorded from non-cortical sites. In the most recent of these, reported at the 1981 ISCEV meeting, data obtained from an hydranencephalic infant were included, confirming the sub-cortical nature of such responses. We have tentatively assumed that these responses relate to geniculate activity. We have recently carried out an extensive series of VEP studies using patterned stimuli, recording simultaneously from cortical and noncortical sites (Oz-Mastoid and Mastoid-Nose). Various stimulus presentation techniques were used, including transient flash/pattern and pattern alternation at various rates.

Marked responses were obtained consistently from the non-cortical montage, under some conditions being nearly equal in amplitude to those obtained from the usual montage. With Mastoid-Nose the major component occurs at 100 msec, this seeming to agree with our earlier findings. More significantly, however, with the Oz-Mastoid results we find two major positive components, at 100 and about 200 msec. These react quite differently to changes in spatial frequency. The latter component, assumed to be related to cortical activity, reacts very strongly to high spatial frequency and very weakly to low spatial frequency, whereas the earlier component reacts strongly to a wide range of spatial frequencies. This finding corresponds with the different results of single-cell studies in the LGN and cortex in recent studies (DeValois, 1982, personal communication).

INTRODUCTION

In a series of papers on color VEPs published by our group we have demonstrated that certain short latency components of the response, which differentiated on the basis of wavelength, have similar latencies when recorded from either the standard occiput to mastoid or from non-cortical sites. Several considerations have led to a tentative assumption that these responses are related to activity in the lateral geniculate and geniculocortical relay.

Several investigators have shown that contour related responses can be obtained from sub-cortical sites. For example, Millidot and Riggs (1970) showed that it was possible to obtain a measure of an eye's refractive state by using a pattern-reversal technique with the ERG as well as with the VEP. Armington and co-workers (1971) also simultaneously obtained pattern responses from VEP and ERG. More recently there has been more specific evidence of pattern processing at the retinal level (Maffei and Fiorentini, 1981; Arden, Vaegan and Hogg, 1982; Vaegan, Arden and Hogg, 1982).

For some time our group has been carrying out research related to pattern processing at various levels of the visual system, using both transient and pattern-reversal procedure. This report will present findings which concern two related issues. First an association between pattern VEP components around 100 msec at both cortical and non-cortical sites. Second the relative importance and significance of both P100 and P200 in the contour specific responses to large and small visual angles.

METHODS AND RESULTS

The Nicolet 1170 was used throughout. Pattern-reversal stimuli were generated by a Nicolet 1006 vision stimulator; brightness at level 3; reversal rate at 2 Hz unless otherwise indicated. Transient pattern obtained with Grass Photostimulator with checkerboard transparencies. The only procedure deviating from the standard was montages which are described below. All subjects were adults with corrected vision of 20/20 or better.

Fig. 1 shows the effect of varying sharpness of the retinal image on the VEP with transient pattern. This procedure is an extension of earlier studies by Harter and White (1968), but here the active electrode is non-cortical over the cheek bone. When the pattern is completely blurred (6 diopters) the response resembles the classic ERG. However, with sharper focus well established contour related responses are seen. At the sharpest focus these non-cortical EP include a definite positive peak at 50 msec, in agreement with the recent work on retinal pattern cited; while two important negative components are seen at 90 and 150 msec. The P90 was called the 'A' component by Harter and White and the 'contour specific component' by Spekreijse, van der Tweel and Zuidema (1973). Notably, however, the non-cortical does not show the second contour specific component identified by Harter and White in the postive peak at 175 msec. As in our color EP, components occurring after 175 or 200 msec are either missing or minimized in non-cortical records. The cortical and non-cortical records show certain systematic relationships but follow different 'rules'. This is particularly marked for the pattern responses.

Early and late components, P100/P200; cortical/non-cortical. Relationships of these components and their cortical/non-cortical correspondences were studied at Oz and at mastoid. Simultaneous responses were obtained with active electrode at each site, varying spatial frequency with reversal at 2 Hz, Figs. 2, 3, 4. Fig. 2 the cortical (Oz-M) record shows a shift in prominence from P100 for large to P200 for small checks, an effect which is not in the

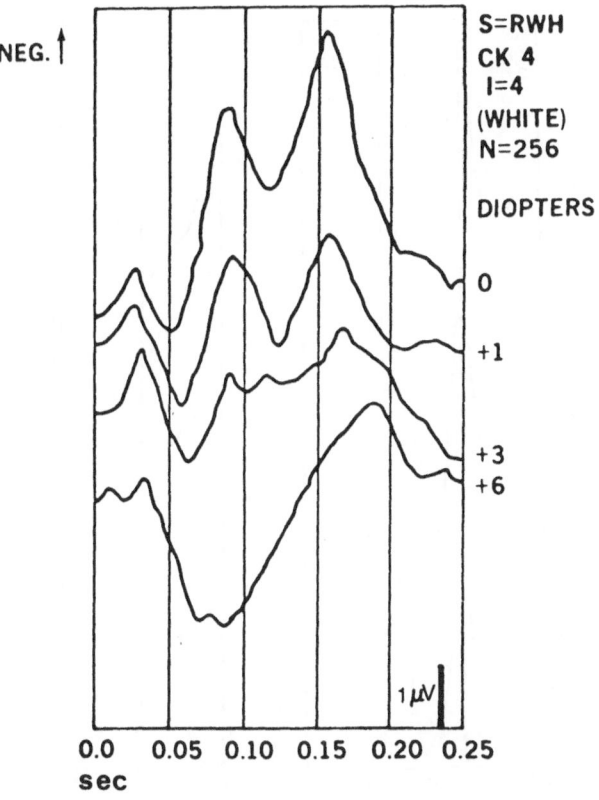

NEG. ↑

S=RWH
CK 4
I=4
(WHITE)
N=256

DIOPTERS

0

+1

+3
+6

1 μV

0.0   0.05   0.10   0.15   0.20   0.25
sec

Fig. 1. Transient pattern presented with active electrode over the cheek bone and reference at the mastoid. Check 4 is the 'optimal size', 14 min of arc.

mastoid (M-nose) record. P100 shows greater agreement at each site, however, than does P200. The non-cortical record shows components later than 50 msec which are usually thought of as exclusively occipital, occurring as late as 200 msec. In Fig. 3 presentation is made to single eyes. At 14′, the optimal size, we expect and find a prominant cortical (Oz-M) P200 which is minimal from the mastoid. Despite correction for 20/20 this subject is missing P200 at the smallest visual angle in OD recording from both sites.

Comparing cortical and mastoid records the latter suggest that the P100 is not a unitary response, but may be related to 2 or 3 sub-components differing with spatial frequency. Non-cortical P100 appears to contribute consistently to this component in Figs. 2 and 3, but in Fig. 4 it is shown that this contribution occurs most clearly in the central visual field. For the cortical response P100 is produced primarily by the lower visual field at each visual angle, but most clearly for the optimal 14′. The LVF should be used in neurological examinations when P100 is of critical concern. This has been found also by Stockard, J. S. (Personal communication).

403

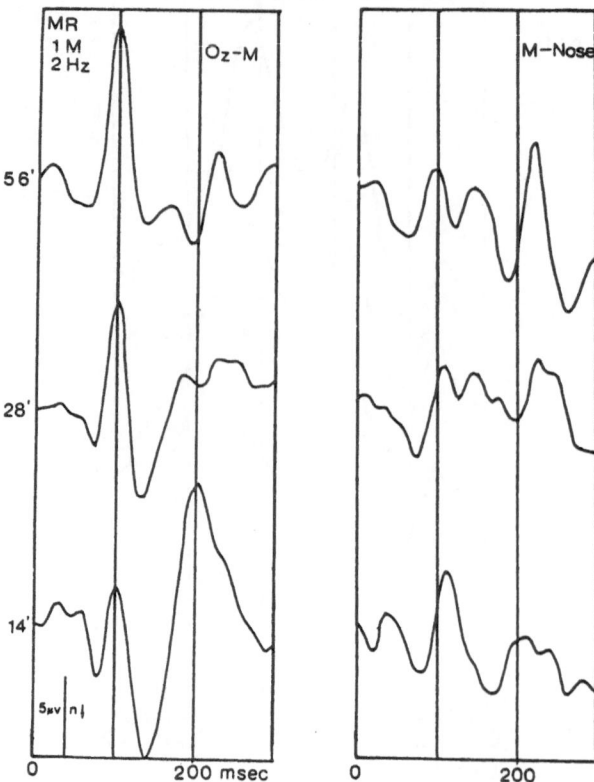

Fig. 2. Binocular presentation of pattern reversal with visual angle at 1 meter: 56', 28' and 14' (min of arc). Simultaneous records were obtained for cortical and non-cortical sites with active electrode at Oz and reference at the mastoid for cortical, and active electrode over the right mastoid and reference on the tipe of the nose for non-cortical.

Cortical/non-cortical components in fast pattern reversal (16.5 Hz). The degree of cortical vs non-cortical function sampled by fast pattern reversal has been examined. Fig. 5 shows clearly that the cortical processing is primarily sampled; the largest amplitude was obtained when the Oz-chin montage was used, about 25% greater than the standard Oz-mastoid montage. Of primary interest is the high spatial-frequency sensitivity of the Oz amplitudes, while the mastoid-active show almost the same amplitude for the full set of check sizes. The occipital response is finely tuned to high spatial frequencies while the sub-cortical is not; a conclusion which is in accord with the studies of De Valois and associates sampling the 'spatial tuning' of single LGN and cortical cells (1977).

Comparison of P100/P200 component as well as single cell LGN/striate spatial tuning. Our work suggests that with the slower pattern-reversal work P100 more consistently than P200 represents non-cortical function and that

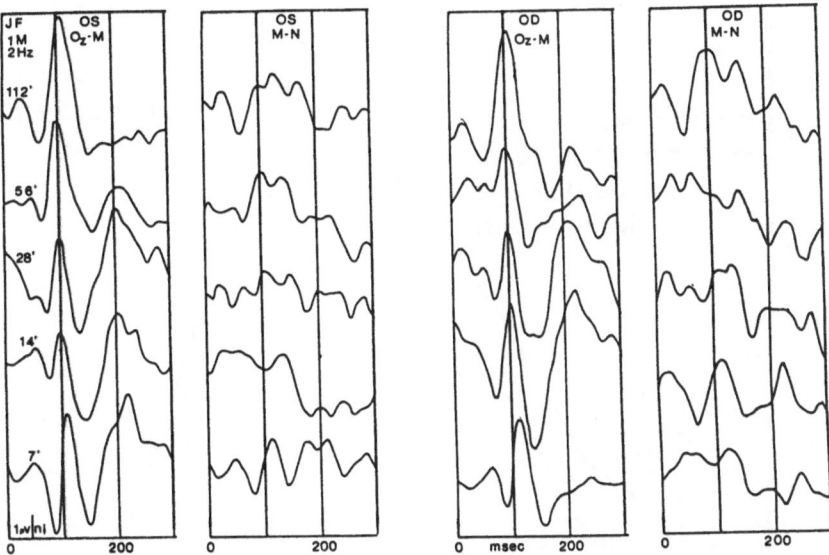

Fig. 3. Pattern reversal presentation at 1 meter for single eyes with recording simultaneous at cortical (Oz-Mastoid reference) and non-cortical (mastoid-nose reference). Visual angle of patterns ranged from 112' to 77' min of arc.

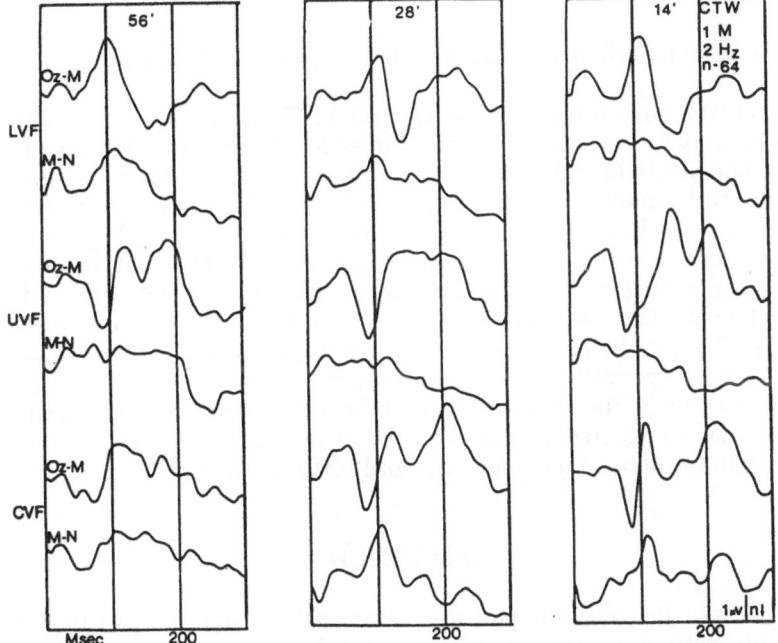

Fig. 4. Binocular presentation of 3 check sizes with pattern reversal and recording simultaneously from cortical (Oz-M) and (M-Nose). Upper, lower and central visual field EPs are presented for each visual angle at 1 meter.

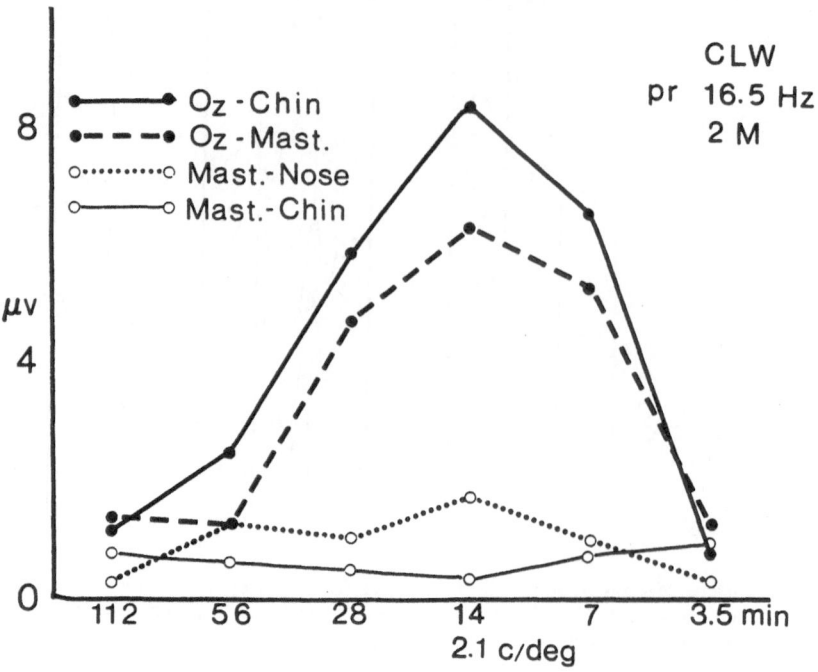

Fig. 5. Cortical and sub-cortical responses to high frequency pattern-reversals.

it is relatively insensitive to spatial frequency. The difference in spatial sensitivity is shown in a diagram in Fig. 6 in which the mean amplitudes of the two components for 10 normal subjects are given, using binocular presentation. P100 includes maximum response obtained in the time zone of 100–120 msec, and P200 was measured at precisely 200 msec. The former is constant over a wide spatial-frequency range while P200 is sharply sensitive to the higher frequencies. The difference at 2.1 c/deg is significant $p < 0.01$ with student t-test for paired observations. In Fig. 6 we have also included findings from DeValois recorded from macaque LGN and striate cortex. The former responded in a fairly equal manner over a wide range of spatial frequencies, while the cortical cells were 'tuned' to specific high frequencies. These data are adapted so that the contrast sensitivity of cells can be compared with the mean amplitude values for P100 and P200.

DISCUSSION

It is believed that the data presented support the hypothesis that for either transient pattern or slow pattern reversal VEP components around 100 and 200 msecs are related to processing occurring at different levels of the visual system. Our earlier suggestions that the activity around 100 msec is

406

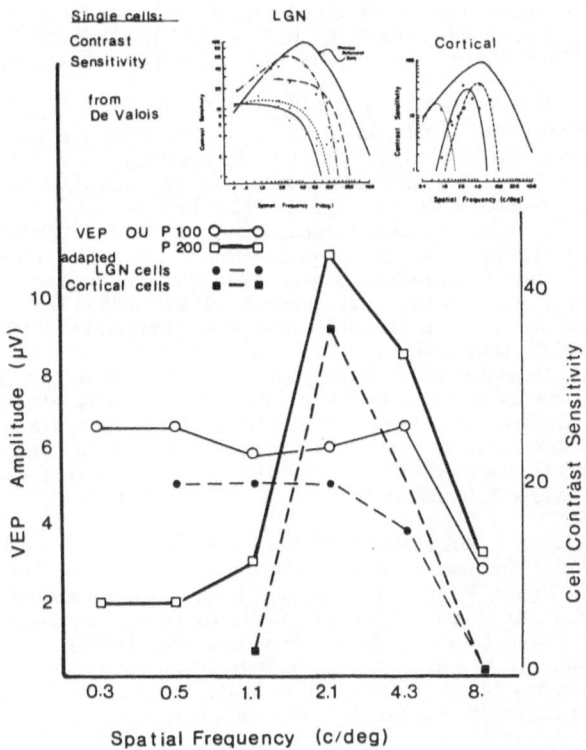

Fig. 6. Mean amplitudes P100 and P200 for normal humans in comparison with cell activity of LGN and striate cortex of macaque.

related to sub-cortical processing, probably in the LGN gain support from the findings of marked functional differences with regard to spatial frequency of cells in the macaque LGN and cortex. The large P100 activity recorded with the active Oz electrode could well be primarily related to activity in the geniculo-striate fibers and not to cortical processing per se. This possibility has been discussed earlier by Creutzfeldt (1973). The observation made by others that P100 tends to occur later when the spatial frequency of the stimulus is increased, appears to be related to the presence of a number of components around 100 msec which react differentially to spatial frequency.

REFERENCES

Arden, G. B., Vaegen and Hogg, C. R. Clinical and experimental evidence that the pattern ERG (PERG) is generated by the innermost retinal layers. Annal. N.Y. Accad. Sci. (1982).

Armington, J. C., Corwin, T. R. and Marsetta, R. Simultaneously recorded retinal and cortical responses to patterned stimuli. J. Opt. Soc. Amer. 61: 1514–1521 (1971).

Creutzfeldt, O. D. and Kuhnt, U. Electrophysiology and topographical distribution of visual evoked potentials in animals. In: R. Jung (Ed.) Handbook of Sensory Physiology, Vol VII/3, Visual centers of the brain. New York: Springer-Verlag, 595–646 (1973).

De Valois, R. L., Albrecht, D. G. and Thorell, L. G. Spatial tuning of LGN and cortical cells in monkey visual system. In: H. Spekreijse and L. H. van der Tweel (Eds.) Spatial Contrast. Amsterdam, North Holland, 60–63 (1977).

Harter, M. R. and White, C. T. Effects of contour sharpness and check-size on visually evoked cortical potentials. Vis. Res., 8: 701–711 (1968).

Maffei, L. and Fiorentini, A. Electroretinographic responses to alternating gratings before and after section of the optic nerve. Science, 211: 953–955 (1981).

Millodot, M. and Riggs, L. A. Refraction determined electrophysiologically: Responses to alternation of visual contours. Arch. Ophthal., 84: 272–278 (1970).

Spekreijse, H., van der Tweel, L. H. and Zuidema, T. Contrast evoked responses in man. Vis Res. 13: 1577–1601 (1973).

Vaegan, Arden, G. B. and Hobb, C. R. Properties of normal electroretinograms evoked by patterned stimuli in man. Doc Opthal. Proc. Series, Vol 31; 19th ISCEV Symposium. Eds. G. Niemeyer and C. Huber. The Hague: Dr. W. Junk, 111–129 (1982).

White, C. T., Kataoka, R. and Martin, J. I. Colour evoked potentials: Development of a methodology for the study of the processes involved in colour vision. In J. Desmedt (Ed.) Visual Evoked Potentials in Man: New Developments. Oxford, Clarendon Press, 250–272 (1977).

White, C. T., White, C. L. and Hintze, R. W. The color evoked potential and comparison of monocular and binocular effects. Int. J. Neurosci., 8: 205–217 (1979a).

White, C. T. and Hintze, R. W. Color evoked potentials: cortical and subcortical elements. In: E. Callaway and D. Lehmann (Eds.) Human Evoked Potentials: Applications and Problems. New York: Plenum Press, 431–442 (1979b).

White, C. T., White, C. L. and Hintze, R. W. Sub-cortical components of the VEP in adults and infants. Docum Ophthal. Proc. Series, Vol 31, Eds. G. Niemeyer and C. Huber. The Hague: Dr. W. Junk, 483–489 (1982).

Mailing address:
University of California Medical Center, San Diego
Department of Pediatrics, H-638-A
University Hospital
225 Dickenson Street
San Diego, California 92103, U.S.A.

STUDIES ON VISUAL LEARNING GAIN BY MEANS OF VEP'S

S. ICHIHASHI AND J. TSUTSUI

(Kurashiki, Japan)

ABSTRACT

Vertex potential (P200) and event related potential (P300) evoked by word stimulation on a TV screen were studied in normal adults and patients with organic or functional disease of the brain and optic nerve.

In normal adults, the effects of the meaningful words (in 3 Japanese letters) on visual evoked potentials (VEPs) with and without the task were compared. The task was to count the numbers of randomly interposed animal names out of the 50 words. In normal adults when watching words with the task, the P300 waves were topographically distinct from the preceding P200 over the centro-parietal scalp.

In patients with organic brain lesions such as cerebral atrophy, components corresponding to the P200 were decreased in amplitude whereas the P300 were not affected by the lesion. The P300 was however affected by whether the subjects had a task solving ability or not. In cases with mental deterioration, the peak latency of P300 conformed to the subjective ability of the task solving. In patients with functional amblyopia and optic nerve disease, prolongation of the peak latency and reduction of the amplitude of P200 occurred when the affected eye was stimulated. However, there was no difference in the latency period of P300 between the normal and affected eye.

Consequently, the P200 was influenced not only by the amount of attention the subjects paid but also by the degree of visual input. On the other hand, the P300 was influenced not by the degree of visual input but by the subject's ability of solving the task.

Therefore, the P300 response is useful for an objective evaluation of visual learning gain.

INTRODUCTION

The late components of visual evoked potentials (VEPs) have been reported as an indicator for psychological activity (1–6). We studied vertex potential

A preliminary report of this subject has been published in the Jap. J. Clin. Ophthal., 34: 873–876, 1980 and the Acta Soc. Ophthalmol. Jap. 86: 587–595, 1982.

(P200) and event related potential (P300) for objective evaluation of the visual learning gain. The P200 and the P300 evoked by word stimulation on a TV screen were studied in normal adults and patients with organic or functional disease of the brain and optic nerve. We elucidate the significance of P200 and P300 components in VEPs.

METHODS

Fourteen neurologically healthy adult subjects and at least 5 patients each with organic or functional disease of the brain and optic nerve were studied. Patients were classified in 4 groups; organic brain lesions, mental deterioration, functional amblyopia and optic nerve disease.

Stimulation words were meaningful words (in 3 Japanese characters) arranged to include various names of common objects and animals as well as some verbs (Fig. 1). They were recorded at intervals of 2 to 3 seconds on a video tape recorder (VTR). These words were continuously projected on a video TV-screen as a series. A trigger pulse could be recorded on a sound track of the VTR when patterns changed.

ひらがな文字

こねこ	だっこ	あそび	ねずみ	さとう
あまい	きつね	からだ	いたい	うさぎ
あせも	かゆい	たぬき	くすり	にがい
いちご	きりん	ばなな	どうろ	わたる
きけん	にげる	ころぶ	くるま	はねる
さかな	めろん	わかめ	さざえ	すいか
おかし	あわび	さいふ	おかね	きっぷ
もうけ	くじら	りんご	するめ	つばめ
おさつ	たかい	やすい	ひよこ	みかん
まぐろ	ぶどう	みやげ	おかき	すずめ

Fig. 1. Stimulation words, the fifty meaningful words in 3 Japanese letters including various names of common objects and animals as well as some verbs.

The subject reclined in a chair 1.0 m from a viewing screen. The spindle electrodes were placed at Cz, Pz and Oz according to the international 10–20 system. The right ear lobe served as reference for monopolar recording. Supraorbital and infraorbital electrodes were applied to the right eye. The vertical EOG was recorded to detect eyeblinks and eye movements. EEG and periorbital potentials were amplified both with a time constant of 0.1 sec and a high cut filter of 25 Hz. Fifty responses were averaged by an averager and recorded on a X-Y recorder.

The effects were compared of the meaningful words on VEPs with and without additional task. The task was to count the numbers of randomly interposed animal names out of the 50 words.

RESULTS

1. Normal adult subjects

The effects of meaningful words on VEPs at Cz with and without the task are shown in Fig. 2. A reproducible VEP was obtained in 10 cases out of 14 cases (71%). Fig. 2 shows the VEPs when watching with and without task. The VEPs at Cz from 10 normal subjects were superimposed. The earlier waves, P200, did not show a significant difference between the two conditions. On the contrary, when subjects count the animal names, P300 elicited typically at Cz.

2. Subjects with organic brain lesion

Reproducible data were obtained in 6 cases out of 12 (50%). We were not able to find P300 waves in all cases with the exception of one case who was able to solve the task. Fig. 3 shows the 18-year-old male who had the ability of the task solving. He had porencephaly and a low density area at the left occipito-parietal region on CT scan, which was, severely atrophied. The P300 waves were found widely distributed cerebral surface. On the other hand, the components corresponding to the P200 wave at O_1 were smaller than those at O_2.

Consequently, in patients with the organic brain lesions such as cerebral atrophy, components corresponding to the P200 were decreased in amplitude but the P300 was not affected by the lesion. P300 was however, affected by whether the subjects had a task solving ability or not.

3. Subjects with mental deterioration

Reproducible data were obtained in 10 cases out of 15 (67%). The VEPs at Cz of the patients with mental deterioration, when watching words with the task were presented in Fig. 4. The latency periods of P200 and P300 were longer in patients than in normal adults. Especially, the peak latency periods of P300, indicated by the triangles, were delayed. The latency periods of P300 waves at Cz in 6 cases with mental deterioration are longer by 2 standard deviations than those of normal controls.

411

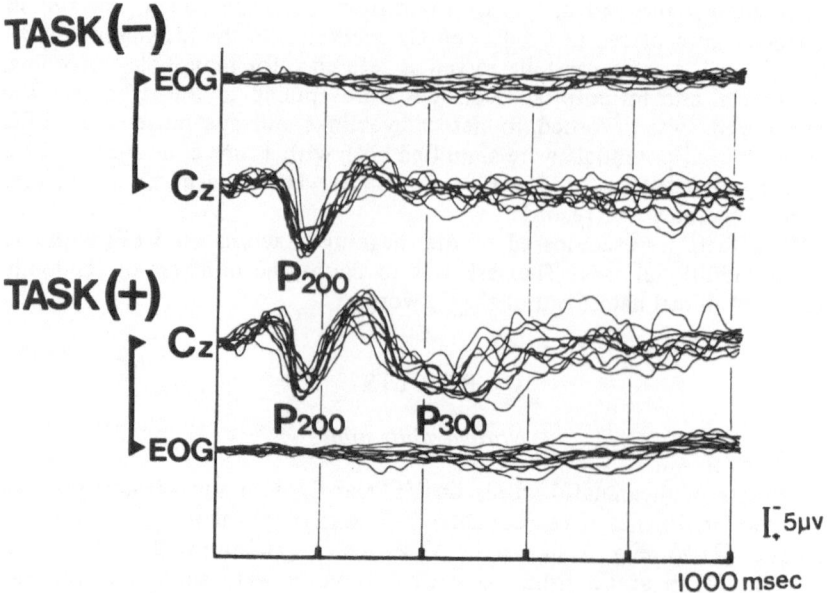

Fig. 2. The VEPs at Cz from 10 normal subjects were superimposed when watching with and without task.

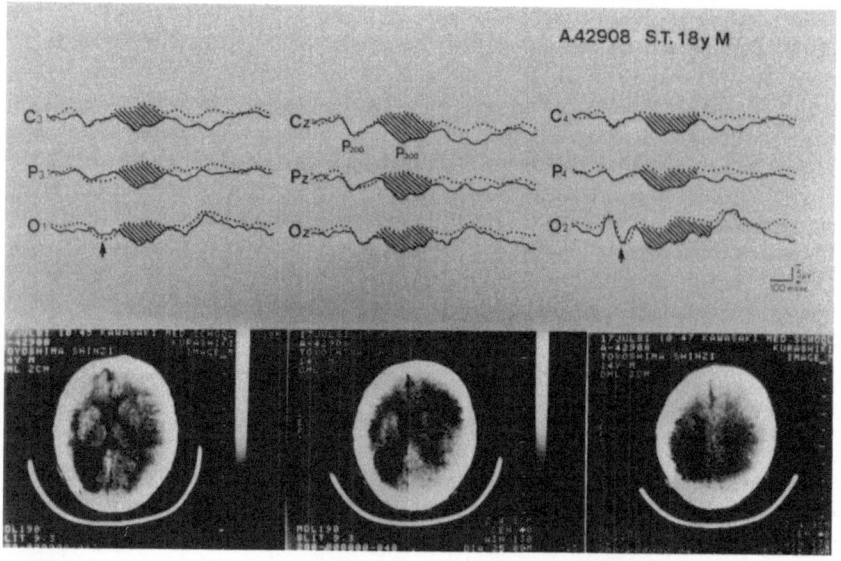

Fig. 3. VEP topography and CT scan in a case of porencephaly of a 18-year-old male. There was a low density area at the left occipito-parietal region in CT scan. Components corresponding to P200 at O_1 were decreased in amplitude, whereas the P300 was not affected at the lesion.

412

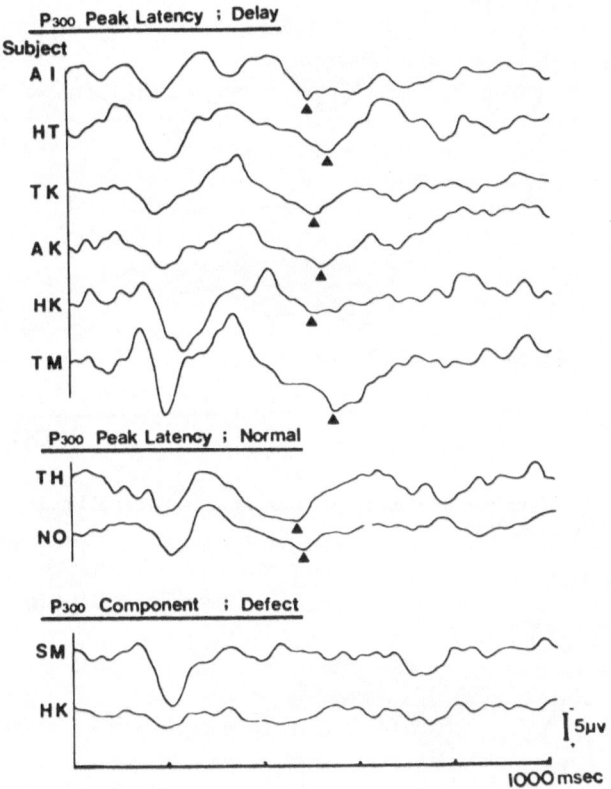

Fig. 4. The VEPs at Cz of patients with mental deterioration when watching words with the task. The latency periods of P300 waves in 6 cases were delayed (upper). 2 cases were within normal limits (middle). There were no P300 components in 2 cases (lower).

Besides that 2 cases were within normal limits and no P300 components were seen in the remaining 2 cases. In mental deterioration, the peak latency periods of P300 waves are influenced by the subject's to solve the task.

4. Subjects with functional amblyopia

Reproducible data were obtained in 5 cases out of 10 (50%). Fig. 5 shows VEPs at Cz to stimulation of either eye in the case of a 9-year-old male with strabismic amblyopia in the right eye. The corrected visual acuity was 0.2 in the right eye and 1.0 in the left eye. The latency of P200 was about 250 msec in the affected eye and 215 msec in the normal eye. The amplitude of the P200 was smaller in the affected eye than that in the normal eye. P300 latency showed no difference between the two eyes. Four other cases of functional amblyopia also showed the same tendency as this case.

413

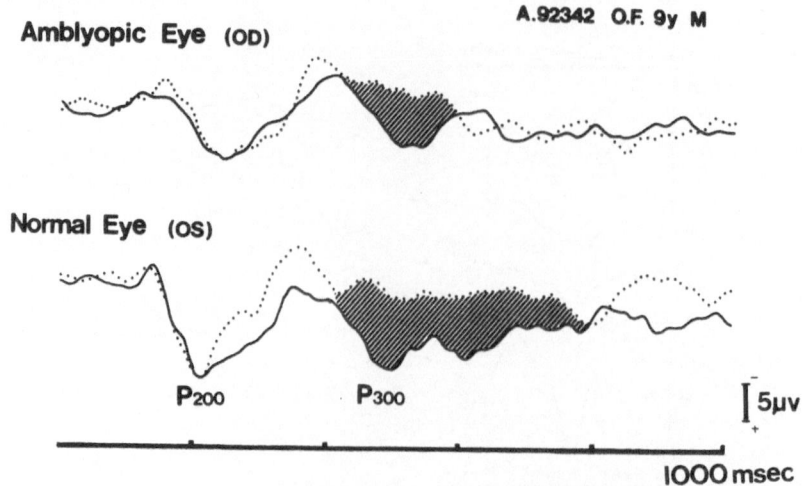

Fig. 5. VEPs at Cz to stimulation of either eye in a case of a 9-year-old male with strabismic amblyopia in the right eye. (see text)

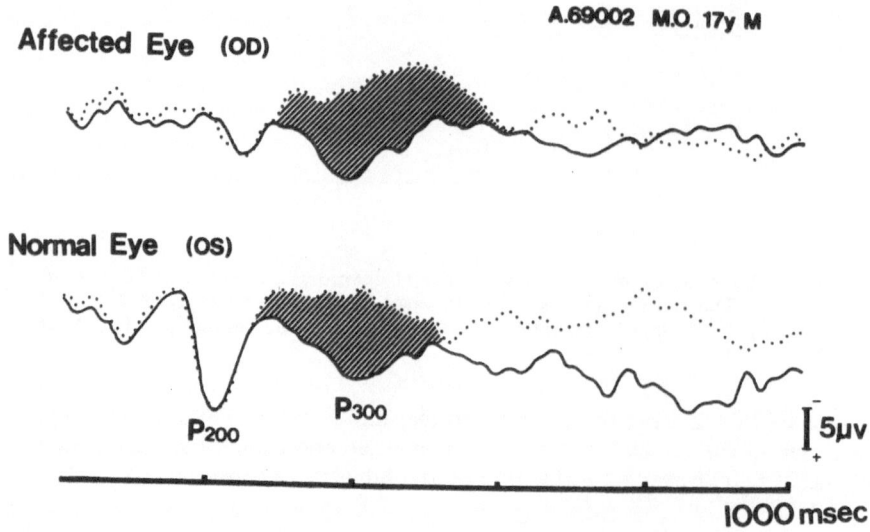

Fig. 6. VEPs at Cz to stimulation of either eye in the case of a 17-year-old male who had a right optic atrophy caused by an optic canal fracture. (see text)

5. Subjects with optic nerve disease

Reproducibility was found in 5 cases out of 7 (71%). Fig. 6 shows the VEPs of a 17-year-old male who had a right optic atrophy caused by an optic canal fracture. His corrected visual acuity was 0.2 in the affected eye and 1.5 in the normal eye. The latency of P200 was extended by about 35 msec and the

414

P200 amplitude was reduced by about 8.0 μV in the affected eye. However, there was no difference in the latency of P300 between both eyes. The group with optic nerve disease showed the same tendency as the group with functional amblyopia.

DISCUSSION

The present study showed a change of the vertex potential (P200) and event related potential (P300) of VEPs in normal subjects and in patients with organic or functional disease of the brain and optic nerve. There were differences between P200 and P300 because intrinsic or extrinsic factors affected them in different ways.

The P200 component in patients with organic brain lesions and mental deterioration showed longer latencies than in normal adults. Since their intelligence quotients were low a reduction of alertness or consciousness might have influenced them. P300 was not appearing in patients who were not able to solve the task.

In patients with functional amblyopia and optic nerve disease, a prolongation of the peak latency and reduction of the amplitude of P200 occurred when the affected eye was stimulated.

On the other hand, components of P300 were not different between the eyes.

In conclusion, the evidence we found in this study showed that P200 must be the first step in the cognitive process of visual attention, and the following P300 seemed to indicate a higher selective process of vision. Moreover P200 was influenced not only by the amount of the subject's attention but also by the degree of visual input. On the other hand, P300 was influenced not by the degree of visual input but by the subject's ability of the task solving.

REFERENCES

1. Davis, H., Osterhammel, P. A., Wier, C. C. and Gjerdingen, D. B. Slow vertex potentials: Interactions among auditory, tactile, electric and visual stimuli. Electroenceph. clin Neurophysiol., 33: 537–545, 1972.
2. Freidman, D., Simson, R., Ritter, W. and Papin, I. The late positive component (P300) and information processing in sentences. Electroenceph. clin. Neurophysiol., 38: 255–262, 1975.
3. Goodin, D. S., Squires, K. C. and Starr, A. Long latency event-related components of the auditory evoked potential in dementia. Brain, 101: 635–648, 1978.
4. Kutas, M., McCarthy, G. and Donchin, E. Augmenting mental chronometry: The P300 as a measure of stimulus evaluation time. Science, 197: 792–795, 1977.
5. Shelburne Jr., S. A. Visual evoked responses to word and nonsense syllable stimuli. Electroenceph. clin. Neurophysiol., 32: 17–25, 1972.
6. Sutton, S., Braren, M., Zubin, J. and John, E. R. Evoked-potential correlates of stimulus uncertainty. Science, 150: 1187–1188, 1965.

Mailing address:
Department of Ophthalmology
Kawasaki Medical School,
Kurashiki, Japan 701-01

PATTERN EVOKED POTENTIAL LATENCY AS INDICATOR OF EARLY AND DELAYED CNS CHANGES DUE TO ANTILEUKEMIA TREATMENT IN CHILDREN

E. MACCOLINI

(Bologna, Italy)

ABSTRACT

Central nervous system (CNS) irradiation and/or intrathecal antineoplastic drugs have strongly reduced meningeal involvement in young patients affected by acute lymphoblastic leukemia (ALL), but they have also produced adverse side effects: a) cranial irradiation has been implicated in the pathogenesis of early CNS defects (self-limited somnolence syndrome), b) the association of cranial irradiation (CI) with intrathecal methotrexate (IT-MTX) seems to give rise to late encephalopathies.

White matter demyelination has been demonstrated in both early and late CNS side effects of ALL therapy. Pattern reversal visually evoked potentials (VEPs) were examined in children affected by ALL in order to test their usefulness in the detection of early and delayed side effects.

Peak to peak amplitude and peak latency of the main positive component (high contrast check-reversal stimulation of different angular size: 80′, 40′, 20′ and 10′) were compared with those of a control group.

The results suggest that:

a) in patients without self limited somnolence syndrome and visual symptons increased VEP latency may occur 40–80 days after CI probably caused by early subclinical CNS changes involving optic pathways,

b) delayed CNS changes (detected by neurological routine examination, EEG, and CAT scan) are correlated to increased VEP latency, even in the absence of visual symptons.

The results, as a whole, show that pattern reversal VEPs are a useful diagnostic aid for screening CNS changes due to CI and IT-MTX in ALL patients.

INTRODUCTION

Central nervous system (CNS) irradiation and/or intrathecal antineoplastic drugs have strongly reduced meningeal involvement in young patients affected by acute lymphoblastic leukemia (ALL), but they have also produced adverse side effects:

a) cranial irradiation (CI) has been implicated in the pathogenesis of early CNS defects (self limited somnolence syndrome: Freeman et al., 1973),
b) the association of CI with intrathecal methotrexate (IT-MTX) seems to give rise to late encephalopathies (Bleyer et al., 1980).

White matter demyelination has been demonstrated in both early and late CNS side effects of ALL therapy (Lampert et al., 1959; Rider, 1963; Freeman et al., 1973; Rubinstein, 1975; Muller et al., 1976; Poplack et al., 1977; Smith, 1979).

A increased pattern reversal VEP latency appears to be closely connected with demyelination of visual pathway even in absence of visual symptoms (Halliday et al., 1973, 1974, 1977; Hennerici et al., 1977).

Pattern-reversal visually evoked potentials were examined in children affected by ALL (and free from visual symptoms) in order to test their usefulness in the detection of early and delayed side effects of CNS treatment.

MATERIALS AND METHODS

Patients. Two groups of ALL patients were studied.

First group: 18 children (6 male and 12 female, between 3 and 11 years of age, mean age 6.9 years) were examined (VEPs recordings, EEG, opthalmological and neurological routine examination) initially and 40–80 days after CI.

Out of these patients 6 (33%) developed symptoms of somnolence, anorexia and EEG changes attributed to the self limited somnolence syndrome.

Second group: 27 children (11 male and 16 female, between 5 and 16 years of age, mean age 9.2 years) underwent VEPs examination, as well ophthalmological and neurological routine examinations and neuroradiological investigations, between 45 and 78 months after CI. Out of these patients 7 (26%) developed late CNS changes which were attributed to the side effects of ALL therapy.

All patients (of both the first and the second group) were free from: a) pathological findings at the routine ophthalmological examination, b) meningeal leukemia, c) peripheral nervous system anomalies.

All children received antileukemia treatment according to protocol #7601 or #7602 (which include prednisone, vincristine, cytosine arabinoside, levo-asparaginase, methotrexate, 6-mercaptopurine) and underwent cranial irradiation (Co 60: 200–2400 R total dose).

Visually evoked potentials. Reversing checkerboard patterns with check sizes of 80′, 40′, 20′ and 10′ were generated on a circular television screen subtending a visual angle of 17° (at the viewing distance of 1 m).

A fixation point was placed at the center of the screen. Reversal frequency was 1 Hz. The mean luminance of the screen was 20 cd/m^2 and the pattern contrast was 0.88. VEPs were recorded bipolarly by Ag-AgCl scalp-electrodes placed at positions O_z, P_z (10–20 system). The right earlobe was grounded. 64 responses were averaged and recorded on an X-Y plotter.

Experiments were performed in a dark room.

Peak to peak amplitude and peak latency of P100 of VEPs following binocular stimulation were evaluated.

In a previous study, pattern-reversal VEPs were recorded in 42 control subjects (20 male and 22 female, between 4 and 17 years of age, mean age 8 years); each subject submitted to 2 recording sessions at intervals ranging from 1 to 90 days. Mean values of P100 amplitude and latency (and their SD) found in both the first and second recording sessions are reported in Table 1.

Table 1. Normal subjects. Mean amplitude (uVolt), mean latency (msec), and their SD, of P100 with different check sizes, found in both the first and the second recording session

	AMPLITUDE				LATENCY			
	1st RECORDING SESSION		2nd RECORDING SESSION		1st RECORDING SESSION		2nd RECORDING SESSION	
	$\overline{X}$	SD	$\overline{X}$	SD	$\overline{X}$	SD	$\overline{X}$	SD
Check size: 80'	14,2	6,8	14,6	6,8	100,5	5,5	99,5	5,4
40'	16,5	6,9	16,6	7,1	102	5,3	104,5	5,6
20'	18,7	6,1	19,1	5,8	105	4,7	101	4,6
10'	15,6	6,7	15	6,2	120,5	7,6	122,5	7,4

The normal deviation ($Zi = X - \mu/\sigma$) of P100 peak amplitude and peak latency (and its probability of being greater than values found in controls) was evaluated in VEP recordings of each patient of the first group (assuming μ and σ values differ between the first and second recording session), and of the second group (comparing them with μ and σ values found in the first recording).

The technique used to record the EEG was with electrode placement according to either the 10—20 system (during the first year of this study) or to the measurements from bony landmarks (Pampiglione, 1976).

The CAT scan was performed by a 1010 CT EMI scan with contrast enhancement when necessary.

RESULTS

First group. No significant anomalies of both amplitude and latency of P100 were found in leukemic patients before treatment.

In 7 patients (39%), the traces recorded 40—80 days after the CI showed an increased ($P < 0.05$) latency as compared with the previous ones (recorded before treatment). This delay was more evident in responses obtained by the checker-board pattern with check sizes of 20' and 10' (Fig. 1).

Out of these 7 cases 4 developed self limited somnolence syndrome symptoms, 3 cases did not.

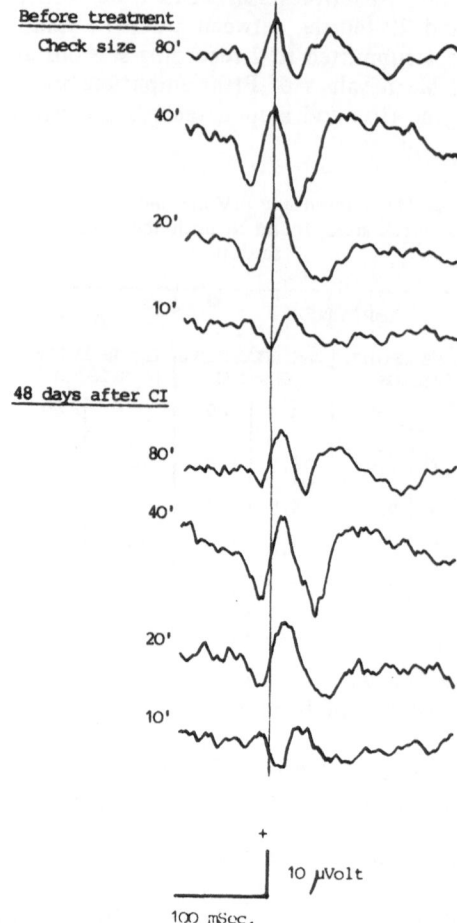

C.L. 10 YRS. (AFFECTED BY ALL)

PATTERN-REVERSAL VEPs

Before treatment
Check size 80'

40'

20'

10'

48 days after CI

80'

40'

20'

10'

+

10 μVolt

100 mSec.

Fig. 1. Pattern-reversal VEPs recorded in a 10 years old boy affected by ALL before and after cranial irradiation.
The P100 latency time appears increased in the traces obtained after CI.
The patient showed the limited somnolence syndrome symptoms (somnolence and EEG changes) at time of the second VEPs recording session.

Second group. No significant anomalies of the P100 amplitude were found.

Latency, on the contrary, was significantly (P 0.05) increased (for all 4 spatial frequencies) in 4 patients (15%), who developed very serious CNS alterations (Figs. 2, 3).

Out of the other 22 patients (free from VEPs anomalies) only 3 developed mild neurologic symptoms: the EEG showed a mild excess of slow components in particular over the posterior regions in 2 cases; one case showed low amplitudes.

420

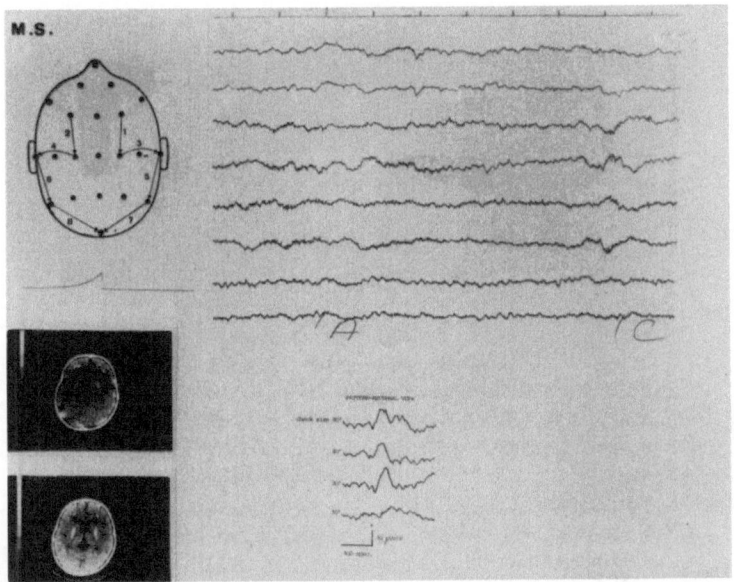

Fig. 2. Examples of correlation between neurophysiological (VEPs and EEG) and neuroradiological findings in two ALL patients, affected by late CNS therapy side effects,
Case a): the child (7 years old) experienced seizures 4 months after CI (at this time the
EEG showed diffuse slow amplitude activity), therefore IT-MTX maintenance therapy
was withdrawn. He was examined 45 months after CI: EEG showed normal activity,
CAT showed white matter isodensity near the frontal horn of lateral right ventricle and
some calcium deposits in the right frontal area.

DISCUSSION

The present study was performed on a limited number of patients, however, some conclusions may be drawn.

The variability of P100 latency found in normals is partially due to experimental conditions: TV stimulating technique (van Lith et al., 1978),
variations in pupillary size (Penne et al., 1981), X-Y plotter on paper recording, etc.

Nevertheless, the finding of increased P100 latency in patients of both
the first and the second group suggests that early and late CNS side effects
of ALL therapy might cause prolonged latencies in pattern-reversal VEPs,
even in absence of visual symptoms.

Moreover VEP delay appeared closely correlated with late CNS changes.
The results, as a whole, suggest that pattern VEPs are a useful diagnostic
aid for screening CNS changes attributed to CI and chemotherapy in ALL
patients.

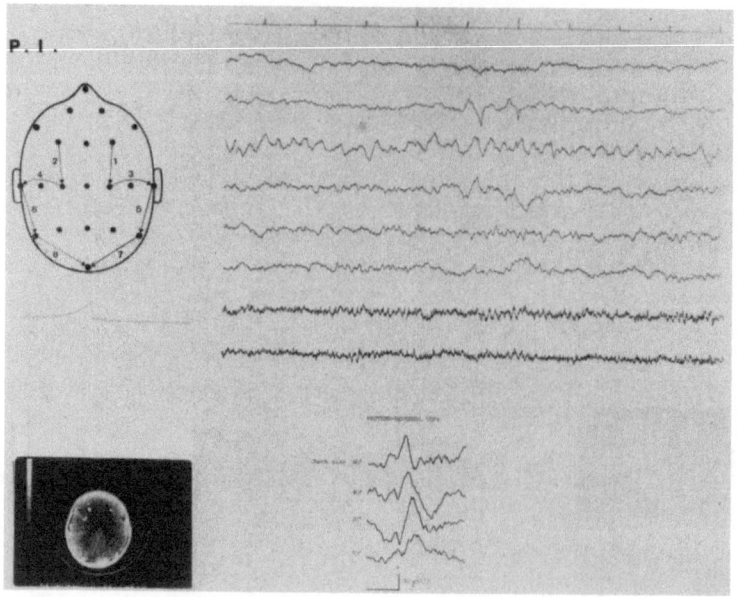

Fig. 3.
Case b): the child (6 years old) received antiepileptic drugs for Jackon epilespy which began 9 months after CI. She was examined 46 months after CI: EEG showed an excess of irregular slow activity of high amplitude in particular over parietal and posterior regions of the right hemisphere, CAT showed calcium deposits in the white matter of both frontal and parietal regions.

REFERENCES

Bleyer, W. A. and Griffin, T. W. White matter necrosis, mineralizing microangiopathy and intellectual disabilities in survivors of childhood leukemia: associations with central nervous system irradiation and methotrexate therapy. In: Gilbert, M. A. and Kagan, A. R. Eds.: 'Radiation damage to nervous system'. Pag. 155–174, Raven Press, New York, 1980.

Freeman, J. E., Hohnston, P. G. B. and Voke, J. M. Somnolence after prophylactic cranial irradiation in children with acute lymphoblastic leukemia. Brit. Med. J., 4: 523–529, 1973.

Halliday, A. M., McDonald, W. I. and Mushin, J. Visual evoked response in diagnosis of multiple sclerosis. Brit. Med. J., 4: 661–664, 1973.

Halliday, A. M., McDonald, W. I. and Mushin, J. Delayed pattern-evoked responses in progressive spastic paraplegia. Neurology, 24: 360–361, 1974.

Halliday, A. M., McDonald, W. I. and Mushin, J. Visual evoked potentials in patients with demyelinating disease. In: Desmedt, J. E. (Ed.) Visual evoked potentials in man: new developments. Clarendon Press, Oxford: 438–449, 1977.

Hennerici, M., Wenzel, D. and Freud, H. J. The comparison of small-size rectangle and checkerboard stimulation for the evaluation of delayed visual evoked responses in patients suspected of multiple sclerosis. Brain, 100: 119–136, 1977.

Lampert, P. W. and Dawies, R. L. Delayed effects of radiation on the human nervous system: 'early' and 'late' delayed reactions. Neurology, 14: 912–917, 1964.

Lampert, P. W., Tom, M. and Rider, W. D. Disseminated demyelination for the brain following Co^{60} gamma radiation. Arch. Pathol., 68: 222–330, 1959.

Lith, G. H. M. van, Henkes, H. E. and Marle, G. W. van. Projector of TV as a pattern stimulator. In: Tazawa, Y. (Ed.) Proc. of 16th ISCEV Symposium, Morioka, 1978. pp. 201–206, Jpn. J. Ophthalmol., Tokyo, 1978.

Muller, S., Bell, W. and Seibert, J. Cerebral calcifications associated with intrathecal methotrexate therapy in acute lymphocitic leukemia. J. Pediatr., 88: 650–653, 1976.

Pampiglione, G. Some anatomical considerations upon electrode placement in routine EEG. Proceedings of the electrophysiological Technologists Associations, 7: 1, 1976.

Penne, A. and Fonda, S. Influence of pupillary size on P100 latency time of pattern-reversal VEP. In: Spekreijse, H. and Apkarian, P. A. (Eds.) Visual pathways electrophysiology and pathology Proc. of 18th ISCEV Symposium, Amsterdam, 1980. (Doc. Ophthal. Proc. Series, 27: 255–262, 1981).

Poplack, D. G., Peyelan-Ramu, N., Pizzo, P. A. and Di Chiro, G. Abnormal computed to mography (CT) scans in children with acute lymphocitic leukemia (ALL). Proc. Am. Ass. Cancer Res., 28: 554–560, 1977.

Rider, W. D. Radiation damage to the brain: a new syndrome. J. Cancer Assoc. Radiol., 14: 67–69, 1963.

Rubinstein, L. J., Herman, M. M., Long, T. F. and Wilbur, J. R. Disseminated necrotizing leucoencephalopathy with calcifications of treated central nervous system leukemia and lymphoma. Cancer, 35: 291–305, 1975.

Smith, B. Brain damage after intrathecal methotrexate. J. Neurol. Neurosurg. Psychiatry, 38: 810–815, 1979.

Mailing address:
Department of Ophthalmology
University of Bologna
Via Massarenti 9
Bologna, Italy 40138

CLINICAL APPLICATION OF HYPNOTIC-INFLUENCED VEP

A. TABUCHI, S. ICHIHASHI AND S. KAWASHIMA

(Kurashiki, Japan)

ABSTRACT

A clinical application of hypnotic-influenced VEP was investigated comparing the awake VEP with the hypnotic-VEP. Hypnotics used were chloral hydrate; chloral hydrate and trichlorethyl phosphate, or barbiturates; phenobarbital sodium and pentobarbital calcium.

In hypnotic-VEPs from 13 normal children, with chloral hydrate or barbiturates, a prolongation of the peak latency of the negative wave (N90) and the positive wave (P120) was observed.

The difference in amplitude of N90–P120 was decreased in the hypnotic-VEP under chloral hydrate, but increased, named P120 enhancement, under barbiturates.

Characteristics of the VEP induced by barbiturates in 18 children with various kinds of visual disturbances were classified into 4 types as follows, type I; normal awake VEP and existence of P120 enhancement, type II; normal awake VEP but no P120 enhancement, type III; abnormal awake VEP and existence of P120 enhancement, and type IV; abnormal awake VEP without P120 enhancement. The P120 enhancement in the hypnotic-VEP corresponded well with a good visual prognosis. By means of simultaneous analysis of the awake VEP and hypnotic-VEP, the prognosis of a visual disorder can be interpreted more precisely than ever before.

INTRODUCTION

The effect of hypnotics on the visual evoked potential (VEP) was studied for the following two reasons: first, VEP under hypnotics is ordinarily used for infants and unconscious persons, but the effect of hypnotics on it is unknown and therefore it can not be readily interpreted; secondly, the electrophysiological significance of VEP itself may be evaluated, if the change of VEP can be analyzed based on the pharmacological activities of hypnotics. The authors have discussed the conditions of examination of hypnotic-VEP on normal subjects and those with visual disturbances (6, 7). In this study, the clinical application of the hypnotic-VEP is reported.

Doc. Ophthal. Proc. Series, Vol 37, ed. by H.E.J.W. Kolder
© 1983 Dr W. Junk Publishers, The Hague/Boston: Lancaster

MATERIALS AND METHODS

The subjects were 13 normal children (1 to 13 years of age; mean, 5.2 years) and 18 children with various kinds of visual disturbances (3 months to 10 years of age: mean, 4.6 years).

The hypnotics used were chloral hydrate (Escre®) in a dose of 30—50 mg/kg, monosodium trichlorethyl phosphate (Tricloryl®) in 0.8—1.0 cc/kg, phenobarbital sodium (Wakobital®) in 2 mg/kg, and pentobarbital calcium (Ravona®) in 50—100 mg. For the stimulation, a 0.5 or 1 Joule Xenon strobe light was applied at 1 Hz from a distance of 30 or 50 cm. The electrodes of Ag-AgCl were placed at O_1 and O_2 or Oz, and at Cz according to the International 10—20 method. A reference electrode was placed at A_2 and a ground electrode on the forehead. The evoked responses were obtained from bilateral or unilateral ocular stimulation (closed eyes on awakening) and 50 responses were averaged by the multi-purpose biophysical data processor (SM61)(Sanei Sokki, Tokyo) and recorded on a X-Y recorder. The time constant was 0.1 sec and the high pass filter was 25 Hz. The sleep stages were defined according to Dement and Kleitman's classification of the sleep EEG (5).

RESULTS

1. Normal group

Chloral hydrate was given to 5 children and barbiturate to 8 children. Fig. 1 showed a case of the VEP under chloral hydrate and barbiturate respectively. In order to make clear the differences between the two kinds of hypnotics, the negative wave around 90 msec, N90, the subsequent positive wave around a 120 msec latency, P120, and the difference in amplitude of N90—P120 were observed. Waves of N90 and P120 usually correspond to those of N70 and P120, but in this study, the latency period and the difference in amplitude were both prolonged and decreased respectively because of young subjects, recording with closed eyes and a 25 Hz high pass filter.

The latency period of N90 and P120 was 8.5 ± 10.2 msec (mean ± SD) and 122.6 ± 16.4 msec respectively, and the difference in amplitude of N90—P120 was 17.1 ± 9.3 μV in the awake VEP of all subjects. In Fig. 2, the latency period of both N90 and P120 at each sleep stage was represented using the value on awakening as 100%. The latency period of both N90 and P120 gradually increased depending on the depth of sleep induced by both hypnotics. In Fig. 3, the difference (dB) in amplitude of N90—P120 is presented taking the value on awakening as 0. The difference in amplitude tends to decrease under chloral hydrate while an increase was observed under barbiturates. The increase was named P120 enhancement.

2. Visual disturbance group

In all of 18 cases with visual disturbances, the hypnotic-VEP was induced by barbiturates. Table 1 shows the diagnoses and the clinical course of vision:

426

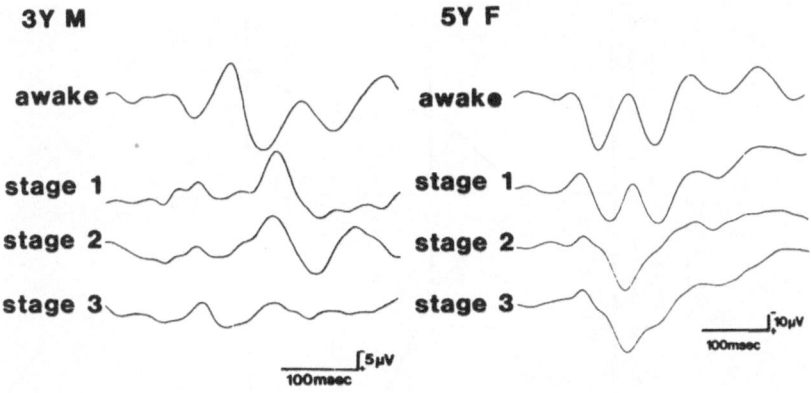

CHLORAL HYDRATE   **BARBITURATE**

Chloral hydrate 500mg   **Phenobarbital sodium 50mg**
Flash-VEP 1J 1Hz 50cm N:50 **Flash-VEP 1J 1Hz 50cm N:50**

3Y M   **5Y F**

awake   awake

stage 1   stage 1

stage 2   stage 2

stage 3   stage 3

Fig. 1. Hypnotic-influenced VEP in normal children: left; 3 yr male, Escre[®] 500 mg, right; 5 yr. female, Wakobital[®] 50 mg.

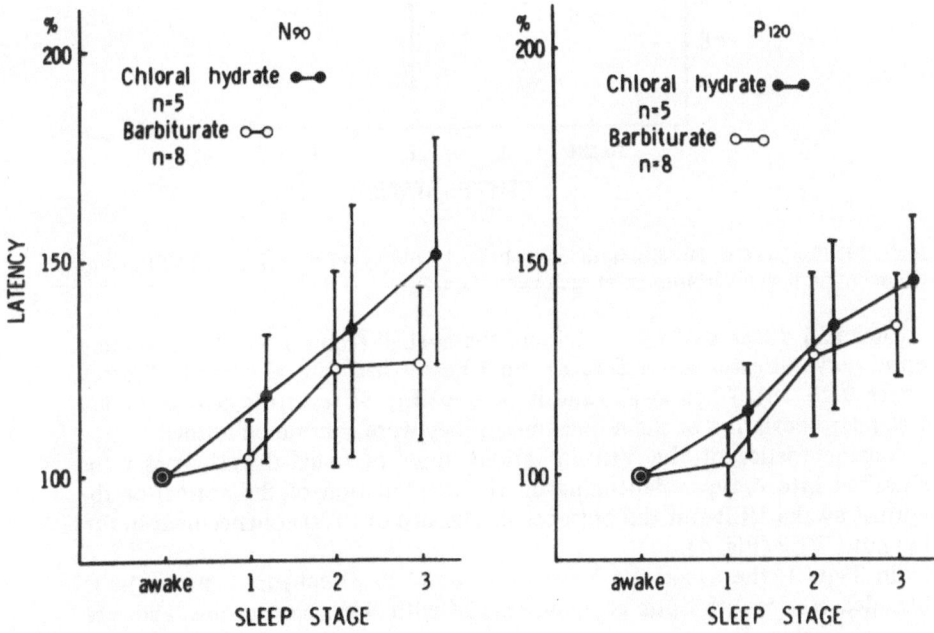

Fig. 2. Peak latency period of N90 and P120 in the hypnotic-influenced VEP under chloral hydrate and barbiturates at each sleep stage.

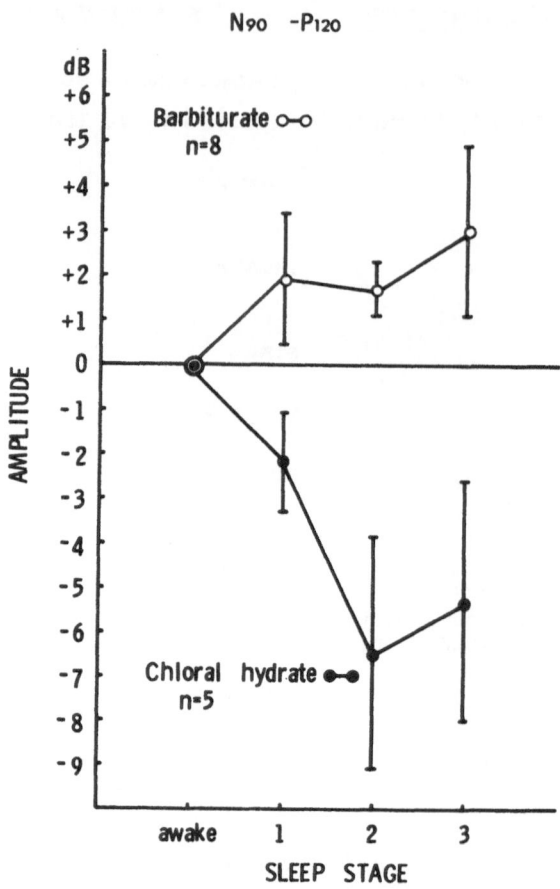

N90 -P120

Fig. 3. Differences in amplitude of N90–P120 in the hypnotic-influenced VEP under chloral hydrate and barbiturates at each sleep stage.

4 cases had diseases of the eyelid and the eyeball (cases 1 to 4), 4 cases had optic nerve diseases (cases 5 to 8) and 10 cases had central nervous diseases (cases 9 to 18). When awake and hypnotic-VEPs were within plus or minus 1 standard deviation of the normal mean, they were considered normal.

Characteristics of the VEP in various kinds of visual disturbances were classified into 4 types depending on the combination of the normal or abnormal awake VEP and the presence or absence of P120 enhancement in the hypnotic-VEP (Fig. 4).

In Type I, the awake VEP was normal and P120 enhancement exists. It included case 5 with optic atrophy, case 14 with Down's syndrome, and case 15 with strabismic amblyopia. Normal cases usually belong to this type.

In Type II, the awake VEP was normal but P120 enhancement did not exist. Case 8 with optic neuropathy, case 17 with anisometropic amblyopia, and case 18 with hystery showed these tendencies.

428

Table 1. Clinical data from 18 patients and their visual prognosis

Case	Age(y)	Sex	Clinical diagnosis	Visual prognosis
1 N. K.	3/12	F	R) Blepharoptosis	?
2 N. S.	2	F	R) Corneal dermoid	RV = ? ⟶ L. S. LV = ? ⟶ 1.5
3 H. Y.	5	M	R) PHPV	RV = HM ⟶ HM LV = 1.5
4 T. A.	7	M	R) Vitreous hemorrhage	RV = L. S. ⟶ L. S. LV = 1.5
5 E. H.	6/12	F	B) Optic atrophy	?
6 N. I.	3	M	R) Optic nerve hypoplasia	RV = 0.03 ⟶ 0.03 LV = 1.0
7 T. C.	8	M	L) Optic neuropathy	RV = 1.5 LV = 0.1 ⟶ 0.5
8 Y. K.	10	F	L) Optic neuropathy	RV = 0.1 ⟶ 1.0 LV = 1.2
9 K. F.	10/12	M	Hydrocephalus	?
10 N. I.	1	M	Cerebral blindness	?
11 M. H.	3	F	Cerebral palsy	?
12 S. I.	3	F	Cerebral palsy	?
13 M. S.	4	M	Cerebral blindness	?
14 Y. I.	5	F	Down's syndrome	?
15 Y. T.	6	F	Strabismic amblyopia	RV = 0.1 ⟶ 0.9 LV = 0.1 ⟶ 0.9
16 E. H.	8	F	Strabismic amblyopia	RV = 0.05 ⟶ 0.6 LV = 1.5
17 Y. I.	8	F	Anisometropic amblyopia	RV = 1.5 LV = 0.2 ⟶ 1.2
18 K K.	8	M	Hysteria	RV = 0.2 ⟶ 1.2 LV = 0.2 ⟶ 1.2

In Type III, the awake VEP was abnormal but P120 enhancement exists. It included cases 1, 3 and 4 with eyelid and eyeball diseases, cases 10 and 13 with cerebral palsy, cases 11 and 12 with cortical blindness and case 16 with strabismic amblyopia.

In type IV, the awake VEP was abnormal and P120 enhancement did not exist. Case 2 with corneal dermoid, cases 3 and 7 with optic nerve disease, and case 9 with hydrocephalus, belong to this type.

DISCUSSION

The hypnotic-VEP induced by chloral hydrate shows each wave gradually decreases depending on the depth of sleep. These hypnotics act on the cortex pharmacologically; depression of the VEP in an early stage of sleep will be

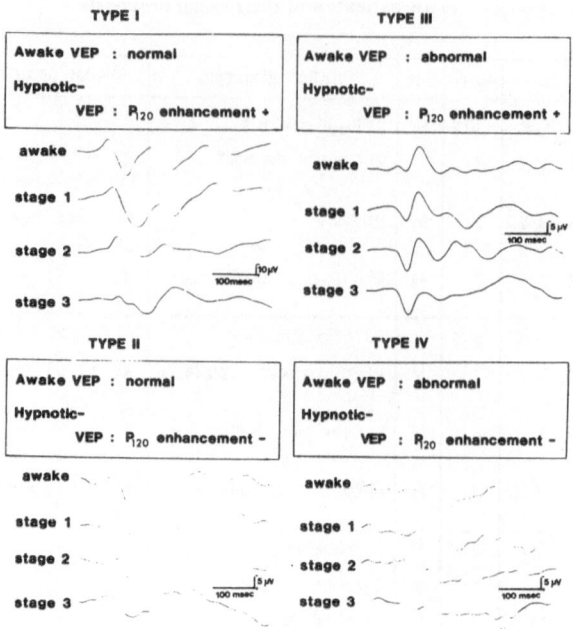

Fig. 4. Four types of hypnotic-influenced VEP under barbiturates in visual disturbances: left above; normal awake VEP and existence of P120 enhancement, case 15. Left below; Type II, normal awake VEP but no P120 enhancement, case 8. right above: Type III, abnormal awake VEP and existence of P120 enhancement case 11. right below: Type IV, abnormal awake VEP and no P120 enhancement, case 9.

due to the fact that the visual cortex of the occipital lobe is first affected. When using barbiturates, normal cases show the characteristic phenomenon of P120 enhancement. It can be used clinically. In this study, it was difficult to reveal clearly the characteristics of the hypnotic-VEP based on the location of the lesion in cases with visual disturbance. P120 enhancement was, however, suggested to relate to the severity of the disease and the prognosis of the visual acuity more than the location of the lesion. Type I, in which the awake VEP is normal and P120 enhancement exists, has a good prognosis. In case 15 with strabismic amblyopia the visual acuity recovered from 0.1, before treatment, to 0.9 after treatment.

Two cases (5 and 14) were also thought to have a good visual prognosis. The cases with Type II, which show normal awake VEP and no P120 enhancement, also recovered good visual acuity. In these cases, neurons in the visual pathway do not show any organic change. The effect of barbiturate hypnotics on the cortex appeared early and strongly. Changes were similar to those described above with chloral hydrate. P120 enhancement could not be induced. In Type III which has an abnormal awake VEP and P120 enhancement, the neurons in the visual pathway do not show any organic change, only functional change. The visual prognosis is good. In Type IV with abnormal and reduced the visual input to the visual cortex, suggests organic

430

disturbance of the visual pathway and/or cortex. Accordingly the visual prognosis is the worst.

The clinical application of hypnotic-VEP is rarely reported, and only one report is available by Tsutsui (9). He recognized the increase of the VEP similar to that reported here in amblyopic eyes after intravenous injection of amobarbital. However, some papers reported the influence of anesthetics on the VEP in normal cases (1, 2, 4, 8), the influence of barbiturates is similar to that observed in this study, and particularly a change corresponding to the P120 enhancement is reported. The mechanism of the occurrence of P120 enhancement has not been clarified; however, as barbiturates are considered to act on the reticular formation in the brain stem, P120 enhancement will be recognized when the central nervous control is eliminated from that part. In a recent study (10), barbiturates were considered to depress selectively the excitatory postsynaptic potential (EPSP).

The evoked potential is a summation of EPSP and inhibitory postsynaptic potential (IPSP) according to the hypothesis of Creutzfeld et al. (3).

In the evoked potential, the negative wave is EPSP and the positive one is IPSP related. The P120 enhancement is therefore a phenomenon in which EPSP is suppressed by barbiturate and IPSP become predominant; thus, even in the cases whose awake VEP are abnormal, when the suppression of some synapses is removed and P120 enhancement will appear (Type III). The visual prognosis is generally good in cases with P120 enhancement. The disturbance of the visual pathway can be classified to be organic or functional based on this phenomenon.

By means of simultaneous analysis of the hypnotic- and awake VEP, the visual prognosis of a visual disorder can be interpreted more precisely than ever before. In addition, in the cases of non-cooperative infants or unconscious patients, the hypnotic-VEP is especially useful because the existence of P120 enhancement can still be determined.

ACKNOWLEDGEMENT

The authors are grateful to Professor Jun Tsutsui for his supervision and the members of Physiological Function Center of Kawasaki Medical School for their cooperation.

REFERENCES

1. Abrahamian, H. A., Allison, T., Goff, W. R. and Rosner, B. S. Effects of Thiopental on human cerebral evoked responses. Anesthesiology 24: 650–657, 1963.
2. Cigánek, L. The EEG response (evoked potential) to light stimulus in man. Electroenceph. Clin. Neurophysiol. 13: 165–172, 1961.
3. Creutzfeldt, O. D. and Kuhnt, U. The visual evoked potential: Physiological, developmental and clinical aspects. Electroenceph. Clin. Neurophysiol. Suppl. 26: 29–41, 1967.
4. Domino, E. F., Crossen, G. and Sweet, R. B. Effects of various general anesthetics on the visually evoked response in man. Anesth. Analg. 42: 735–747, 1963.
5. Ohkuma, T. (ed.) Clinical electroencephalography (2nd) p. 113, 1970, Igaku-shoin, Tokyo.

6. Tabuchi, A., Ichihashi, S. and Kawashima, S. Hypnotic-influenced VEP. Jpn. Rev. Clin. Ophthalmol. 76: in press.
7. Tabuchi, A., Ichihashi, S. and Kawashima, S. Hypnotics effect on VEP. Jpn. Rev. Clin. Ophthalmol. 76: in press.
8. Takeshita, H. Anesthesia and evoked response. Clin. Encephal. 14: 125–134, 1972.
9. Tsutsui, J. Visually evoked response of the occipital scalp in pharmacological treatment of amblyopia. Ophthalmology (proceeding of the XXI International Congress, Mexico, D.F., 1970), Excerpta Medica International Congress Series, No. 222: 1344–1348.
10. Yamamura, H. (ed.) Basic and clinical neuro-pharmacology, p. 13–15, 1973, Shinko Koeki, Tokyo.

Mailing address:
Department of Ophthalmology
Kawasaki Medical School,
Kurashiki, Japan 701-01

432

COMPLEX STRUCTURED STIMULI FOR VECP

V. MISZALOK AND M. BUNKRAD

Freie Universität Berlin, Augenklinik Charlottenburg

Director: Prof. Dr. J. Wollensak

The use of centrally symmetric stimuli (computer generated) reduces markedly lid and oculomotoric artifacts and subjective fatigue effects. Such patterns are presented and the results discussed.

ASYMMETRIES OF VECP SCALP DISTRIBUTION EVOKED BY NASAL AND TEMPORAL HEMIRETINAL STIMULATION IN ESOTROPIC PATIENTS

K. YANASHIMA, A. RUNNE, Y. KAKISU AND M. BOPP

Tokorozawa, Japan, Frankfurt M./Bad Nauheim, F.R.G.

To identify the site of suppression in esotropia, steady state VECP evoked by pattern stimulation of the nasal and temporal hemiretina were recorded horizontally on the scalp. While normal subjects exhibited a similar scalp distribution of VECP signals evoked by stimulation of the nasal and temporal hemiretina, patients with esotropia showed bigger amplitudes with nasal than with temporal hemiretinal stimulation. By contrast, sensitivity measurements along the horizontal meridian determined by a Tübinger perimeter indicated in esotropia higher sensitivity in the temporal hemiretina. At the retinal level, no difference of amplitudes was found in the pattern ERG to stimulation of the nasal and temporal hemiretina. From these findings we conclude the site of suppression in the visual cortex beyond area 17.

THE VISUAL ELECTRICALLY EVOKED POTENTIAL (VEEP): STEADY STATE RESPONSES

G. K. BIJL

Department of Neurophysiology, University of Groningen, Bloemsingel 10, 9712 KZ Groningen, The Netherlands

The electrical stimulation of the visual system (through electrodes placed near an eye) is perceived as a modulation of the brightness of the visual field (flicker) when the current is alternating. The extent of this modulation depends on the frequency and intensity of the current and on the brightness level. In general the current has to be rather large so that artifacts in the recording of the VEEP cannot be avoided and the VEEP will be obscured by them. Even with the use of our rotatable stimulating electrode (previously described) we could only record properly after the current is switched off. Fortunately, due to the latency of the VEEP, frequency and phase characteristics can be obtained this way. Results of these and other measurements will be shown and discussed.

NOTES ON FOURIER METHODS IN VISION RESEARCH

L. H. VAN DER TWEEL, O. ESTEVEZ AND J. P. M. PIJN

Laboratory of Medical Physics, University of Amsterdam
(Amsterdam, The Netherlands)

ABSTRACT

In this paper a number of problems is discussed that arise when applying Fourier methods to distributions of light. It is shown that the 'non-negative' nature of light represents a serious constraint both in analysis and synthesis problems; in fact, the simplest analysis of a signal in terms of Fourier harmonics can not be carried out completely in physical Fourier components. Attention is also drawn to the abuse of Fourier concepts for the analysis of two-dimensional patterns (like checkerboards) and it is argued that these patterns are better characterized directly in the space-domain. Finally, some attention is given to problems associated with phase relations and it is argued that phase is a very important variable since it carries most of the information about place. It is concluded that the correct use of Fourier theory, be it as an analysis tool or as a theoretical framework for visual perception, requires careful consideration of the basic constraints imposed among other things by the physical nature of light.

INTRODUCTION

As more and more researchers are using the ideas and methods of Fourier analysis and synthesis (FAS) to describe and study spatial patterns, it seems timely to examine some of its basic principles and their consequences for research in vision.

The main problem we will try to elucidate here concerns the relation between the theoretical aspects of Fourier Analysis and the physical constraints imposed by the nature of light. Besides we will also examine some consequences of applying Fourier concepts for the build up of the visual world because this may contribute to the understanding of the various theories and experiments in visual processing.

One of the basic considerations of this paper, indeed the root of the first problem we want to treat, stems from a more or less trivial observation: there is no negative light, which is simply a consequence of the fact that energy can not be negative. This has important implications for the application of FAS in visual research for, contrary to what in general is possible with electrical signals, there is no way to cancel non-coherent illumination. Therefore physically realisable procedures of FAS must consist of positive components. The restrictions that follow from this fact in the application of e.g. spatial FAS are worth being examined since they are not always obvious.

SOME BASIC FACTS OF FOURIER ANALYSIS

Fourier theory is essentially a *mathematical* tool that allows one to represent a function of time or space as a sum of harmonic functions — popularly known as sine waves — each with a certain amplitude and a specific phase relation with respect to a given origin. For completeness sake it should be mentioned that in order to perform FAS with regard to a given wave shape certain mathematical requisites must be fulfilled; for most physical situations this will be the case.

There are two mathematical idealizations usually made in Fourier theory: a phenomenon can be considered to be a *single* event, and is then called a 'transient', or it can be considered to be *repetitive* or periodically recurrent, and often referred by the unfortunate name 'steady state'. In nature though, neither of the two situations occurs, and certainly not within the time span of the phenomena in which one is usually interested in the laboratory: a true transient or 'once-in-a-lifetime' event is scientifically not seizable, its existence involves both minus and plus infinite! On the other extreme, no real phenomenon can be truly repetitive, partly for the same reason why the true transient does not exist, and partly because exact periodicity is also not realizable due to the ubiquitous presence of noise in nature.

These two idealizations are nevertheless useful as approximations to real phenomena. The prerequisite is then that the total time span or space range with which we deal is large relative to that of the 'transient', or that the 'periodic' phenomenon has begun long enough before we started observing it. In spatial FAS this means either one single pattern in a very large empty field or a repetitive pattern that extends well past our field of observation and in which the variation of the period is relatively small. The advantage of analyzing 'transient' and 'periodic' shapes is that they can be handled by respectively the Fourier Integral or resolved into the Fourier Series.

While most computations of this kind are nowadays carried out in digital computers, one must not forget that, given enough time, all numerical calculations can be carried out using nothing more than paper and pencil. This is not a trivial remark: much too often is the process of computation just because it is performed by a physical machine, confused with a physical process; but it is not: it is still 'pencil and paper' and its laws are those of mathematics, not of physics.

Let us now take the simple, but illustrative example of analyzing (and synthesizing) a periodic square wave, as is shown in Fig. 1. It can be seen that this wave shape can be thought to consist of the harmonic functions:

$$A_n \sin 2\pi nft$$

with $n = 2p + 1$, and $p = 0, 1, 2$ etc.

440

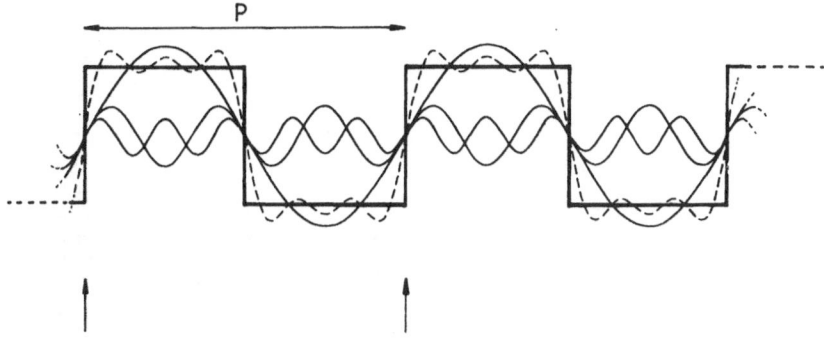

Fig. 1. The first three harmonics of a square wave and their sum (dashed). Note that the amplitude of the fundamental is larger ($4/\pi$) than that of the square wave taken as 1. The overshoot in the sum does not diminish in size when higher harmonics are added but moves towards the steep flanks of the square wave (Gibb's phenomenon).

The origin $t = 0$ is taken at a positive going discontinuity (indicated by the arrows). The Fourier series is given in Fig. 2A. Note that for the *graphical* construct the number of periods is irrelevant. However, restricting the number of periods changes the Fourier representation drastically. This is (schematically) indicated in the Figs. 2B and C, where the Fourier transform of respectively 2 and 1 periods are presented; the spectra are now continuous. The broadening in each case (one or two periods) is constant for all harmonics and depends on the number of periods: the more periods involved the smaller the frequency bands; in other words the higher the harmonic the more selective the representation.

There is a revealing demonstration of Fourier Analysis invented by Anstis (1975). Fig. 3 (A, B, C) can be used to understand the principle. The reader should best make a slide (or as an alternative a transparency) of each of the figures with the silhouettes and project these through a system of parallel glass rods of some 3 mm diameter acting as cilinder lenses (Fig. 4). This will smear out the silhouettes in one direction and leave them more or less intact in the other one. A simpler, somewhat less efficient method, is to make use of a 'maddox' well known in ophthalmological clinics (if possible remove the usually present red filter) and look directly at the figures. It is advised to make a black mask just leaving the silhouettes exposed. Using one of the described techniques Fig. 3A shows a 100% contrasty sine wave grid. Fig. 3B is the approximate representation of a square wave as can be judged by measuring the amplitudes of the silhouetted sinusoidal harmonics. They are 1, 1/3, 1/5 etc. (For typographical reasons we have restricted this to the 21st harmonic). In this technique it is easy for instance to take out the fundamental of a square wave as one can do following Fig. 3C, and then get the (wrong) impression that, in a way, a fundamental-period grid is present. Fig. 3D represents a sawtooth, we will find the period P, P/2, P/3 in the latter.

Now we come to our basic problem especially with regard to spatial FAS; observe that, although each of the component silhouettes (Fig. 3) is made

441

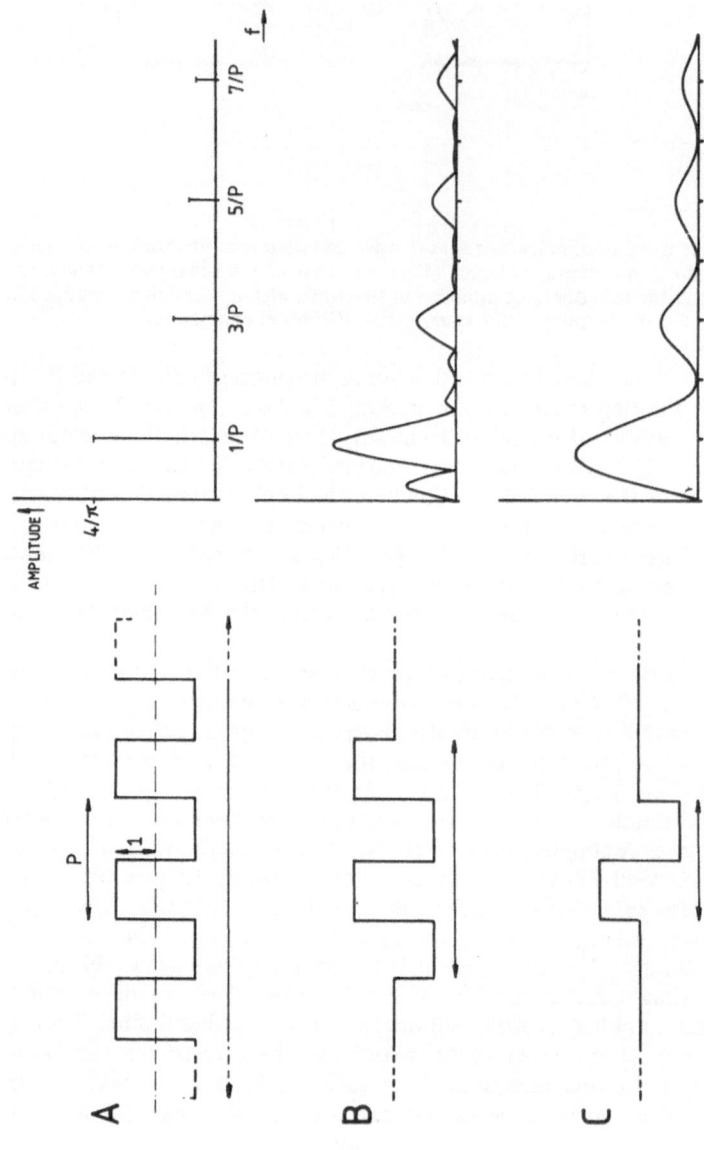

Fig. 2. Fourier amplitude spectra of A) a periodic square wave, B) two periods and C) one square wave as a transient. A has a line spectrum, B and C are represented by continuous spectra. Note that in each representation the width Δf around the original harmonics is constant and decreases for a higher number of periods (B versus C). This means a constantly increasing sharpness of representation f/Δf for increasing order of harmonic. The scaling is adapted for illustrative purposes.

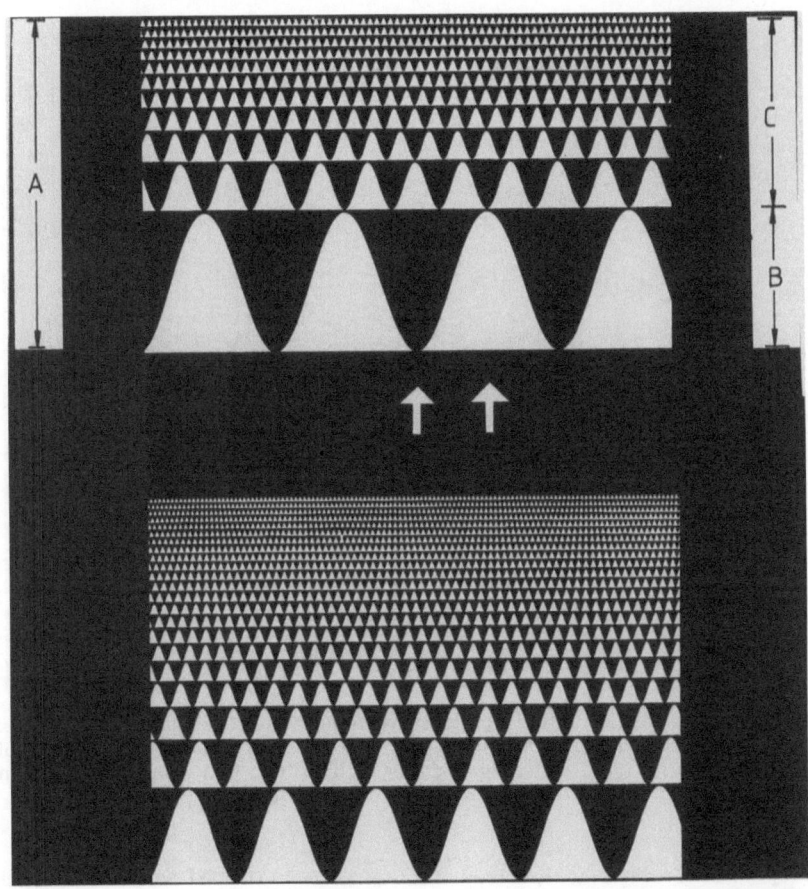

Fig. 3A, B, C. If this composition of silhouettes (A) of harmonic functions according to Fig. 1 is stretched in the vertical direction by means of the device of Fig. 4, a square wave is seen. If by means of a black paper the sine wave (B) is isolated, a 100% contrast sine wave grating is produced; if only the fundamental is covered (C) a square wave minus the fundamental is produced.

Notice the diminished contrast of the square wave due to the obligatory positive average of each composing function. For typographical reasons and to obtain enough contrast the number of harmonics is restricted.

Fig. 3D. Representation of a sawtooth. Now also even harmonics are included.

of black and white, yielding 100% contrast, the synthesized wave shape has a much lower contrast. The reason is simply that, as said, once light is present it can not be cancelled and therefore the components alternatively dilute further the contrast of the resulting shape. If the situation at the two arrows is taken as an example the sum in a vertical direction gives the extremes that will be reached. For the left arrow this sum will be composed of the series $0 + 1/3 + 0 + 1/7 + ..$ etc.; for the right one this will be $1 + 0 + 1/5 + 1/9 + ...$ etc. The effect is that $L_{right} - L_{left}$ remains near to the value 1,

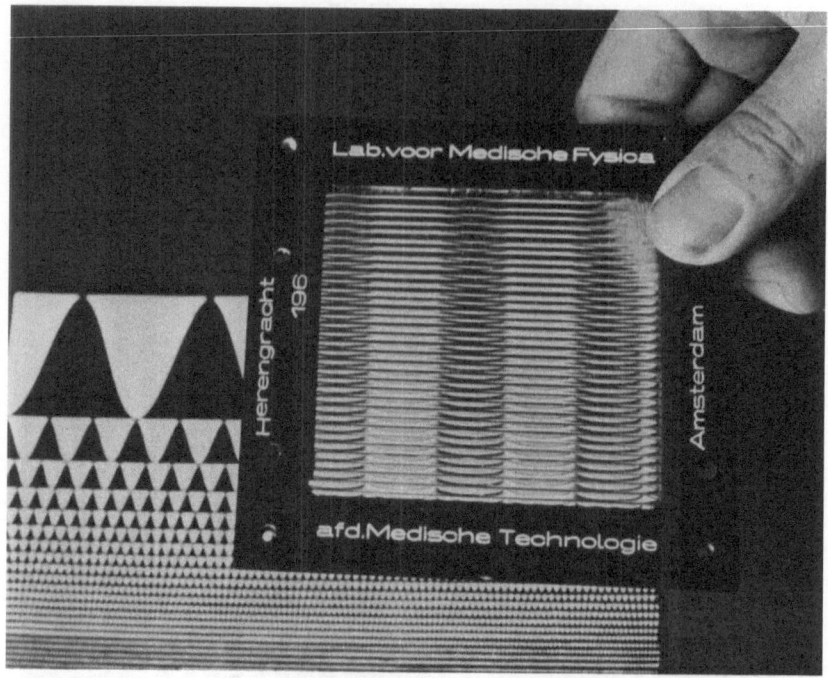

Fig. 4. Device for Anstis' optical Fourier synthesis consisting of 33 glassrods of approximately 3 mm diameter. Notwithstanding the primitive optics of the device and the problems involved in the construction and printing of the silhouetted figures, the definition of the squares is very satisfactory if slide projection is performed.

asymptotically reaching it, but at the cost of the contrast as conventionally defined by

$$\frac{L_{max} - L_{min}}{L_{max} + L_{min}}$$

This approaches zero with the inclusion of more and more harmonics. In the frequency domain all this is equivalent to the addition for each harmonic of its spatial average. An extreme case is that of a 100% contrast square wave grid: such grid cannot be synthesized using light, because its fundamental (first harmonic) has an amplitude of $4/\pi$, which is larger than 1 and therefore requires negative light. One could think that this problem can be avoided by using a contrast less than 100%. But this is wrong as well, as we shall now demonstrate.

To understand this synthesis problem imagine a stimulation-response experiment in which our aim is to compare the responses to a complex grating with the responses to its seperate components. Let us consider the Fourier Series of a M% grid:

$$I_{av}[1 + (4/\pi)(M/100)(\sin \omega t + 1/3 \sin 3\omega t + 1/5 \sin 5\omega t + \ldots)]$$

If we want to synthesise this with sinusoidal grids the problem is that we can not make physically the AC terms separately, because of the no-negative light constraint. We have to add to each AC term a DC at least equal to the amplitude. At first sight one would think that the general DC term could take care of that. But this is *not* the case: to the first harmonic we have to add at least $I_{av}.4/\pi.M/100)$, to the third 1/3 of this, to the fifth harmonic 1/5 etc. But the series $1/3 + 1/5 + 1/7 + \ldots$ does not converge.

However if we restrict for this hypothetical experiment only to the fundamental and the third harmonics, then an infinite number of combinations of contrast for the two composing grids is possible. What one intuitively, but in principle wrongly, would do is to take the fundamental and third harmonics both with the average level of the original square wave, in which case the contrast would be decreased at physical addition. A better way is then probably to take the two harmonics at half the DC level but at double contrast, in which case the final mixture correctly reaches the desired contrast.

For a linear system any combination will work but then the whole problem is not very interesting; on the other hand the more non-linear the system is the more caution should be taken and the trickier the problem is.

The vital point of the above discussion is that a full and complete FAS cannot be physically carried out with spatial patterns and this has also strong implications for the corresponding models one can postulate for visual operations. In fact the DC component that each harmonic function has to carry with it means a highly complicating factor.

Another interesting consequence of the 'no negative light' principle is the following. In an electrical signal a fundamental with an amplitude larger than the original can be realized by (passive low-pass or resonant) filtering Optically there is, in the case of a periodic square wave shape, no way of performing such a filtering; neither is high-pass filtering possible. For instance, removing the higher harmonics by blurring reduces at the same time the overall maximal contrast; the spatial DC level (average) remains constant.

A sine wave grating is, by the way, the only grating that retains its intensity distribution by simple blurring; the only change is reducing the amplitude (contrast).

With respect to blurring there is an important difference between the time and space domains involved, which arises from the asymmetry of time. Time has an inherent direction, while space doesn't. In the time domain this means that every physical filtering that affects the amplitudes also introduces a phase shift, while in the space domain left and right are treated equally. If we blur a line this generally gives a symmetrical distribution around the site of the line, i.e. the phases at that place of the components are preserved, while smoothing a short pulse in time always gives a displaced maximum.

THE CHECKERBOARD PROBLEM

We turn now our attention to 'checkerboards', which have become quite useful and popular in pattern EP studies. If we use the Anstis method to project a checkerboard (Fig. 5), placing the (composite) cylinder lens in front

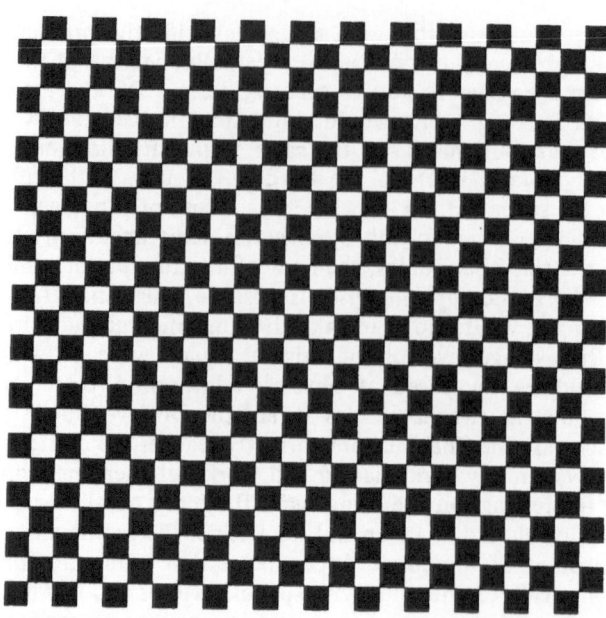

Fig. 5. If the cylinder lens device is applied to the checkerboard the main directions that produce an one-dimensional grating can easily be demonstrated. In particular the 45° direction gives a clear picture.

of the projecting lens, we see that smearing the image in the vertical or horizontal direction produces an homogeneous gray field (for an ideal checkerboard; in practice and due to imperfections the border lines can still be seen). This result is easy to understand, since for every white square there will be also a black one and the net result is gray. Actually, the cylinder lens is acting as a kind of spatial filter selecting those spatial components perpendicular to its axis, and we see in our experiment that a checkerboard does not have any components corresponding to (twice) the checker size. For this reason the use of 'Fourier' terminology i.e. spatial frequency as a specification for checkerboard patterns should be discouraged. On the other hand, if the lens is tilted 45° either side one sees at once gratings appearing with triangular contrast profiles corresponding to the maximum of the checkerboard contrast. Each of these two perpendicular triangular gratings contains a fundamental grid with a period equal to $\sqrt{2}$ times the check size and an amplitude of $4/\pi$, and the higher odd harmonics of this fundamental with their corresponding diminishing modulations (1/9, 1/25 etc). Fig. 6 demonstrates how this comes about. It can be seen that only in certain directions (1:1, 1:3 etc) a triangular grating will result. Furthermore, rotating the cylinder lens system e.g. from ratio 1:1 to 1:3 will not change the direction of the image of 45°, but its contrast will diminish to zero (Fig. 6C). At further rotation the next direction will emerge, initially with a low contrast, (Fig. 6D) etc. Apart from the absence of a fundamental with a period of twice the check size, there is also no harmonic relation between the frequencies that *are* present (e.g. the frequencies in Fig. 6B and D); obviously

446

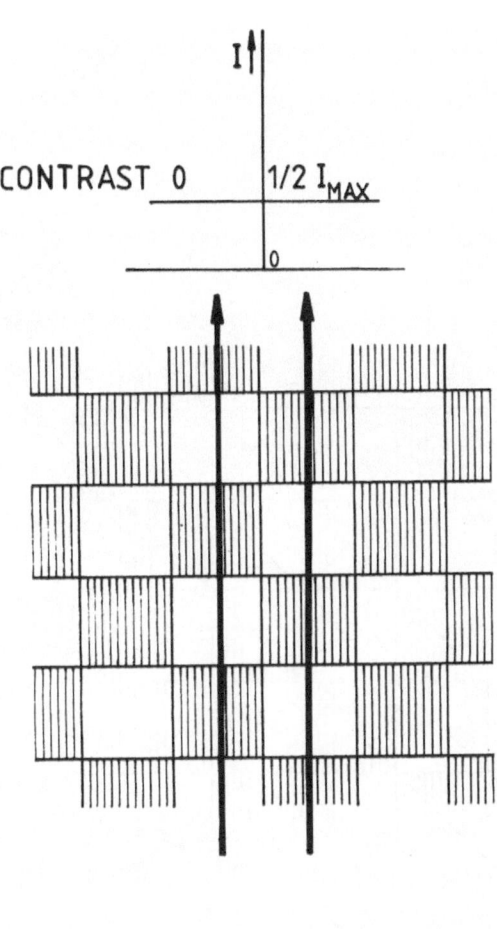

A

Fig. 6. Theoretical luminance distribution with application of cylinder lenses under various angles to a checkerboard pattern.
A) There is no net result, the projection field will be homogeneous. B) A triangular distribution with identical top contrast as the original checkerboard will be obtained. According to Fourier Analysis the fundamental for the 45° direction is $8/\pi^2$ for a black and white pattern. C) Again a net result of zero is obtained. All black and white checks are included in equal numbers. D) In this case is indicated that at the maxima and minima out of every 3 squares, 2 will cancel. The maximum contrast is now 1/3 but the spatial frequency is $1/5 \sqrt{10}$ which bears no harmonic relations to any other.

check size is the relevant parameter. Not only is a checkerboard, in FAS, an extremely complex object, but it can also not be composed or decomposed as such of physical sinusoidal gratings for the same reasons explained as for the one-dimensional case.

447

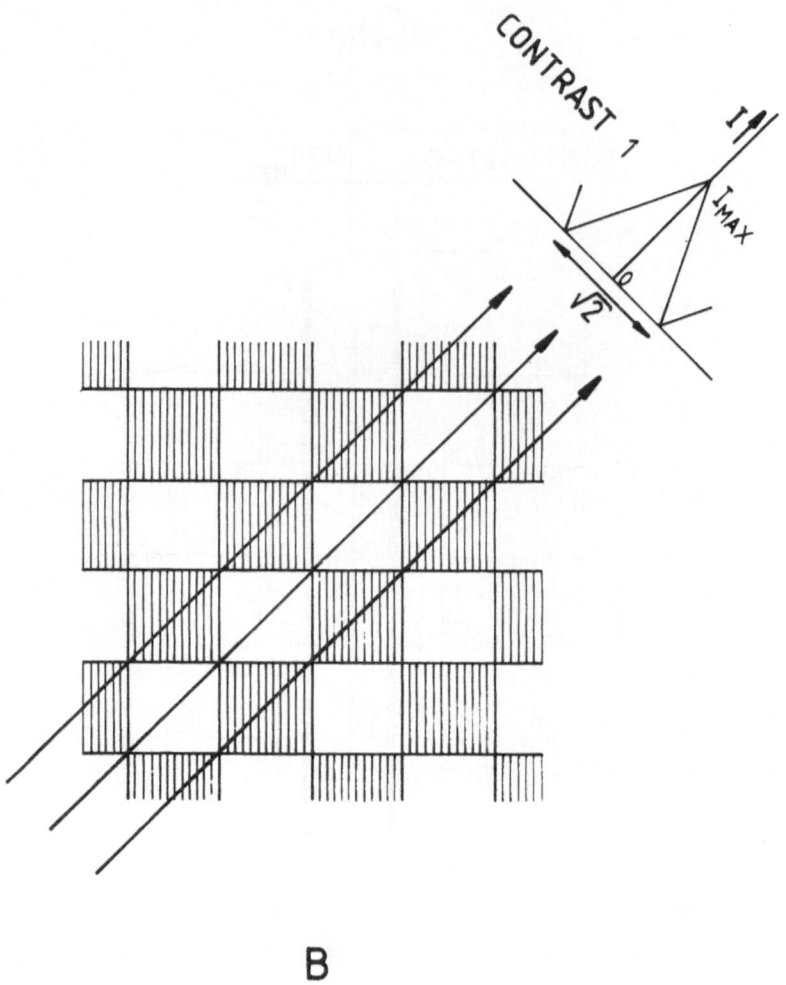

B

Fig. 6B.

PHASE

The next problem concerns the phases of the components in spatial FAS. As we know, the mathematical reconstruction of a shape from its Fourier components requires knowledge of both the amplitudes and phases at all frequencies. A rather trivial, yet not unimportant, case is when a transport delay τ or a translation D in place is present. This does not influence the shape, nor the amplitude representation in the Fourier transform. The phase shift due to such a delay τ or distance D will, as a natural consequence, be proportional to the frequencies involved: $\phi = 2\pi f\tau$, respectively $2\pi fD$. Note that ϕ will include a certain number of whole periods (n.2π) if τ or D

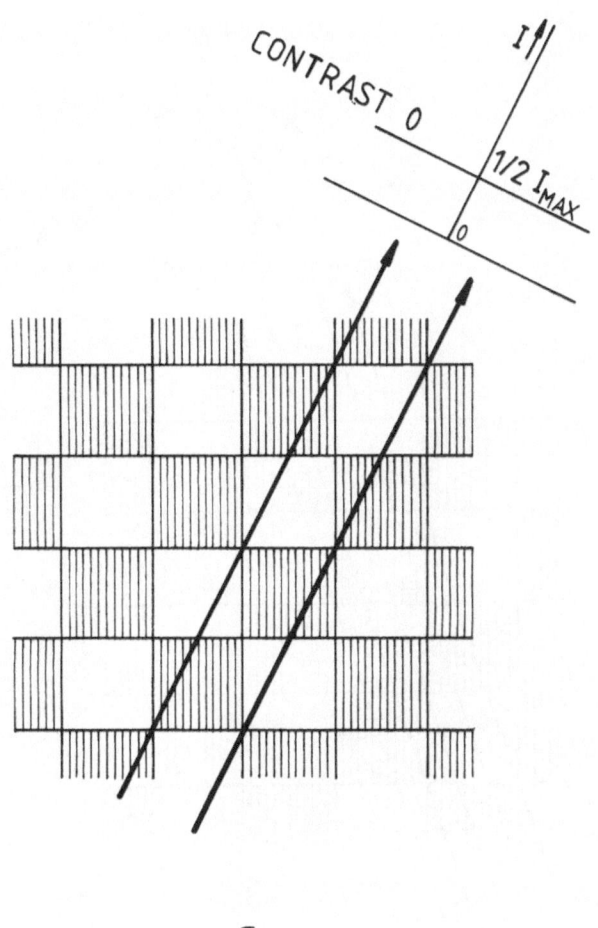

Fig. 6C.

exceeds 1/f. In procedures to determine τ or D from phase shifts, knowledge of n is imperative.

Other kinds of phase shifts, however, may be disastrous Fig. 7 shows how drastically a periodic square wave and the corresponding square wave grid on a cathode ray screen change in shape if the various harmonics are shifted in phase, but at unchanged amplitudes. This is, for the time dependent signal producing the grating, physically realizable by electronic methods, contrary to changing amplitudes when obligatory phase shifts, as we said before,* have to occur. It is interesting to note that in Fig. 7B the top-top excursion by far exceeds that of the original square wave. As soon as electrical

*If the two wave shapes of Fig. 7 are produced acoustically no difference will be heard as was already known to Helnholtz.

449

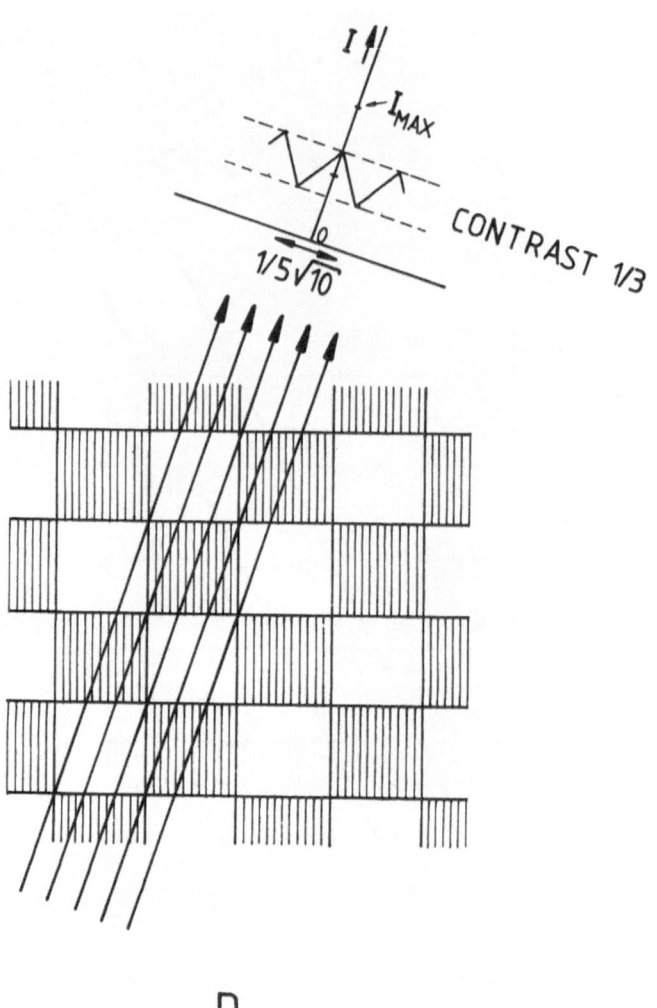

D

Fig. 6D.

signals are involved the constraints due to the physical nature of light fall away.

If spatial FAS is considered one can maintain that in the frequency domain it is phase and phase relations that spatial vision is mainly about, amplitude being relatively unimportant. This is the same as saying that in the spatial domain it is the POSITION of every detail in an image that conveys most of the visual information. In the choice of what types of representation lie at the basis of visual processing the above considerations may play a significant role.

In conclusion we hope to have shown that the Fourier concepts applied to light distributions, be it in space be it in time, require special care

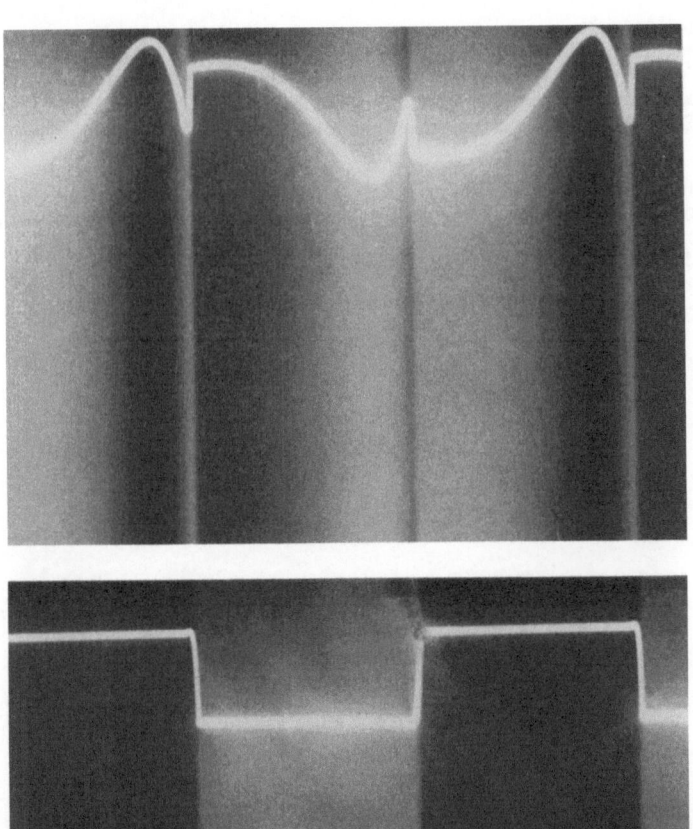

Fig. 7. The square wave intensity grid is generated on a CRT screen. With an all pass phase shifting filter a very different picture emerges demonstrating the importance of phase in the visual world.

particularly because of the limitations due to the fundamental non-negative nature of the signal.

REFERENCES

Anstis, S. M. & Comerfort, J. P. A simple method of projecting Mach bands, color mixtures and variable contrast sine wave gratings. Beh. Res Methods and Instrumentation 1975 Vol. 7, 283–287.

Anstis, Stuart. Luminance profiles demonstrate nonlinearities of brightness perception. Beh. Res Methods and Instrumentation 1976 Vol. 8 (5), 427–436.
Kelly, H. D. Pattern detection and the two-dimensional Fourier transform: flickering checkerboards and chromatic mechanisms. Vision Res. 1976 Vol. 16, 277–287.
MacKay, D. M. Strife over visual cortical function. Nature, 1981 Vol. 189, 117–118.

Mailing address:
Laboratory of Medical Physics
University of Amsterdam
Herengracht 196
1016 BS Amsterdam
The Netherlands

AN ELECTRONICALLY-INDUCED PULFRICH ILLUSION AS A QUANTITATIVE MEASURE OF VISUAL DELAY AND STEREOPSIS

L. TYCHSEN AND H. S. THOMPSON

(Iowa City, Iowa, U.S.A.)

ABSTRACT

A Pulfrich illusion of elliptical rotation in depth was created by presenting two illuminated circles of light to each eye separately. The circles moved in tandem horizontally on an oscilloscope which was equipped with an adjustable relative phase delay. Following the introduction of an unpredictable delay by the examiner, the subject was asked to flatten the illusion by turning a dial that varied the delay linearly. We produced an artificial 'lesion' in healthy subjects by placing neutral density filters in front of one eye and found close agreement of the visual delay measured on the Pulfrich device with that measured by dichoptic double flash or pattern visual evoked potential. Subjects with only coarse stereopsis due to strabismus had no trouble seeing the illusion, though their skill at discerning the point of no phase delay was about half as good as that of the normal group. The Pulfrich delay in patients with optic neuritis was comparable to the pattern visual evoked potential delay if the fellow eye was normal and the scotoma of the involved eye did not straddle a large portion of the horizontal meridian of the visual field.

INTRODUCTION

A difference in stimulus intensity between the two eyes produces a difference in conduction time between the two optic nerves: the signal from the brighter eye moves faster than the signal from the dimmer eye. The brain sometimes interprets this as a difference in time and sometimes as a difference in space. For example, if simultaneous flashes are presented separately to the two eyes (dichoptically) it may appear that the flash to the dimmer eye occurred later. In the case of pendular motion in the frontal plane, darkening one eye by a filter or by damage to the optic nerve makes the object appear to follow an elliptical path in depth (Fig. 1). This spatial illusion was described by C. Pulfrich in 1922 (1) and numerous investigators have since adapted it to clinically detect optic nerve delay (2–10, review 11).

Whereas the Pulfrich illusion is induced in the healthy by producing a brightness difference which is interpreted as a spatial difference, we devised

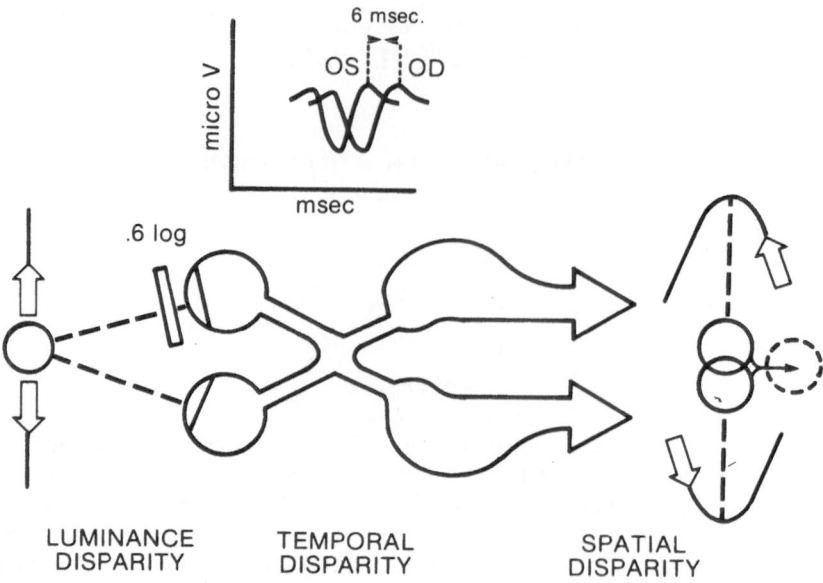

LUMINANCE   TEMPORAL   SPATIAL
DISPARITY   DISPARITY   DISPARITY

Fig. 1. A cartoon showing an oscilloscope tracing (above) of the visual evoked potential phase delay created by a neutral density filter in front of the right eye. The neutral density filter produces a Pulfrich illusion of elliptical rotation in depth; the target actually moves only horizontally in the frontal plane.

a technique (a variation of which we then discovered had been done by Rushton (12)) which does the reverse – at least partially. We produced a phase-delay electronically which induced a Pulfrich illusion, then we offset the illusion with a brightness disparity created by a neutral density filter.

Judging from the literature, delays measured by Pulfrich techniques have, on the whole, correlated poorly with the visual evoked potential, while methods such as dichoptic double flash have correlated well. It has been suggested that temporal judgments required by the double flash are psychophysically simpler than combined judgments of time and space required to appreciate motion in depth (13). This dichotomy may be based on differences in the complexity of the underlying neural circuitry. Microelectrode recordings from animals – as far forward as the retinal ganglion cell (14–16) and as far back as the occipital cortex (17) – suggest that there are parallel, but discrete, neural channels subserving separate visual functions. Distinct sensitivities to changes of brightness, color, contrast, spatial frequency, orientation, and movement have also been demonstrated by human evoked potential experiments (18). The same optic nerve lesion may cause different degrees of impairment in each channel, and this explanation has been invoked to account for the inaccuracy of most Pulfrich techniques, along with the claim that these techniques require fine stereopsis (13, 18).

As shown in the Venn diagram (Fig. 2), though others have made two-way clinical comparisons of temporal disparity (visual evoked potential delay or dichoptic double flash delay), brightness disparity (log filter), and phase disparity (estimated depth of the Pulfrich illusion) we decided to address

454

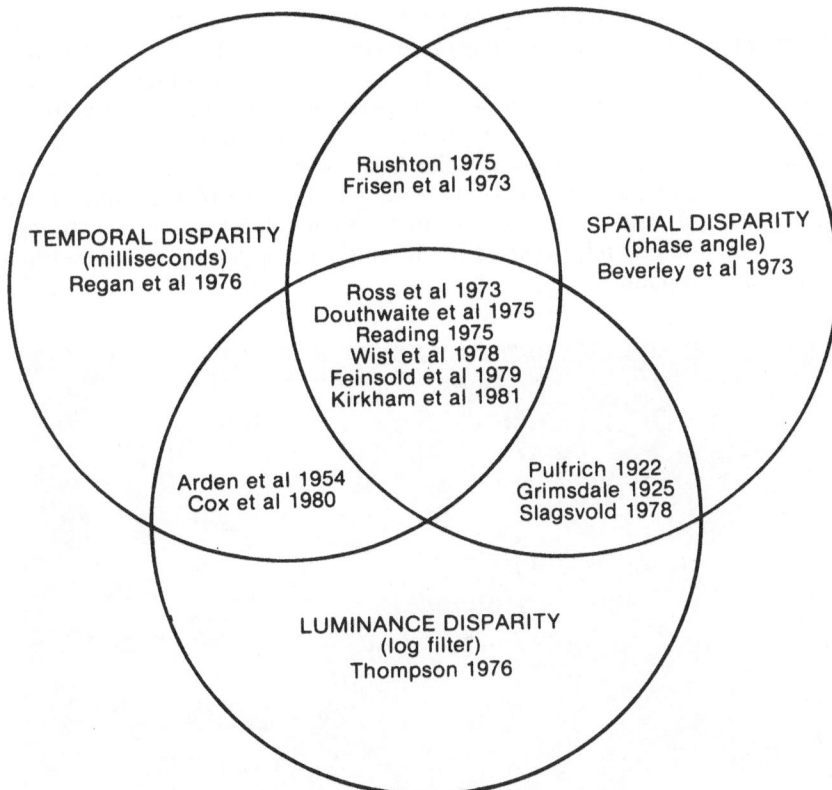

Fig. 2. A Venn diagram cataloging previous studies which have compared temporal disparity, spatial disparity, and luminance disparity.

these issues by a quantitative comparison of three techniques. A neutralization-of-delay method was used with the Pulfrich and double flash devices; that is, an artificial decrease in brightness to one eye was offset by an electronic delay to the fellow eye. Pattern visual evoked potential delay was used as our standard. Drawing on the preceding arguments, we anticipated that the two psychophysical methods would yield different delays to the same drop in brightness. To determine if subnormal stereopsis impaired the usefulness of the device, we tested a group of subjects with strabismus, and compared their Pulfrich delay with a standard measure of stereoacuity.

METHODS

Eight normal volunteers, wearing + 3.00 spectacles, dichoptically viewed two circles of light on a gridded dual-beam oscilloscope screen with an overall luminance of 2.5 ft-cd. Each circle subtended 1.3 deg of visual angle and moved through a horizontal excursion of 6 deg (produced by a sinusoidal

455

signal generator at a frequency of 1.0 Hz) at a peak velocity of 15 deg/sec. By turning a control dial, the subject linearly retarded the phase of the light ball viewed by the right or left eye. This resulted in alternating crossed and uncrossed disparity seen as either clockwise or counterclockwise elliptical rotation in depth, depending upon which eye viewed the lagging target. The examiner turned an identical dial in a forced match test requiring the subject to counteract appropriately with his dial in order to flatten the ellipse. Without being instructed to do so, each subject adopted a strategy whereby they alternately reversed the leading and lagging eyes while settling toward the null point.

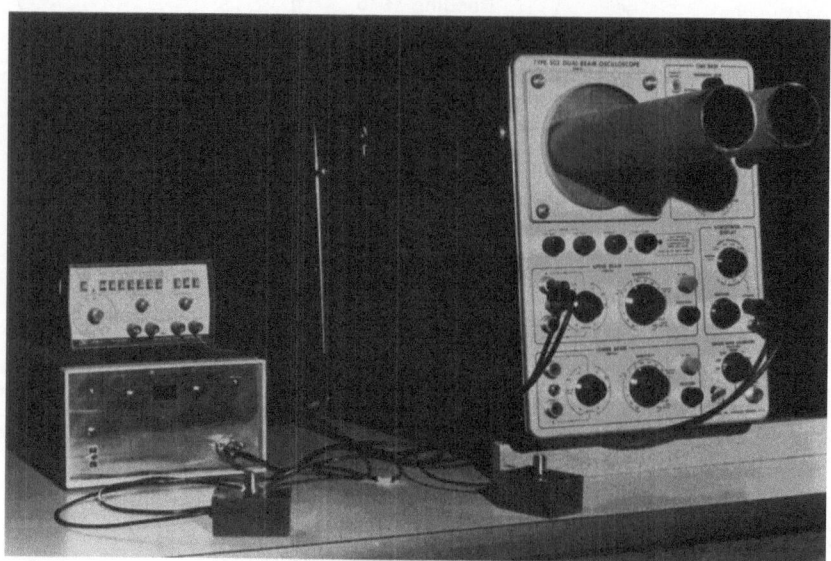

Fig. 3. The Pulfrich device consisting of two viewing tubes attached to a dual beam (i.e. dual target) oscilloscope. The signal generator sits atop the relative phase delay device. The latter is adjusted by the hand-held controls: one for the examiner and one for the subject.

Following a two minute warm-up session each subject was tested at four luminance disparity levels created by neutral density filters: 0.3, 0.6, 0.9, and 1.2 log units held before one eye. The subject was asked to flatten the ellipse within 15 seconds of an unpredictable deviation introduced by the examiner. Ten readings (appearing on a digital display to the nearest millisecond of phase lag) were recorded at each filter value.

A separate experiment was conducted on one subject employing a dichoptic double flash device. This consisted of two panel-mounted green light-emitting diodes (luminance 1.9 ft-c) at the end of two viewing tubes. The stimuli subtended 1.1 deg of visual angle and projected 2.0 deg temporal to the foveas with the subject fixating a cross created by fusion of a horizontal bar viewed by the right eye and a vertical bar viewed by the left. Paired 3.0 msec pulses were delivered sequentially by a Grass S8 stimulator.

With a filter placed before the right eye the subject turned a dial to vary the delay of the pulse to the left eye. Ten trials were recorded at each of the four filter densities to determine the mean minimum millisecond delay necessary to produce an illusion of simultaneity.

The delay neutralized by a given density filter in these two experiments was compared with the pattern visual evoked potential delay produced by the same filters (19).

To test the usefulness of the device in those with impaired stereopsis we recruited five small-angle esotropes who met the following criteria: a) a minimum visual acuity of 20/25 in each eye, with best correction, b) no greater than one Snellen acuity line difference between the two eyes, and c) strabismus with less than eight diopters of shift to the single-cover test (or no shift to the four diopter base-out prism test). The Titmus Optical Stereotest was administered under room illumination at the standard distance of 40 cm. The subjects were then required to find the null point of the Pulfrich device over ten trials as described above.

RESULTS

Naive subjects, given two minutes practice, could consistently reset the phase lag to a mean of 0.6 msec (two standard errors = 1.2 msec). Long periods of viewing did not lead to appreciable tiring. Discrimination was best above 0.66 Hz and below 1.5 Hz (Fig. 3). This frequency 'window' allowed a high target velocity and thus the greatest interocular disparity but was not so fast that it lead to defoveating errors of smooth pursuit (which would impair fine disparity discriminations).

Fig. 4 is a graph of Pulfrich phase delay in milliseconds versus log filter, dichoptic double flash delay versus log filter, and visual evoked potential latency delay versus log filter. The Pulfrich and evoked potential ranges shown are two standard errors (double flash = deviations) above and below the means and have been adjusted for the luminance difference between the oscilloscope screen and the video screen. The slopes of the regression lines agree closely (Pulfrich 15.8 msec/log unit, double flash 16.8 msec/log unit, evoked potential 18.6 msec/log unit). Though the double flash line is derived from a single subject it is comparable to that calculated from the data of Arden and Weale (20)(about 15 msec/log unit).

None of the strabismus subjects had difficulty appreciating the illusion, though their discriminatory skill, as judged by the standard error from the Pulfrich null point, was about half that of the normal group. Those with strabismus attained an overall mean 0.8 msec (two standard errors 3.1) of zero phase-delay. Fig. 5 is a graph of arc seconds of Titmus stereoacuity vs. the magnitude of the standard error of the Pulfrich end point measurement in milliseconds ($r = 0.902$, $p < 0.05$). Subjects with crude stereopsis tolerated progressively larger deviations from the Pulfrich null point than did subjects with fine stereopsis.

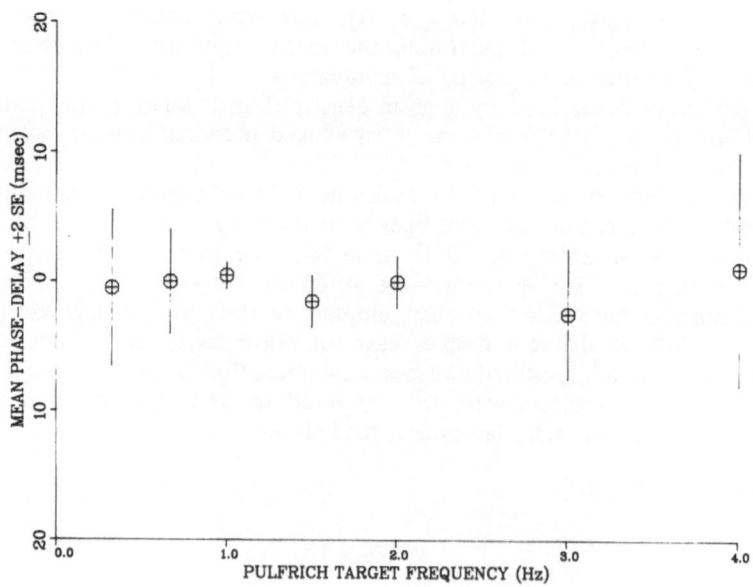

Fig. 4. A graph of mean phase-delay ± 2 standard errors, in milliseconds, versus Pulfrich target frequency. Deviations from the Pulfrich null point (the point of zero phase delay) were seen best at a target frequency of about 1.0 Hertz.

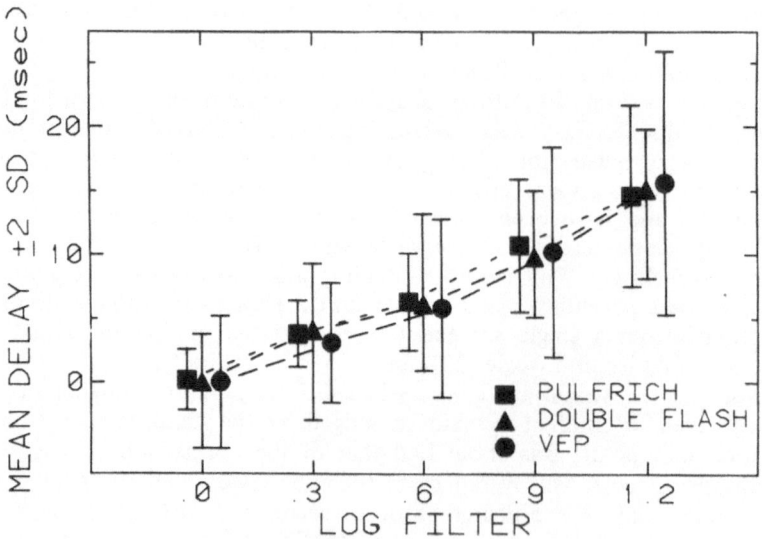

Fig. 5. A plot of mean delay ± 2 standard deviations, in milliseconds, versus the density of the neutral filter placed before the eye (in log units). The Pulfrich device, the dichoptic double flash, and the pattern visual evoked potential agree closely.

458

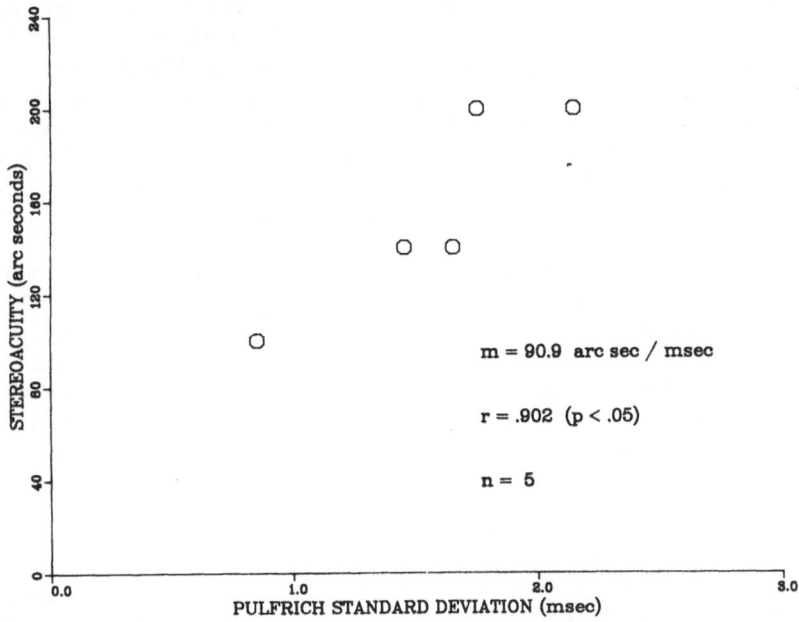

STEREOACUITY (arc seconds)

PULFRICH STANDARD DEVIATION (msec)

$m = 90.9$ arc sec / msec

$r = .902$ $(p < .05)$

$n = 5$

Fig. 6. A graph of Titmus stereoacuity in arc seconds versus the standard deviation of the Pulfrich device in milliseconds. Subjects with fine Titmus stereoacuity appreciated small deviations from the Pulfrich null point, while those with coarse stereoacuity required larger deviations.

DISCUSSION

Our subjects performed better than Rushton's in their ability to resolve the Pulfrich null point. This may be attributed to our use of: a dual-beam oscilloscope without interposed mirror optics; large, circular, sharply delineated targets; an edge-lighted grid serving as a strong reminder of the location of the true frontal plane; and smooth tracking of the target, ensuring continuous foveal 'sampling' of fine phase disparities.

The close agreement among the three methods of measuring delay used in the present study suggest that temporal judgments and spatial judgments share a common neural 'delay-processor', and differences in difficulty between the double flash psychophysical task and the Pulfrich psychophysical task are unimportant. That question answered we are conducting a trial to test the device's clinical utility. We can make only tentative assertions based on the study of five patients with optic neuritis, nevertheless, close agreement with the visual evoked potential delay appears to be achieved if: a) the visual acuity is at least 20/50 in the impaired eye, b) the fellow eye is normal, and c) there is no large, dense scotoma straddling the horizontal meridian, which would preclude stereopsis.

All of our subjects seem to enjoy themselves (many commented that it was like playing a video-arcade game) and we encountered no progressive stereo-insensitivity or marked stereo anomalies (21). Regan and Beverley have reported a phenomenon of stereo-fatiguing in pyschophysical experiments involving visual phase-disparities (22, 23). They propose a model of cerebral phase-disparity detector neurons in which separate neuronal pools, sensitive to either crossed or uncrossed disparity, tire when stimulated continuously. The strategy used by our subjects of crossing zero from one direction to the other and reducing the disparity with each successive pass, may prevent fatiguing of a given pool of cortical disparity detectors.

We believe the Pulfrich device is competitive with the dichoptic double flash and the visual evoked potential for detecting subtle conduction delays in normal subjects who have had one eye artificially disadvantaged by a neutral density filter. Given the restrictions stated above it may also be useful for quantifying delay in patients with optic nerve disease. The device can serve, with or without adaptation (e.g. converting the targets to cartoon figures for children), as an alternative method of measuring stereoacuity.

REFERENCES

1. Pulfrich, C. (1922) Die Stereoskopic im Dienste der Isochromen und hetereochromen Photometrie. Naturwissenschaften 10: 533, 569, 598, 714, 735, 751.
2. Grimsdale, H. (1925) A note on Pulfrich's phenomenon with a suggestion on its possible clinical importance. Br J Ophthal 9: 63.
3. Frisen, L., Hoyt, W. F., Bird, A. C. and Weale, R. A. (1973) Diagnostic uses of the Pulfrich phenomenon. Lancet 2: 385.
4. Reading, V. M. (1973) An objective correlate of the Pulfrich stereo-illusion. Proc. Roy Soc Med 66: 1044.
5. Ross, J. (1974) Stereopsis by binocular delay. Nature 248: 363.
6. Douthwaite, W. A. and Morrison, L. C. (1975) Critical flicker frequency and the Pulfrich phenomenon. Am J. Optom Physiol Opt 52: 745.
7. Burde, R. M. and Gallin, P. F. (1975) Visual parameters associated with recovered retrobulbar optic neuritis. Am J Opthal 79: 1034.
8. Wist, E. R., Hennerici, M. and Dichgans, J. (1978) The Pulfrich spatial frequency phenomenon: a psychophysical method competitive to visual evoked potentials in the diagnosis of multiple sclerosis. J Neur Neurosurg Psych 41: 1069.
9. Slagsvold, J. E. (1978) Pulfrich pendulum phenomenon in patients with a history of acute optic neuritis. Acta Ophth 56: 817.
10. Kirkham, T. H. and Coupland, S. G. (1981) Multiple regression analysis of diagnostic predictors in optic nerve disease. J Canad Sci Neurol 8: 67.
11. Sokol, S. (1976) The Pulfrich stereo-illusion as an index of optic nerve dysfunction. Sur Ophth 20: 432.
12. Rushton, D. (1975) Use of the Pulfrich pendulum for detecting abnormal delay in the visual pathway in multiple sclerosis. Brain 98: 283.
13. Regan, D., Milner, B. A. and Heron, J. R. (1976) Delayed visual perception and delayed visual evoked potentials in the spinal form of multiple sclerosis and in retrobulbar neuritis. Brain 99: 43.
14. Enroth-Cugell, C. and Robson, J. G. (1966) The contrast sensitivity of retinal ganglion cells of the cat. J Physiol Lond 198: 517.
15. Ikeda, H. (1980) Visual acuity, its development and amblyopia. J Roy Soc Med 73: 546.
16. Kruger, J. (1981) The difference between X- and Y-type responses in ganglion cells of the cat's retina. Vis Res 21: 1685.
17. Barlow, H. B. (1982) David Hubel and Torsten Wiesel: Their contributions towards understanding the primary visual cortex. Trends Neurosci, May, p. 145.

18. Regan, D. (1979) New visual tests in multiple sclerosis. In: Topics in Neuro-ophthalmology, p. 219. Editor: Thompson, H. S., Williams and Wilkins, Balt.
19. Cox, T. A., Thompson, H. S., Kolder, H. E. and Snyder, J. (1981) The visual evoked response latency in optic neuritis. In: Doc. Ophthal. Proc. Series, Vol. 27, p. 247. Editor: Spekreijse, H. and Apkarian, P. A., W. Junk Publ., Boston.
20. Arden, G. B., and Weale, R. A. (1954) Variations of the latent period of vision. Proc Roy Soc B 142: 258.
21. Richards, W. (1970) Stereopsis and stereoblindness. Exp Brain Res 10: 380.
22. Beverley, K. I. and Regan, D. (1973) Evidence for the existence of neural mechanisms selectively sensitive to the direction of motion in space. Jour of Physiology 235: 17.
23. Regan, D. and Beverley, K. I. (1973) Disparity detectors in human depth perception: evidence for directional selectivity. Science 181: 877.

Mailing address:
Department of Ophthalmology
The University of Iowa
Iowa City, Iowa 52242, U.S.A.

EYE TRACKING PERFORMANCE AND ATTENTION IN PSYCHOTIC PATIENTS

S. I. ANDERSSON

(Lund, Sweden)

ABSTRACT

The pendular eye tracking performance of a group of psychotic patients (9 schizophrenics, 8 cycloid psychotics and 2 manic-depressive psychotics), tested on two different occasions a week apart, was studied, using electro-oculography. An electronic pendulum involving a light of constant speed was employed, there being two different tasks, a less attention demanding task (red light only) and a more attention demanding task (pressing a button when the light turned to green at short, irregular intervals). Signal/noise ratio, 2nd to 6th harmonics, deviation area and microtremor rate were calculated, as were measures of the effect on these of the attention demands of the task and of the time spent at the task. Schizophrenics were found to differ from the other two psychotic groups in their overall tracking performance, cross validating in part results of an earlier study. Differences here were obtained on the initial test only. This was seen to reflect phasic change or improvement in the cycloid psychotics. There was an overall tendency, as already shown in the earlier investigation, for performance to be better under more attention demanding conditions, certain measures with high reliability. Microtremor appeared rather sensitive to particular aspects of the tracking task.

Since the rediscovery of deviant smooth pursuit eye movements in schizophrenics (Holzman, Proctor and Hughes, 1973), several studies have demonstrated eye tracking to be deviant in schizophrenics as compared with normals and other subjects (e.g., Holzman, Proctor, Levy, Yasillo, Meltzer and Hurt, 1974; Cegalis and Sweeny, 1979). Inferior eye tracking, however, has been reported in other patient-groups as well, for example in affective psychotics (Shagass, Amadeo and Overton, 1974). Interestingly enough, Shagass et al. (op. cit.) found that facilitating attentional effort through the introdution of unsystematic numeric information shown on the oscillating target improved performance considerably, both for patients and non-patients.

An earlier investigation (Andersson, 1983) indicated that schizophrenics (n = 13), cycloid psychotics (n = 9),[*] and normals (n = 4) could be

---

[*]The category of cycloid psychosis stems from the work of Leonhard (1957, 1979), according to whom cycloid psychotics display a phasic course, where recovery after an episode may be complete. Leonhard indicates the condition to be easily misclassified as schizophrenia and treated inappropriately.

distinguished rather well in terms of pendular eye tracking performance. Results of cluster analysis coupled with the use of criterion values for indices based on such pendular eye tracking measures as noise/signal ratio, deviation area, Fourier harmonics and microtremor yielded correct classifications in all but four cases. Patients' performance was found, for most measures, to be considerably better at a more attention-demanding than at a less attention-demanding eye pursuit movement task.

The present study, involving methodology very similar to that of the earlier investigation, concerned two major questions: (a) whether the results of the earlier investigation could be verified using a different group of subjects, representing a sample of all the testable psychotic patients available at a psychiatric hospital during a given period; (b) whether the results obtained would be reliable in the sense that the findings of two testings a week apart would be the same or similar.

METHOD

Recording procedure

Details of the methods and procedures employed are to be found in Andersson (1983); in the present investigation only the results of one of the two pendulae employed earlier is reported, namely the saw-tooth pendulum, in which the 'moving' light travels at a constant speed. This pendulum has special light diodes which can light up either red or green, the moving spot being red most of the time but becoming green for short irregular intervals. The task involves three periods of tracking. During the first period (60 sec) the target is red. During the second period, in which there are 180 sec of tracking following a 60 sec pause, the stimulus color changes temporarily from red to green at irregular intervals, subjects being instructed to press a button each time the light changes to green; a green segment, when it occurs, comprises 1/4 of the 'swing' of the pendulum in one direction or the other. The third tracking period, 60 sec in length following a 30-sec pause, involves (as did the first) a red pendular stimulus only. In contrast with the earlier investigation (Andersson, 1983) all subjects except those who had been discharged from the hospital prior to the second testing were tested twice, the second testing being approximately one week after the first.

Eye movements were registered in the AC mode with an electrooculographic technique, using a mingograph (a Beckman R-511A Dynograph Recorder). The preamplifier of the mingograph drove a Tandberg (TIR) FM tape recorder operating at a 3 3/4 IPS; it was RC-coupled to balance out DC offset voltage, with a high pass filter (cut-off frequency 0.16 Hz) and a low-pass filter (cut-off frequency 30 Hz) for noise reduction. Calibration was obtained by having the subject shift his gaze several times between the two endpoints of the pendulum.

Subjects

Nineteen psychotic patients remitted to S:t Lars Psychiatric Hospital in Lund for short-term therapy were tested. All were informed of the nature of the testing procedure and gave their informed consent. The patients were a subsample of those available during a three month period, only patients judged testable by the staff, lacking signs of organic brain disease, and not treated with electric shock therapy during at least the three previous months being tested. The sample consisted of eight cycloid psychotics (4 men, 4 women; mean age 26.6 with S.D. 5.6), two manic-depressive psychotics (both men; ages 27 and 50), and nine schizophrenics (5 men, 4 women; mean age 30.9 with S.D. 9.3). The subcategorization of the schizophrenics was as follows: 4 hebephrenics, 3 paranoids, 1 undifferentiated and 1 non-regressive, the latter according to the criterion of Nyman (1978). The combined cycloid psychotic and manic-depressive psychotic group had a mean age of 29.0 with S.D. 8.9. The mean time of current hospitalization was 8.5 days (S.D. 8.7), there being no notable differences between the three groups in this respect. All subjects had completed at least nine years of formal education. All except one (the non-regressive schizophrenic) were receiving phenothiazine derivates or related substances (derivates of thioxanthene or butyrophenone). In addition, two cycloid psychotics and one manic-depressive psychotic had received lithium citrate; the latter patient and one cycloid psychotic had been given benzodiazepine derivates; also, five cycloid psychotics and two schizophrenics were receiving anticholinergic drugs. The four subjects who were tested only once due to their discharge from the hospital before a second testing could be carried out consisted of two cycloid psychotics, one hebephrenic schizophrenic and the undifferentiated schizophrenic.

Measures obtained

Processing of the data from any given subject followed Andersson (1983) and was carried out for each of four different 30-sec segments of the total tracking task separately, each such 30-sec segment comprising 12 cycles (or slightly more than this) of the pendulum. Periods 1–4 involve successive portions of the pendular task – Period 1 representing the initial 30 seconds of the first of the two red-light-only tasks, Period 2 the initial 30 seconds of the red-and-green-light tracking tasks, Period 3 a 30-sec segment of the latter task commencing 90 seconds after the end of Period 2, and Period 4 the initial 30 seconds of the second red-light-only tracking task. Tape-recorded signals were digitized at a rate of 8,200 sampling points for each 30 second period. Data-processing involved computing eye position P from electrical voltage V at each of the sampling points through solving the differential equation $dV/dt = a \cdot dP/dt - b \cdot V$, where dV/dt represents change in V over time. A correction employed for drift consisted in subtracting from V its mean value within each cycle. Each 30 sec recording was shortened to exactly 12 cycles, a preliminary Fourier analysis being used in identifying cycles here. A more thorough Fourier analysis was also carried out. The following measures were obtained for each of the four periods:

(1) *Signal/noise ratio*. The ratio between the sum of the squared amplitudes of the 2nd, 3rd, 4th, 5th and 6th harmonics, on the other hand, and the

465

squared amplitude of the major wave (1st harmonic) on the other. For a subject following the movements of the pendulum closely, this measure would be low.

(2) *The 2nd, 3rd, 4th, 5th and 6th harmonics.* the ratio of the respective higher harmonic factor (i.e., 2nd, 3rd, 4th, 5th and 6th harmonic factor) to the 1st harmonic factor. With perfect tracking the values would be 0 for the 2nd harmonic, 0.111 for the 3rd, 0 for the 4th, 0.040 for the 5th and 0 for the 6th harmonic.

(3) *Deviation area.* The area between the two curves describing the movements of the pendulum and of the subject's eyes, respectively. If the subject followed the pendulum closely, this measure would be low.

(4) *Microtremor rate.* $(d(tot)-d(eff))/d(eff)$, where $d(tot)$ represents the total distance and $d(eff)$ the 'effective' distance the eye covered, and where $d(tot)$ and $d(eff)$ represent the sum of all small eye movements as measured through recording eye positions at 3.66 msec intervals, and at intervals nine times larger (33 msec), respectively.

For each such measure, a summary measure of the subject's *overall tracking performance (OTP)* during the four periods together was calculated. In addition, two types of difference score, *Dif-1* and *Dif-2*, were obtained for each of the measures (1) to (4) above, following Andersson (1983). *Dif-1*, the difference $(1 + 4)-(2 + 3)$, where the numbers here refer to the successive periods, indicates the effect on eye tracking performance of changing from the less attention-demanding conditions (red-light-only) to the more demanding (changing light color). *Dif-2*, the difference $(1 + 2)-(3 + 4)$, represents the effect of practice. Using these summary measures, comparisons were made between the schizophrenic (S) and the cycloid-manic-depressive (CD) groups, the latter group comprising both the cycloid psychotic (C) and the manic-depressive (D) patients. For the fifteen persons tested twice, comparisons were made between A and B for all the above measures. Statistical tests were all two-tailed.

RESULTS

Significant differences between the S and the CD groups were found on two of the overall tracking performance (OTP) measures, in both cases for A only. CD tended here to have more extreme signal/noise ratios ($p < 0.01$, Moses test) and higher deviation area ($p < 0.02$, Mann-Whitney U-test) than S. Similar differences were obtained in comparing S with C. The results for deviation area ($p < 0.05$, Mann-Whitney U-test) concurred with those of the earlier investigation (Andersson, 1983), whereas those for signal/noise ratio concurred only in part. The earlier study had shown signal/noise ratios to be higher for C than for S. Although in the present investigation, the signal/noise ratios of C tended instead toward the two extremes ($p < 0.01$, Moses test), the three subjects with the highest signal/noise ratios (also when the D group is considered) all belong to the C group.

466

Concerning Dif-1 and Dif-2 scores, no clear differences between the psychotic groups were found, quite in agreement with the results of the earlier investigation. At the same time, these difference scores revealed general tendencies for the psychotic group as a whole in various of the measures:

For signal/noise *ratio*, performance was found to be better generally under more than under less attention-demanding conditions (i.e., Dif-1 scores were predominantly positive), both for A (15 +, 4 −, $p < 0.02$, χ^2 − here as in the following), as in the previous study, and for B (12 +, 3 −, $p < 0.05$). These results appeared reliable, only 2 of 15 subjects showing a different sign (+ or −) on the two occasions tested.

Regarding the Dif-1 scores for the various *harmonics*, performance (assessed relative to the ideal values listed above) was found, for the *4th* harmonic, to be better under the more demanding conditions (14 +, 4 −, $p < 0.02$, in A; 10 +, 5 −, n.s., in B), whereas for the *5th* harmonic the opposite results were obtained, (5 +, 14 −, $p < 0.05$, in A; 3 +, 12 −, $p < 0.05$, in B). Both results are in agreement with those of the earlier investigation. No consistent or significant tendency could be found for the *2nd* harmonic, as it was in the earlier study, for performance to be better under the more attention demanding conditions. Regarding Dif-2 scores, no significance was obtained for the different harmonics, although a non-significant tendency toward improvement over time was found for the *4th* harmonic, both for A and B, in weak agreement with the significant tendency of this sort obtained in the previous study.

Concerning *deviation area*, no significant tendency was found, as it had been in the earlier investigation, for performance to be better under the more attention demanding conditions, although results in A did point in this direction (13 +, 6 −, n.s.). Also, comparing A and B, results for the individual subjects appear to be reliable, 13 of the 15 subjects who were tested on both occasions showing the same type of tendency during A and B. (7 + +, 6 − −). All four of the subjects who were discharged from the hospital after A showed better performance under the more attention demanding conditions.

The general finding of eye tracking performance improving under the more attention demanding conditions is illustrated by the curves (of a staircase form in Periods 1 and 4) obtained for a cycloid psychotic (Fig. 1), whereas the less usual finding of performance deteriorating under the more attention demanding conditions is illustrated by the curves of a hebephrenic schizophrenic (Fig. 2).

Microtremor rate tended to be higher under the more attention demanding conditions (17 +, 2 −, $p < 0.001$, for A; 9 +, 6 −, n.s., for B). Dif-2 scores showed microtremor rate to decrease over time, both in A (14 −, 5 +, $p < 0.05$) and in B (12 −, 3 + , $p < 0.05$).

DISCUSSION

Results of the present study provide cross-validational support for many of the findings of the earlier investigation (Andersson, 1983). Both deviation

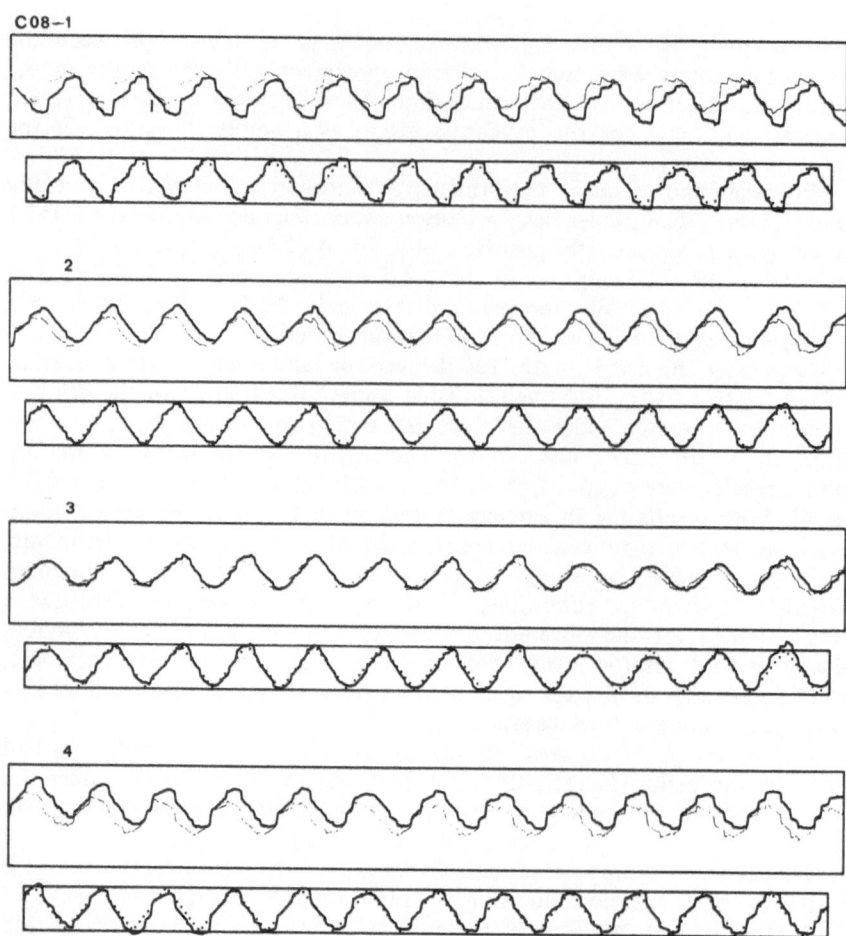

Fig. 1. Eye-tracking pattern in a cycloid psychotic during Periods 1–4. Periods 1 and 4 = red light only, Periods 2 and 3 = intermittent occurrence of segments where the light is green. The lower, more abbreviated record from each period has been corrected for drift and shortened to 12 cycles. Thin curve = initially registered voltage; thick curve = eye position; dotted, saw-tooth curve = stimulus (light) position. An improvement in eye tracking performance under the more attention-demanding conditions (Periods 2 and 3) is evident.

area and signal/noise ratio differentiated clearly enough between cycloid psychotics (or the combined group of these and manic-depressive psychotics) and schizophrenics. The signal/noise ratio measure appeared somewhat enigmatic, since in the previous investigation cycloid psychotics showed poorer performance, whereas here they showed more extreme performance (high or low), as compared with schizophrenics. The differentiation found on either measure was obtained only on the first test (A). This may be due, as the work of Leonhard (1957, 1979) would suggest, to phasic changes on the part of the cycloid psychotics. The phasic change here may have been

468

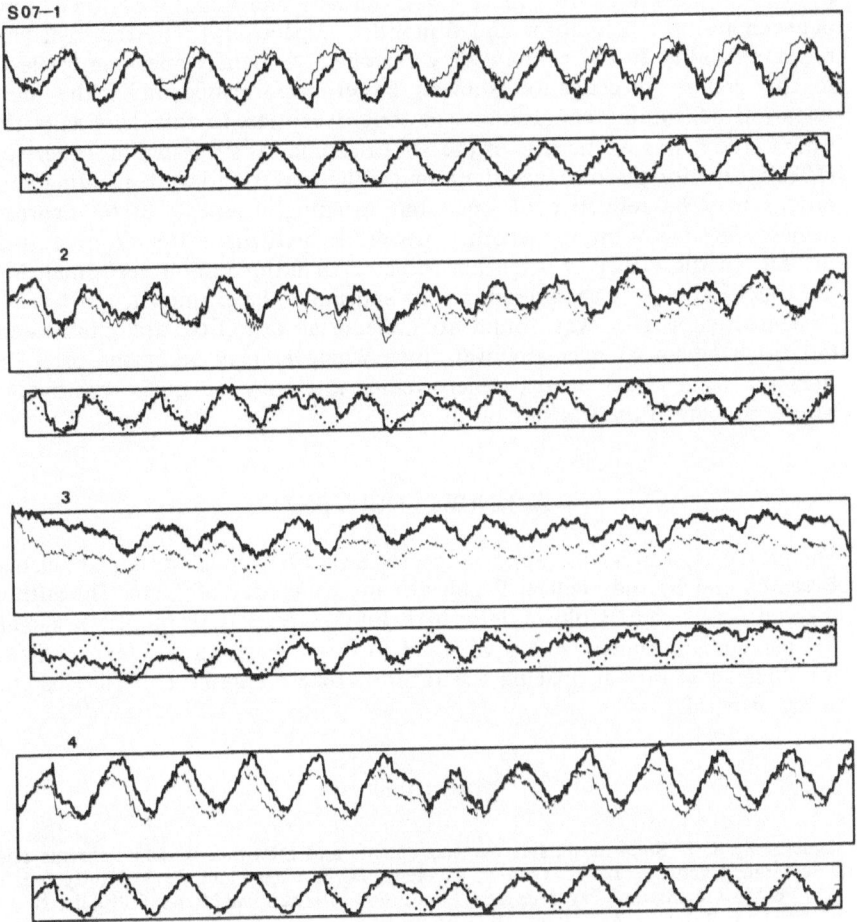

Fig. 2. Jagged eye tracking pattern in a schizophrenic patient (cf. Fig. 1). A deterioration in eye tracking performance under the more attention-demanding conditions (Periods 2 and 3) is evident.

largely that of improvement, since in terms of deviation area the cycloid psychotics shifted between A and B from being worse in performance than schizophrenics to not differing from them. A crucial investigation in future work would involve following changes in the eye tracking performance of cycloid psychotics and schizophrenics during a more extended period, with shorter intervals between testing.

No differentiation between the psychotic groups could be shown as regards the effect of variations in the attention demands of the task or in the time spent at the task. Scores indicative of the former (Dif-1 scores) showed a high degree of reliability from the first to the second test occasion for the deviation area and signal/noise ratio measures. This accords roughly with findings of Holzman et al. (1973) and Shagass et al. (1974), who with other eye-tracking measures than those employed here and a longer period of time between testings (2 months and 6 months, respectively) reported high test-retest reliability in the patients they examined. Generally speaking, patients in the present investigation showed better performance under the more attention demanding conditions. The lone exception to this, here as in the earlier study, was in the case of the 5th harmonic. As suggested in Andersson (1983), superior performance there under the less attention demanding conditions may be reflective of small but meaningful aspects of task performance. The question of whether psychotic patients differ from normal subjects in the effect of attention demands or fatique upon performance is not touched upon by the present results and should be examined.

Microtremor rate was found to increase as cognitive strain increased, but nevertheless to decrease over time. Whatever may lie at the basis for this, the results suggest that microtremor rate may be quite sensitive to various aspects of the tracking task.

ACKNOWLEDGEMENT

The present research was supported by the Swedish Council for Social Science Research and by the Medical Faculty of the University of Lund. The author is grateful to Robert Goldsmith for his helpful comments, to Birgitta Rorsman for her encouragement and advice and to Göran Franzén and Mårten Gerle for their generosity in placing the facilities of S:t Lars Psychiatric Hospital at my disposal.

REFERENCES

Andersson, S. I. Smooth pursuit eye movements and attention in schizophrenia and cycloid psychoses. In: R. Groner, C. Menz, D. F. Fisher and R. A. Monty (eds.), Eye Movements and Psychological Functions: International Views. Hillsdale, N. J.: Lawrence Erlbaum Associates, 1983 (in press).

Cegalis, J. A. and Sweeny, J. A. The effect of attention on smooth pursuit eye movements of schizophrenics. Journal of Psychiatric Research, 1981, 16, 145−161.

Holzman, P. S., Proctor, L. R. and Hughes, D. W. Eye-tracking patterns in schizophrenics. Science, 1973, 181, 179−181.

Holzman, P. S., Proctor, L. R., Levy, D. L., Yasillo, N. J., Meltzer, H. Y. and Hurt, S. W. Eye-tracking dysfunctions in schizophrenic patients and their relatives. Archives of General Psychiatry, 1974, 31, 143−151.

Leonhard, K. The Classification of Endogenous Psychoses (5th ed.). New York: New York: Irvington Publishers, 1979. (Originally published as Aufteilung der endogenen Psychosen, 1957).

Nyman, G. E. The clinical picture of non-regressive schizophrenia. Nordisk Psykiatrisk Tidsskrift, 1975, 29, 249−258.

Shagass, C., Amadeo, M. and Overton, D. A. Eye-tracking performance in psychiatric patients. Biological Psychiatry, 1974, 9, 245−260.

Mailing address:
Department of Psychology
Lund University
Paradisgatan 5, S-223 50 Lund
Sweden

CHROMATIC STIMULATION IN PARTIAL ACHROMATOPSIA

W. R. BIERSDORF AND A. WEISS

Department of Ophthalmology, University of South Florida and Veterans Hopsital, Tampa, Florida 33612, USA

Male patients with blue cone (pi)$_1$ monochromatism from two families exhibiting x-linked recessive inheritance were studied. A two-beam optical stimulator was used to provide high intensity chromatic stimulation in Maxwellian view. Both ERG and psychophysical spectral sensitivities were obtained. Under photopic conditions, the patients showed maximum psychophysical sensitivity in the blue region about 440 nm with sensitivity dropping off rapidly with increasing wavelengths. ERG sensitivity was also maximal in the short wavelengths, although not exactly the same as the visual sensitivity. Under blue adaptation, both visual and ERG sensitivities were a close match to the standard scotopic (rod) curve.

AUTHORS INDEX

SUBJECT INDEX

Acidosis
 ERG, perfused eye, 41
Albinism, human
 EOG, 361
 Oculomotor behavior, 361
Amblyopia
 Pattern ERG, 273
Aminodipic acid
 ERG, 51
Analog filtering, 247
Aortic arch syndrome
 EOG, 175
 ERG, 175
Apple II
 Electrophysiology use, 199
 Pattern stimuli, 217
 VEP/ERG, 209
Arterial occlusion
 ERG, 65

Barbiturates
 VECP, 425
Blue cone monochromatism
 ERG, 471
 Spectral sensitivities, 471

C-wave
 Acidosis, 41
 Amplitude, 21
 Anesthesia affect, 57
 Canine, 57
 Components, 21
 Diabetic retinopathy, 169
 EOG comparison, 159
 Human, 151
 Origin, 159
 Retinal detachment, 191
 Retinal disease, 159
 Species dependent, 57
 Variability, 151
Canine
 ERG, 57

Chloral hydrate
 VECP, 425
Chloroquine toxicity
 Color vision, 121
 EOG, 121
 EOG, 301
 ERG, 301
Color vision simulator, 253
Computer assisted electrophysiology
 Microcomputers, 199
Computer program, 193
Computer-assisted analysis
 Electroretinogram, 231
 Intensity-response functions, 231
Congenital Stationary Night Blindness
 ERG, 347
 Oscillatory potentials, 347

Diabetes mellitus, early
 ERG, 351
Diabetic retinopathy
 C-wave, 169
 EOG, 143
 ERG, 169
 Fast Oscillations, 143
Digital filtering, 247
Drusen, dominant
 EOG, 105

Electrical evoked potential, 437
Electro-oculogram
 Acidosis, 41
 Aortic arch syndrome, 175
 Best's disease, 93
 Carbon dioxide, 41
 Chloroquine Toxicity, acute, 301
 Development, 81
 Diabetic retinopathy, 143
 Diamox response, 115
 Drusen, dominant, 105
 Fast oscillation, 105
 Fast oscillation, 137

THE INTERNATIONAL SOCIETY FOR CLINICAL
ELECTROPHYSIOLOGY AND VISION (ISCEV)

(formerly The International Society for Clinical Electroretinography
(ISCERG)

TEN YEAR CUMULATIVE INDEX
1972–1981

Preface

This ten year cumulative index of the ISCERG/ISCEV Symposia is divided into an author and subject section. Each author is listed with the volume and first page number. Subjects were divided by primary topic and multiple subtopics, all alphabetised, with the volume and first page number. Because a cursory review was made of each article from the ten years, topics may have been chosen that may differ from the emphasis that the author would have selected. If this occurred, I hope that no grievous errors have been made.

One problem developed in listing the volume numbers for the Morioka Symposium in that the proceedings were not published in the Documenta Ophthalmologica Proceeding Series; in order to establish a uniform numbering system, THE SYMPOSIUM NUMBER WAS USED AS THE VOLUME NUMBER. The key to the volume numbers is listed on the next page.

The membership of ISCERG/ISCEV can look with pride at the fine work and research that have been performed by members in the field of visual electrophysiology. I hope that this cumulative index will be supportive in on-going projects, and will allow for member's work to be cited more often by other members in future scholarly works.

I would like to thank Miguel Palos and Debby Leja for their technical assistance in preparing this index.

John R. Heckenlively, M.D., Editor
International Society for Clinical Electrophysiology and Vision
Los Angeles, California

KEY TO VOLUME NUMBERING IN INDEX

Vol. 10 = ISCERG Symposium X, 1972 (Los Angeles) Junk Doc. Ophthalmologica Proc. Series Vol. 2
Vol. 11 = ISCERG Symposium XI, 1973 (Bad Nauheim) Junk Doc. Ophthalmologica Proc. Series Vol. 4
Vol. 12 = ISCERG Symposium XII, 1974 (Clermont-Ferrand) Junk Doc. Ophthalmologica Proc. Series Vol. 10
Vol. 13 = ISCERG Symposium XIII, 1975 (Kibbutz Ginossar) Junk Doc. Ophthalmologica Proc. Series Vol. 11

Vol. 14 = ISCERG Symposium XIV, 1976 (Louisville) Junk Doc. Ophthalmologica Proc. Series Vol. 13

Vol. 15 = ISCEV Symposium XV, 1977 (Ghent) Junk Doc. Ophthalmologica Proc. Series Vol. 15

Vol. 16 = ISCEV Symposium XVI, 1978 (Morioka) Japanese Journal of Ophthalmology Supplement

Vol. 17 = ISCEV Symposium XVII, 1979 (Erfurt) Junk Doc. Ophthalmologica Proc. Series Vol. 23

Vol. 18 = ISCEV Symposium XVIII, 1980 (Amsterdam) Junk Doc. Ophthalmologica Proc. Series Vol. 27

Vol. 19 = ISCEV Symposium XIX, 1981 (Horgen-Zurich) Junk Doc. Ophthalmologica Proc. Series Vol. 31

Please note: the volume numbers in the index do *not* correlate with the Documenta Ophthalmologica Proceeding Series numbering.

INDEX OF SYMPOSIUM AUTHORS

481

485

INDEX OF SYMPOSIUM SUBJECTS

491

499